Psychiatry - Theory, Applications and Treatments

Psychiatry on the Edge

PSYCHIATRY - THEORY, APPLICATIONS AND TREATMENTS

Additional books in this series can be found on Nova's website under the Series tab.

Additional e-books in this series can be found on Nova's website under the e-book tab.

Psychiatry - Theory, Applications and Treatments

Psychiatry on the Edge

Ronald William Pies, M.D.

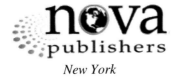

New York

Copyright © 2014 by Nova Science Publishers, Inc.

All rights reserved. No part of this book may be reproduced, stored in a retrieval system or transmitted in any form or by any means: electronic, electrostatic, magnetic, tape, mechanical photocopying, recording or otherwise without the written permission of the Publisher.

For permission to use material from this book please contact us:
Telephone 631-231-7269; Fax 631-231-8175
Web Site: http://www.novapublishers.com

NOTICE TO THE READER

The Publisher has taken reasonable care in the preparation of this book, but makes no expressed or implied warranty of any kind and assumes no responsibility for any errors or omissions. No liability is assumed for incidental or consequential damages in connection with or arising out of information contained in this book. The Publisher shall not be liable for any special, consequential, or exemplary damages resulting, in whole or in part, from the readers' use of, or reliance upon, this material. Any parts of this book based on government reports are so indicated and copyright is claimed for those parts to the extent applicable to compilations of such works.

Independent verification should be sought for any data, advice or recommendations contained in this book. In addition, no responsibility is assumed by the publisher for any injury and/or damage to persons or property arising from any methods, products, instructions, ideas or otherwise contained in this publication.

This publication is designed to provide accurate and authoritative information with regard to the subject matter covered herein. It is sold with the clear understanding that the Publisher is not engaged in rendering legal or any other professional services. If legal or any other expert assistance is required, the services of a competent person should be sought. FROM A DECLARATION OF PARTICIPANTS JOINTLY ADOPTED BY A COMMITTEE OF THE AMERICAN BAR ASSOCIATION AND A COMMITTEE OF PUBLISHERS.

Additional color graphics may be available in the e-book version of this book.

Library of Congress Cataloging-in-Publication Data

ISBN: 978-1-63117-699-9

Published by Nova Science Publishers, Inc. † New York

CONTENTS

Foreword vii
    Cynthia M.A. Geppert, MD, PhD, MPH

Preface ix

Chapter 1   The Philosophical and Scientific Foundations of Psychiatry   1
*Ronald William Pies, MD, Sairah Thommi
and Nassir Ghaemi, MD, MPH*

Chapter 2   Psychiatric Diagnosis and the DSM Debates   67

Chapter 3   Grief, Depression, and the Bereavement Controversy   103

Chapter 4   Psychiatry in Crisis   131

Chapter 5   Psychiatry and Humane Values   163

Author Contact Information   187

Index   189

FOREWORD

It is a great honor that my mentor and friend, Ron Pies, MD, accepted my offer to write a foreword to his first collection of essays and other writings published in *Psychiatric Times,* over nearly 25 years.

The eighteenth century philosopher Jean Jacques Rousseau one wrote, "When God made me he broke the mold." Leaving aside the egoism of self-attributing the saying, this collection of essays and other writings amply demonstrates that this idiom is a perfect description of Ron Pies, MD. The expression applies to Dr. Pies and his work in two important senses. The first meaning is that of being unconventional, in the most constructive import of the concept. Moral imagination is a hallmark of the career of Dr. Pies, recapitulated in this thought provoking series of commentaries. Dr. Pies, like Socrates, is a psychiatric gadfly who has spent a lifetime questioning the assumptions of psychiatry, such as the reification of the DSM; exploding the reductionist myths of the "chemical imbalance" theory of psychiatric illness; and courageously and compassionately challenging the complacency of our professional self-formulations, as he responds to the perennial critics of psychiatry.

The second meaning of the Rousseau quote-- "being unique"--applies to Ron Pies, MD more than to almost any other figure in psychiatry in the last century. The phrase "Renaissance physician" is overused and superficially understood. Yet when employed with historical accuracy as referring to a polymath who aspires to bridge science and philosophy in one mind, this defines Dr. Pies and the body of work that is offered in this volume. Dr. Pies is at once a serious psychopharmacologist; a gifted poet; a Judaic scholar; a medically astute psychiatric physician; and a psychiatric ethicist, grounded in the Greek and Judaic heritage of virtues and values. In his own creative terminology, Dr. Pies is a member of a rapidly vanishing species, not just in psychiatry but also in all of medicine and even scholarship at large: a *polythetic pluralist.*

The title of this collection of 46 essays concisely articulates the overarching theme of Pies' thought: Psychiatry is "on the edge" of losing its distinctive identity--its cutting edge, if you will--and falling into a vacuous cultural milieu of commercially induced conflicts of interest and regnant biological positivism, like much of the rest of American medicine and society. To regain its edge—or, as Ron Pies puts it in a brilliant, two-part critique, "How American Psychiatry Can Save Itself"--practitioners must draw upon the many neglected sources that form the "edges" of our calling: ancient religious traditions like those of Buddhism and Judaism, regarding the difference between grief and major depression; and philosophers like the stoics and pragmatists, pointing toward "a Third Way" of understanding the diagnostic categories of mental illness.

Over years of empathic and erudite pages, Dr. Pies has recalled us to the prophetic dimension of psychiatry, in a voice that speaks wisely and bravely about contemporary ethical and social dilemmas; for example, gun violence, internet-based scholarly discourse, and the right to health care.

Readers of this collection who know Dr. Pies as the editor-in-chief emeritus of *Psychiatric Times* will enjoy having so many of his most salient pieces collected in one book. Those who are new to his unparalleled breadth of knowledge and depth of humanism will be inspired to explore further his 12 books, hundreds of articles, commentaries, and blog postings. But all who dip or dive into the waters of "Psychiatry on the Edge" are assured that the thirst for wisdom we all seek and seldom find these dry days will be quenched.

Cynthia M.A. Geppert, MD, PhD, MPH

PREFACE

To say that psychiatry is "on the edge" these days is to say something both troubling and hopeful—and that is really the crux of the essays in this book. Indeed, a psychiatrist facing the current state of the profession might well echo Charles Dickens, in the first lines from *A Tale of Two Cities*:

> *"It was the best of times, it was the worst of times, it was the age of wisdom, it was the age of foolishness, it was the epoch of belief, it was the epoch of incredulity, it was the season of Light, it was the season of Darkness, it was the spring of hope, it was the winter of despair, we had everything before us, we had nothing before us..."*

To begin with the "worst of times": a psychiatrist prone to searching the internet for items on psychiatry might well wind up, in very short order, with a bad case of reactive depression. There is so much online misinformation about the current state of psychiatry—its mission, nature, and accomplishments—that the public's skepticism and cynicism is not hard to understand. Thus, in an article for Scientific American, Jeffrey A. Lieberman, President of the American Psychiatric Association, commented on the baneful effects of anti-psychiatry groups:

> "This relatively small "anti-psychiatry" movement fuels the much larger segment of the world that is prejudiced against people with disorders of the brain and mind and the professions that treat them. Like most prejudice, this one is largely based on ignorance or fear–no different than racism, or society's initial reactions to illnesses from leprosy to AIDS. And many people made uncomfortable by mental illness and psychiatry, don't recognize their feelings as prejudice. But that is what they are...For this reason, I am especially shocked when other clinicians—psychologists, social workers, even, in some cases, primary care docs who would rather just dispense psychiatric meds themselves—side with anti-psychiatry forces without realizing these people are "against" them, too. These strange anti-mental health bedfellows include a series of contemporary psychiatrists and psychologists who have fashioned platforms for self-promotion from their critical positions on psychiatry and DSM-5." [1]

I fully concur with Dr. Lieberman's assessment. And yet, it would be a mistake to see the public's sometimes low opinion of psychiatry solely in terms of anti-psychiatry rants and rhetoric. The wellsprings of public discontent are darker and deeper. Dr. Lieberman himself notes that,

"There is historical fear of mental illness, stemming from when these diseases were viewed first as demonic possessions and later as character or moral defects, before we had any scientific understanding for the biological basis of, say, schizophrenia, bipolar disorder, autism or Alzheimer's disease...[Moreover] I do not overlook the checkered history of psychiatry itself. It's a relatively new discipline which branched from neurology in the 19th century, whose early practitioners were alienists and analysts, superintendents of asylums and Freudian therapists. But, at the time, asylums were little more than humane warehouses, and Freudian theory turned out to be a brilliant fiction about personality and behavior. When psychiatry did make its first forays into medical treatment, it used crude instruments like strait jackets, cold packs, fever induction, insulin shock therapy and psycho-surgery. The underlying theories for the causes of these illnesses at the time were also wrong; it was largely about blaming the parents."

Contributing to public animus toward psychiatry are several troubling trends, which I take up in my essays on "How American Psychiatry Can Save Itself." Among these are psychiatry's sometimes inappropriately close ties with the pharmaceutical industry in recent decades; the declining use of psychotherapy in the average psychiatric practice; and—perhaps most important-- the low level of understanding, among the general public, of how psychiatric treatments benefit those who suffer with mental illness. Another exacerbating factor was the troubled "roll out" of the DSM-5, during which the public was not sufficiently informed or prepared for some of the most controversial changes—particularly the elimination of the so-called "bereavement exclusion" from the criteria for major depressive disorder. (I take up this controversy in a number of essays and defend the DSM-5's decision—but not necessarily the public educational process that should have preceded that decision).

Finally, in my essay titled, "Can Psychiatry be Both A Medical Science and A Healing Art? The Case for Polythetic Pluralism", I describe what I call, "...the continued ideological divide that has bedeviled psychiatry for decades." : This was the focus of anthropologist Tanya Luhrmann, in her book, *Of Two Minds*. There she describes the dueling models of biomedical science and pharmacotherapy, on the one hand; and psychodynamics and psychotherapy, on the other. Despite many attempts at harmonizing these two paradigms, much division within the profession remains, probably exacerbated by economic forces that have discouraged psychiatrists from providing psychotherapy.

In short, the reader would not be mistaken in concluding that psychiatry's position "on the edge" is a perilous one—but such a conclusion is only half the story. Dickens, after all, alluded to an "age of wisdom", a "season of Light", and a "spring of hope." There is much in the evolution of modern psychiatry that speaks to such optimism. While not the focus of the essays in this collection, the impressive gains psychiatry has made in the neurosciences is surely something we can celebrate. True, our growing understanding of the brain abnormalities that underlie schizophrenia or bipolar disorder has not yet been "translated" into practical and effective treatments, and many of our current treatments are only modestly effective. But I believe we are on the "edge" of critical discoveries that will eventuate in useful treatments for the most common and serious psychiatric disorders.

Furthermore, neuropsychiatric research is beginning to move beyond the traditional neurotransmitters toward newer and more innovative approaches—a good example is the recent use of the NMDA receptor antagonist, ketamine, for rapid relief of refractory major depression. [2] Research in mood disorders is increasingly focusing on synaptic connections, neural networks, and gene products, such as BDNF (Brain Derived Neurotrophic Factor) which regulates synaptic plasticity. These sophisticated approaches are a far cry from the canard of the "chemical imbalance theory", so often imputed to psychiatry by its uninformed critics (see "Psychiatry's New Brain-Mind and the Legend of the "Chemical Imbalance")

But "biology" is only a part of the story, and only one reason for optimism. There is the larger issue of how psychiatry is striving for an integrated and holistic approach to mental disorders and their treatment. Yes, I'm all too familiar with the conventional narrative: "Psychiatry, these days, is nothing but writing out prescriptions, after a 15-minute appointment!" But I think this is more of a caricature than a valid characterization of the field as a whole. Unfortunately, it is true that there has been a steep decline (1996-2005) in the number of psychiatrists who provide psychotherapy to all of their patients, according to a 2008 study; however, the same study found that nearly 60% of psychiatrists continue to provide psychotherapy to at least some of their patients. [3] Furthermore, new therapies, such as Dynamic deconstructive psychotherapy for Borderline Personality Disorder; as well as briefer forms of therapy, are now being used effectively.

Even more fundamentally, many "thought leaders" in psychiatry have continued to advocate a broad-based understanding of mental illness and its treatment, incorporating biological, psychosocial, and even psychoanalytic insights. And, many of us are also seeking ways to integrate spiritual and humanistic elements into psychiatric treatment. As I note in one of the essays, psychiatry is blessed with a number of "pluralistic unifiers", such as my *Psychiatric Times* colleagues Nassir Ghaemi, Steve Moffic, James Knoll, Glen Gabbard and Cynthia Geppert—to mention just a few. I note that, "These clinician-scholars have refused to buy into the Manichean world of the "splitters"; rather, they espouse a scientific-humanistic perspective that comfortably embraces both molecules and motives." ("Is Psychiatry Now a House). Another examplar of this unifying impulse is the Nobel prize-winning psychiatrist and neuroscientist, Dr. Eric Kandel. In his book, *Psychiatry, Psychoanalysis and the new biology of mind*, Kandel paints a picture of the "new" psychiatry, in which psychoanalytic and biological constructs complement and reinforce one another. And, in a seminal work titled, *Philosophy of Psychopharmacology*, Dr. Dan J. Stein looks at psychotropic medication in the broad context of "self", psychotherapy, and medical ethics. [5] I am heartened by these trends, though I acknowledge that these thought leaders sometimes seem to be "swimming against the tide".

In short, it is indeed a time when psychiatry stands "on the edge"—of promise and peril, progress and regress. Much will depend on the younger generation of psychiatrists, and how willing they are, in James Knoll's words, to "awaken and return to the path" [6]—the path of professional pride, Hippocratic values and humanistic sensibilities. It is my hope that these essays may serve, in some small way, as guideposts along that path.

ACKNOWLEDGMENTS

I have been writing for, and involved with, *Psychiatric Times* since the days when founder and then Editor, John L. Schwartz MD, published my very first contribution to the paper, in 1985—a short story titled, "Hyman Gleeber Buys a Friend." The paper has undergone many changes since then, including its recent transformation to an "online" (as well as print) publication. Nevertheless, *Psychiatric Times* has continued to fulfill its original role as a publication primarily "by psychiatrists, for psychiatrists." At the same time, the paper has become more inclusive, often showcasing the work of historians, sociologists, and psychologists. The essays in this collection are drawn from my contributions to *Psychiatric Times*, over roughly the past decade. Many have been revised slightly from their original versions, in order to reflect new developments in the field, such as the release of the DSM-5.

I was privileged to have served as Editor-in-Chief, from 2007-2010, and was succeeded by my friend and colleague, James L. Knoll IV, MD. The editorial staff has also changed over the years, and I was blessed with their support and encouragement over the past nearly 30 years. In particular, I would like to thank Leo Cristofar, Susan Kweskin, Laurie Martin, Natalie Timoshin, Arline Kaplan, HeidiAnne Duerr and Cortney Mears for their assistance, editing and support over the years. Thanks also to Cindy Flaum, Vice President, Clinical Publishing, at UBM Medica, for her support and encouragement. My special thanks go to Dr. Dan J. Stein, for his careful reading of my manuscript; and to Dr. Cynthia Geppert, for her kind willingness to provide a foreword. I also appreciate the support of Nadya S. Gotsiridze-Columbus, at Nova Science Publishers, for her willingness to foster the publication of these essays. My thanks go, as well, to Chantelle Marshall, for her excellent editing and formatting of the first draft.

I also want to thank many friends, colleagues and teachers for their generosity in reading and commenting on many of my columns. I have tried to acknowledge these individuals at the end of specific essays, but I would like to mention, with special thanks, the following individuals: Nassir Ghaemi, Glen Gabbard, Elissa Ely, Sasha Helper, Michael Schwartz, Mantosh Dewan, Paul Summergrad, Robert Gregory, Bob Daly, Gene Kaplan, Chetan Haldipur, John Manring, Roger Greenberg, Sid Zisook, Kathy Shear, Vic Camillo, Manuel Mota-Castillo, Henry Lothane, Boris Vatel, Dan Pistone, Steve Moffic, Sharon Packer, Joe Pierre, Tony Stern, Bob Levin, Tim Thornton, Derek Bolton, Mel Gray, Max Fink, Mike Sperber, Peter Kramer, Doug Berger, Hannah Decker, Erik Midelfort, Jim Phelps, Jim Phillips, Allen Frances, John Grohol, Richard A. Friedman, Barney Carroll, Greg Eghigian, Rich Berlin, David Hemenway, Garen Wintemute, David Osser, David Harnett, Peter Buckley, Richard Balon, Alan Stone, and Psychiatric Times Editor-in-Chief, James L. Knoll IV. (My sincere apologies to those friends and colleagues I have inadvertently omitted-- and I'm sure there are many!).

Finally, thanks to Dr. Diane P. Toby and Harvey E. Pies for their encouragement over the years-- and special thanks to my wife, Nancy L. Butters, for tolerating my long hours bent over the keyboard, and for helping me keep my perspective on the many controversies and conundrums that arose during my tenure as Editor-in-Chief.

REFERENCES

[1] Lieberman JA: DSM-5: Caught between Mental Illness Stigma and Anti-Psychiatry Prejudice. Scientific American| May 20, 2013 Accessed at: http://blogs.scientific american.com/mind-guest-blog/2013/05/20/dsm-5-caught-between-mental-illness-stigma-and-anti-psychiatry-prejudice/

[2] Duman RS. Neurobiology of stress, depression and rapid actiing antdepressants: remodeling synaptic connections. *Depress Anxiety.* Mar 10,2014.
[3] Mojtabai R, Olfson M. National trends in psychotherapy by office-based psychiatrists. Arch Gen Psychiatry. 2008;65:962-970. - See more at: http://www.psychiatrictimes.com/articles/psychotherapy-alive-and-talking-psychiatry#sthash.abuIUzd5.dpuf
[4] Kandel ER: *Psychiatry, Psychoanalysis and the new biology of mind.* American Psychiatric Publishing, Washington DC, 205.
[5] Stein DJ, *Philosophy of Psychopharmacology,* Cambridge University Press, 2008.
[6] Knoll JL: Psychiatry: Awaken and Return to the Path. Psychiatric Times, March 21, 2011.Accessed at: http://www.psychiatrictimes.com/couch-crisis/psychiatry.

Chapter 1

THE PHILOSOPHICAL AND SCIENTIFIC FOUNDATIONS OF PSYCHIATRY

GETTING IT FROM BOTH SIDES: FOUNDATIONAL AND ANTI-FOUNDATIONAL CRITIQUES OF PSYCHIATRY

Ronald William Pies, MD, Sairah Thommi and Nassir Ghaemi, MD, MPH

Western institutional psychiatry has been the target of numerous social, philosophical, and scientific critiques over the past century, sometimes lumped together as manifestations of antipsychiatry [1]. In actuality, psychiatry's critics have proceeded from two widely divergent sets of assumptions, though they have generally reached similar conclusions. Both foundational and antifoundational critiques have had the effect of discrediting and marginalizing psychiatry and of delegitimizing psychiatric diagnosis and nosology.

Foundational and Anti-Foundational Philosophies

Foundational philosophies hold that we can reliably and validly describe a coherent, objectively measurable or discernible reality, whether one considers the world as a whole or specific aspects of it, such as the classification of disease. Logical positivism is a specific manifestation of the foundational worldview and regards all genuine knowledge as based on logical inference grounded in observable facts; indeed, only empirically verifiable statements are regarded as meaningful by logical positivists [2].

The best-known foundational critique of psychiatric diagnosis comes from Thomas Szasz [1, 3]. In essence, Szasz argued that we know that real (genuine) disease entails the presence of pathological lesions or abnormal pathophysiology [1, 2]; we know that supposed "diseases" such as schizophrenia do not consistently demonstrate such objectively verifiable abnormalities; therefore, we know that schizophrenia (and similar psychiatric fabrications) cannot be genuine, ontologically real diseases [3].

In contrast, anti-foundational philosophies and philosophers assert that there are no objectively demonstrable truths; rather, there are only various perspectives or narratives that cannot be privileged as uniquely or objectively true. Although there is no fully satisfactory definition of postmodernism, we consider anti-foundational critiques of psychiatry a subset of postmodern philosophies, most of which tend to subvert, negate, or delegitimize the Western rational-empirical tradition. Thus, the postmodern theorist, Francois Lyotard, denies the legitimacy of "grand narratives"—essentially, cultural myths that merely serve ". . . to mask the contradictions and instabilities that are inherent in any social organization or practice" [4]. Western science, in the postmodern view, tends to be associated with coercive power and oppression.

Michel Foucault's analysis of psychiatry is perhaps the archetypal anti-foundational critique. Foucault holds that psychiatric medicine has merely fabricated a set of pseudo-objective technical terms—"delusions," "paranoid," "acute schizophrenia," etc.—and imposed this linguistic framework on a largely powerless group of social misfits. According to Foucault, these unfortunates—labeled "insane" or "mentally ill" by psychiatrists—have been denied their own "discourse" and made to conform to the collective discourse (the episteme [systems of understanding]) of psychiatric medicine [5]. There is some degree of convergence between Foucault's claims and those of Szasz, in so far as both castigate institutional psychiatry for its supposed coercive or authoritarian practices; however, there are substantial underlying differences between Szasz and Foucault, and Szasz, who died in 2012, never considered his views to be an example of "antipsychiatry."

Fallacies of Foundational Critiques: Szasz

Szasz's positivist view of disease is inconsistent with most of the history of clinical medicine and with many modern-day philosophers of medicine [6, 7]. It is only in the past century or so that physicians have begun to understand diseases in terms of their biological causes. Indeed, even today, we recognize many conditions as diseases or disorders while having a very limited understanding of their causes or pathophysiology (e.g., various forms of atypical facial pain, primary torsion dystonia, chronic fatigue syndrome) [6, 7]. In light of the suffering and incapacity associated with these conditions, it seems perverse to argue that they will not become real diseases until we can identify specific histological or pathophysiological abnormalities. Ironically, several biomarkers or endophenotypes, such as abnormal smooth pursuit eye movements and enlarged cerebral ventricles, have been consistently associated with schizophrenia—a condition Szasz has variously characterized as a "myth" or "metaphor" [8].

We would argue—borrowing Ludwig Wittgenstein's term—that the "family resemblance" most characteristic of entities called diseases is the presence of *intrinsic suffering and substantial incapacity* [6, 7]. Although knowledge of a condition's histology, pathophysiology, and etiology is extremely helpful in devising diagnostic tests and treatment strategies, such knowledge is not necessary for the ascription of disease (etymologically, "dis-ease," connoting discomfort).

Fallacies of Anti-Foundational Critiques: Foucault

Michel Foucault argues that all disciplines—whether scientific, legal, political, or social—operate through a system of self-legitimizing texts and linguistic conventions. Truth, therefore, cannot be absolute and claims of objectivity are impossible. More specifically, Foucault maintained that the definition and treatment of insanity constitutes a form of social control. In his classic, Madness and Civilization, Foucault held that involuntary confinement of those deemed insane is really a coercive attempt to confine and marginalize madness [5].

Foucault's analysis may shed light on how differing epistemes affect society's management of mental illness, but it does not impugn the ontological reality of mental illness or the immense suffering it causes. Furthermore, following Foucault's own postmodern logic, his claims regarding madness must be viewed as merely another episteme, wherein Foucault asserts his own self-legitimizing power and knowledge. Like most postmodern claims, Foucault's argument effectively devours itself.

Finally, whereas Foucault saw himself as a kind of cultural archeologist, he is more accurately viewed as an old-fashioned moralist. Foucault's argument with psychiatric praxis, like Szasz's, is fundamentally hortatory: it implicitly prescribes and proscribes how people ought to behave toward their fellow citizens; e.g., "We should not lock people away merely because they think or behave in ways we don't like!" Foucault's analysis is perfectly respectable and potentially salutary political advocacy, but it is in no sense a scientifically based critique of psychiatry. Indeed, as Ian Hacking observes, "Despite all the fireworks, Madness and Civilization follows the romantic convention that sees the exercise of power as repression, which is wicked" [9].

Diagnosis and Values in Medicine and Psychiatry

It is a truism that psychiatric diagnosis relies on certain kinds of value judgments, and this observation is often used to marginalize psychiatry from the fold of general medicine. We acknowledge the role of values in psychiatric nosology, but we do not regard this as fundamentally different from the invocation of certain values in other medical specialties. Thus, we believe that there is no evaluative difference between the claim, "The coronary arteries should not be clogged with plaque, if you want good physical health," and the claim, "The mind should not be bombarded with auditory hallucinations, if you want good mental health." This is not to say that body and mind are identical constructs; that coronary artery disease and schizophrenia are closely related; or that the two conditions are experientially similar. It is simply to aver that, in all of general medicine, deciding that a condition is an instantiation of disease depends upon certain kinds of value judgments. But while such judgments are involved in defining health and disease, our disease categories are not merely value judgments. The determination that someone suffers from either a general medical illness or a "mental disorder" is a complex judgment and involves facts and values, as well as objectivity and subjectivity.

Consistent with the positivist tradition, psychiatric diagnosis reflects a myriad of empirical observations, such as the nature and quality of the patient's speech, affect, thought processes, psychomotor activity, and cognitive abilities. However, subjective judgment and values determine whether putative abnormalities in these spheres amount to disease.

Nevertheless, as Zachar and Kendler point out, ". . . values do not have to be inchoate, fuzzy, or undefinable. For example, in the DSM-IV-TR appendix, the Global Assessment of Relational Functioning Axis can be seen as an attempt to operationalize psychiatric values" [10].

Conclusion

Although the foundational and anti-foundational traditions differ in their language and claims, both call into question the legitimacy of psychiatric diagnosis and treatment. To this extent, the rubric of antipsychiatry is probably warranted for both. We have argued that both critical traditions are founded on several misapprehensions regarding the nature of disease, the role of values in determining the presence of pathology, and on supposed differences between psychiatry and the other specialties within general medicine.

In order to defend itself—and, equally important, to reform itself—psychiatry must understand the nature of the arguments arrayed against it. Not all such criticisms are antipsychiatry and the profession must remain open to reassessment of its diagnostic methods and categories. Furthermore, as many critics would insist, psychiatric practice must take care to protect the civil liberties and ensure the informed consent of those it treats. However, neither psychiatrists nor the general public should be misled or intimidated by psychiatry's more vituperative critics, whether of the foundational or anti-foundational stripe. Neither group adequately recognizes the immense suffering and incapacity associated with psychiatric illness; and, despite their humanitarian pretenses, neither group provides a demonstrably effective and humane alternative to psychiatric treatment.

Acknowledgments

Dr. Pies is professor of psychiatry at SUNY Upstate Medical University in Syracuse, NY, and clinical professor of psychiatry at Tufts University School of Medicine in Boston, Mass. Ms. Thommi is research assistant in the Mood Disorders Program at Tufts Medical Center in Boston, Mass. Dr. Ghaemi is director of the Mood Disorders Program at Tufts Medical Center in Boston, Mass. A slightly modified version of this piece appeared in the July 1, 2011, issue of *Psychiatric Times*.

References

[1] Schramme T. The legacy of antipsychiatry. In: Schramme T, Thome J, editors. *Philosophy and Psychiatry*. Berlin: de Gruyter; 2004:94-119.
[2] Hanfling O. Logical positivism. In: Shanker S, ed. *Philosophy of Science, Logic, and Mathematics in the Twentieth Century*. New York: Routledge History of Philosophy; 1996:193-213.
[3] Szasz T. *The Myth of Mental Illness*. New York: Paul B. Hoeber; 1961.
[4] Klages M. Postmodernism. 2007. Available from: http://davekitchen.webs.com/ENG%204U/1%20Klages%20-%20Postmodernism.pdf

[5]   Foucault M. *Madness and Civilization*. New York: Vintage Books; 1973.
[6]   Pies R. On myths and countermyths. *Arch Gen Psychiatry*. 1979;33:139-144.
[7]   Pies R. Moving beyond the "myth" of mental illness. In: Schaler JA, editor. *Szasz Under Fire: A Psychiatric Abolitionist Faces His Critics*. Chicago: Open Court; 2004:327.
[8]   Pies R. Psychiatric diagnosis and the pathologist's view of schizophrenia. *Psychiatry (Edgmont)*. 2008;5:62-65.
[9]   Hacking I. The archaeology of Foucault. In: Hoy DC, ed. *Foucault: A Critical Reader*. Oxford: Blackwell Books; 1986:27-40.
[10] Zachar P, Kendler KS. Psychiatric disorders: a conceptual taxonomy. *Am J Psychiatry*. 2007;164:557-565.

For further reading

Ghaemi SN. *The Concepts of Psychiatry*. Baltimore: Johns Hopkins; 2003.

~~~~~~~~~~~~~~~~~

MENTAL ILLNESS IS NO METAPHOR: FIVE UNEASY PIECES

Philosophical problems arise when language goes on holiday—Ludwig Wittgenstein [1]

Falsehood is never so successful as when she baits her hook with truth. . .— Charles Caleb Colton [2]

Is the expression "mental illness" merely a metaphor? If so, does that tell us something about the persons we identify as having a mental illness? Are these individuals merely metaphorically ill? If so, does that make mental illness a myth? To clinicians who deal with devastating psychiatric disorders every day—and to those afflicted with these conditions—these questions may seem like a lot of semantic nonsense. And yet, the notion that mental illness is nothing but a rhetorical device or figure of speech is virtually an article of faith among many critics of psychiatric nosology and practice. These very controversial issues came vividly to light in a recent debate on the *Cato Unbound* website [3].

My aim in this essay is to examine the concept of metaphor and to challenge the claim that locutions such as mental illness and related terms (e.g., sick mind) are merely metaphorical—while acknowledging that they may be metaphorical in certain contexts. I want to approach these issues through 5 interlocking pieces.

The Argument from Ambiguity

You might imagine that the concept of metaphor is perfectly clear, given that critics of psychiatry use the term so confidently [3]. Yet the scholarly literature suggests that metaphor is nearly as complex, contested, and controversial a term as mental illness [4-8]. While an exhaustive discussion of metaphor is not possible in this space, a few points relevant to psychiatry are worth noting.

First of all, what is a metaphor? In high school, most of us learned that a simile was an expressed comparison, such as "strong as an ox." In contrast a metaphor, is an implied comparison, shorn of "like" or "as." So, "half-baked idea" is a metaphor, because it implies that a poorly conceived idea is similar, in some sense, to a pastry that is only half-baked. A more informative definition of metaphor is ". . . a figure of speech in which a word or phrase is applied to an object or action to which it is not literally applicable" [9]; e.g., "Joe had fallen through the trapdoor of deceit." In addition, philosopher Donald Davidson observes that metaphor ". . . makes us attend to some likeness, often a novel or surprising likeness, between two or more things" [6, p. 247]. Thus, in the 19th century, describing the atom as a miniature solar system might have been a metaphor revealing such a surprising likeness.

But what about the utterance, "my husband is a clown." Is that a metaphor? It might be, if the speaker intended to compare her buffoon of a husband to Bozo. But it might not be, if she meant, quite literally, that her husband is employed by Ringling Brothers Circus, dresses up in funny costumes, and entertains children. So, on this view of metaphor, the speaker's *intention* is critical.

And yet, many linguists and cognitive theorists question the sharp distinction between literal and non-literal locutions. Rather, metaphoricity is seen as ". . . a dimension along which statements can vary" [5, p. 10]. Indeed, Davidson argues that there are no strict rules delineating metaphorical from non-metaphorical language, and that ". . . there is no test for metaphor that does not call for taste. . . . So, too, *understanding a metaphor is as much a creative endeavor as making a metaphor*, little guided by rules [italics added]" [6, p. 245].

Some critics of psychiatry write as if using the term mental illness necessarily entails using a metaphor—as if metaphoricity is inherent in words or phrases themselves [3, 10]. But if metaphors are intentional comparisons, how can the locution mental illness be declared a metaphor, without ascertaining the speaker's intention? When reporters for *The New York Times* [11] referred to the "severe mental illness" of James E. Holmes—the accused shooter in the Aurora, Colorado massacre—were they employing a metaphor? When, in the same article, these reporters allude to ". . . *diseases* and disorders like Alzheimer's, schizophrenia and autism . . . [italics added]" were they speaking of diseases only in a figurative sense? I doubt it. I think the reporters were using English in a perfectly ordinary way. And here we need to remind ourselves of philosopher Ludwig Wittgenstein's remark in *The Blue and Brown Books* [1]:

> "It is wrong to say that in philosophy, we consider an ideal language as opposed to our ordinary one. For this makes it appear as though we thought we could improve on ordinary language. But ordinary language is all right."

I'll return to the matter of ordinary language after a brief historical excursion.

The Argument from Linguistic History

If the locution mental illness is merely a metaphor, why does it seem to be used in a literal sense throughout much of recent human history? Similarly, the expressions, "sick soul" and "sick mind" seem to have had a quite literal meaning in much of the history of medicine. Thus, the great medieval physician and philosopher, Maimonides, asks:

> "What is the remedy for those whose *souls are sick*? Let them go to the wise men—who are physicians of the soul—and they will cure their *disease* by means of the character traits that they shall teach them. . . ." (italics added) [12].

Now, if the persons Maimonides references are only metaphorically sick and have only metaphorical disease, why would they need a physician of any kind? Why would they need a cure for a mere metaphorical condition? To be sure, Maimonides probably had something akin to psychotherapy in mind, in referring to modification of one's character traits by physicians of the soul—but a psychological mode of treatment does not negate the phenomenological reality of the person's disease [13]. (Indeed, as I have argued elsewhere, disease [dis-ease] is best understood as the suffering and incapacity experienced by *persons*—not as an isolated property of minds, brains, souls, or bodies [14, 15].)

Similarly, when Shakespeare has Macbeth—watching anxiously as Lady Macbeth sleepwalks—say to the attending physician "Canst thou not minister to a *mind diseased*,/Pluck from the memory a rooted sorrow,/Raze out the written troubles of the brain . . ." (italics added) [16, Act 5, Scene 3], there is no compelling reason to regard the expression, "mind diseased" as a metaphor, rather than as ordinary and literal 16th century English usage. (I am grateful to Shakespearean scholar, Prof. Stephen Greenblatt, for confirming this interpretation; personal communication, August 23, 2012.) Indeed, it is striking that Shakespeare places "mind diseased" in the same context as "troubles of the brain . . . ," suggesting that no sharp distinction was present between disordered minds and troubled brains, in Shakespeare's time^^. Perhaps the subsequent reification of mind-body dualism by Rene Descartes [17] (1596-1650) has contributed to our present conundrum over the relationship between mind and brain—including the claim by psychiatry's critics that minds cannot literally be diseased.

The Argument from Ordinary Language

Psychiatry's critics often insist that when we speak of a sick mind, we are necessarily speaking metaphorically, just as we do when we refer to a sick joke or a sick economy [3, 10]. But are these last two expressions really metaphors? Or do they simply represent our ordinary-language use of subsidiary or secondary meanings of the word "sick"? From this perspective, when we describe a joke as sick, we are not proposing or imagining a comparison with real sickness, such as tuberculosis or cancer. Rather, we are simply applying a colloquial—but well-accepted—secondary meaning of sick to the word "joke."

Thus, the *American Century Dictionary* gives, as a colloquial meaning of sick, the terms *cruel* or *morbid* [18]. A joke at the expense of a crippled, blind elderly person could justly be called sick *not* because we are comparing the wellness-state of the joke with an entity that is actually sick (such as a sick AIDS patient); but because we believe the joke is genuinely cruel or morbid.

On similar grounds, when we describe someone as having a "mental illness" or a "sick mind," we are not ordinarily proposing that the listener perform a *comparison* of some sort, as metaphor entails. We are simply applying an ordinary, albeit non-technical, meaning of illness or sick. For example, one meaning of sick, according to the *Merriam-Webster Dictionary*, is "mentally or emotionally unsound or disordered" [19]. So, too, with the term "disease," for which the *American Century Dictionary* gives the following definition [18]: "unhealthy condition of the body *or mind* [italics added]." This is quite consistent with some definitions of disease found in standard medical texts [20].

Errors Deriving from the Intentional Fallacy

Critics of psychiatry and psychiatric nosology often make claims like, "Mental illness is a metaphor (metaphorical disease)," and "Individuals with mental diseases (bad behaviors), like societies with economic diseases (bad fiscal policies), are metaphorically sick" [21]. They go on to claim that the term mental illness is merely a rhetorical device, or a political strategy [3]. I believe these claims reflect a deep confusion between the locution or expression "mental illness" (sense 1); and the actual state of affairs in the heads of individuals clinically diagnosed with mental illness (sense 2). (The use of the word "heads" helps me avert the perennial mind vs. brain conundrum.)

The failure to distinguish these two senses of mental illness has led to much confusion in the literature, in the form of what philosopher Norman Malcolm has termed "the intentional fallacy" [22]. An example of this fallacy would be a claim such as: "When I refer to 'water,' I intend no reference to hydrogen or oxygen atoms. Therefore, water must in fact be something other than an arrangement of hydrogen and oxygen atoms." Thus, the intentional fallacy involves an unwarranted extrapolation from intentional language to the external world.

Now, it may be perfectly true that when *some* people use the locution, "mental illness," they are in fact speaking metaphorically. They may sincerely *believe*, for example, that mental illness stands in the same relation to real illness as the word "unicorn" stands in relation to real animals. However, it is fallacious to infer that specific individuals diagnosed with, say, schizophrenia are not genuinely ill, diseased, incapacitated, or sick. *Nothing we intend, mean, imply, or believe when we use the locution "mental illness" affects the ontological status—the actuality or "is-ness"—of what is going on in somebody's head, or in his life!* In short, the suffering and incapacity of someone accurately diagnosed with schizophrenia is *ontologically real*—independent of the intentional properties of language.

Another form of the intentional fallacy emerges when critics claim that "mental illness" is a term that ". . . *refers to* the judgments of some persons about the (bad) behaviors of other persons" (italics added) [10]. Let us stipulate, for the sake of argument, that this is so. It doesn't follow that what psychiatrists call mental illness (sense 2) is nothing over and above these disapproved of behaviors, or the judgments rendered about them[++]. As the philosopher Tim Thornton has observed, "The behavior may be essential to grasping the meaning of the word. But it may not be the case that the word refers to the behavior" (personal communication, September 4, 2012).

By analogy: if we posit that the term "migraine headache" refers to a doctor's *judgments* regarding a set of pain-related behaviors—e.g., the patient complains bitterly of left-sided head pain, winces, squints, places ice packs on his head, cries "Owwww!"—it does not follow that migraine headache *is nothing over and above the doctor's judgments*, or the set of pain-related behaviors being judged. Migraine may, as a matter of ontological and etiological fact, entail certain reversible changes in vascular nerves, inflammatory substances in the brain, etc. This ontological claim holds, whether such physiological findings have actually been confirmed.

Errors Arising from a False Dilemma

Finally, critics of psychiatry sometimes construct a sophistical and quite fallacious trap for psychiatrists. They create an apparent dilemma, by arguing thus:

Schizophrenia is not a real disease, because real disease requires a demonstration of clear and consistent neuropathology or pathophysiology [proposition 1], and this has never been convincingly demonstrated for schizophrenia [proposition 2]. But, if neuropathology or abnormal physiology should someday be demonstrated in persons said to have schizophrenia, then schizophrenia will obviously not be a *mental* illness—because minds cannot contain lesions—but a *brain* disease, like Alzheimer's Disease [proposition 3]. Now, consistent neuropathology either (a) cannot (now) be shown for persons said to have schizophrenia, or (b) may someday be shown. Therefore, schizophrenia is either (now) not a real disease; or may someday be shown to be a *brain* disease. Therefore, the claim that schizophrenia is a real disease or a *mental* illness is necessarily false.

This dodgy argument—which I have condensed from several sources**—is trivially fallacious on several levels [3, 10]. First, as I have already argued, the term "disease" need not entail the presence of abnormal pathoanatomical or pathophysiological findings [proposition 1]. Second, if there is (ontologically) "no such thing" as schizophrenia, there is no way, even in principle, that schizophrenia can "someday" reveal consistent brain pathology. (If there is no such thing as a unicorn, there is no empirical study that "someday" could show a unicorn to be a horse!)

An additional fallacy is seen in proposition 3: it is simply *not* the case that a condition necessarily ceases to be a mental illness simply because its putative etiology has been traced to neuroanatomical or pathophysiological abnormalities. Once again, we are sorely in need of *ordinary language*. When we say, in ordinary conversation, that Jones has a "mental illness," we are not necessarily positing some immaterial entity called "mind" or "mentality," which—to be sure—would be incapable of containing material lesions or neuropathology. We may mean simply that Jones's particular form of suffering and incapacity *expresses itself in the sphere of thought, cognition, mood, or reality-testing*—usually as some combination of impairments in these domains. We may additionally mean that these impairments render it difficult or impossible for Jones to secure his "prudential interests;" e.g., Jones is unable to secure his own safety, avoid serious injury, achieve enduring relationships, or hold down a job [23].

Finally, with respect to proposition 2: I believe it is simplistic and misleading to insist that no consistent neuropathological abnormalities have been linked to schizophrenia or other serious psychiatric illnesses—alas, a canard credulously accepted by many psychiatrists. In fact, one recent study concluded that, "Enlarged ventricles and reduced hippocampal volume are *consistently* found in patients with first-episode schizophrenia" (italics added) [24]. (The literature far exceeds the scope of the present article but is reviewed in other publications [24-26].)

Conclusion

The concept of metaphor is too ambiguous and unstable to provide a sound basis for criticizing psychiatric nosology or the concept of mental illness. The locution, mental illness, may sometimes be used metaphorically, but need not be; nor must it denote something immaterial or metaphysical. In ordinary language, mental illness may refer to pronounced suffering and incapacity in the sphere of thought, mood, cognition, and reality testing; and to the resultant inability to secure one's prudential interests. There is nothing metaphorical in such affliction, and nothing mythical in the construct of psychiatric disease.

Notes

^^ In his preface the new edition of *The Myth of Mental Illness* [10], Thomas Szasz MD analyzes these same passages from *Macbeth*, focusing on the doctor's conclusion that the mad person "must minister to himself." Szasz sees this as evidence that, for Shakespeare, Lady Macbeth's madness was a consequence of her "internal rhetoric," which must be cured with therapeutic internal rhetoric. But even supposing this interpretation is correct, it does not impugn my claim that the phrase "mind diseased" was to be taken literally, not metaphorically, in Shakespeare's time; and, indeed, that it may still be taken literally in our time.

For more on metaphor and mental illness in the 16th century, see Bridget Gellert Lyons' book, *Voices of Melancholy* [27]. Lyons highlights the risk of assuming that we can confidently recognize figurative language in Elizabethan writing. For example, in *Macbeth*, the statement, "The grief that does not speak/Whispers the o'er fraught heart and bids it break" (IV,iii) is not merely or simply a metaphor; rather, the locution ". . . is based on the belief that the heart of a bereaved sufferer who could not unburden himself by speech was *literally* oppressed and suffocated by [bodily] humours. . . ." (italics added) [27]. Thus, Lyons identifies ". . . the physiological basis of this metaphor. . . ." suggesting that even metaphorical utterances may be grounded in putative physical abnormalities.

++ I believe Prof. Tim Thornton argues along roughly the same lines as I do, when he writes:

". . . even if mental illness is defined by, or identified through, psycho-social norms, this need not imply that it is identical to or constituted by such deviation. It may be that the illness is the cause of the deviation such that, even though it is picked out by its characteristic effects, it is not identical to them" [28].

**See, for example, Szasz's argument in *Fifty Years After the Myth of Mental Illness*:

"The proposition that mental illness is not a medical problem runs counter to public opinion and psychiatric dogma. When a person hears me say that there is no such thing as mental illness, he is likely to reply: 'But I know so-and-so who was diagnosed as mentally ill and turned out to have a brain tumor. In due time, with refinements in medical technology, psychiatrists will be able to show that all mental illnesses are bodily diseases.' This contingency does not falsify my contention that mental illness is a metaphor. It verifies it: The physician who concludes that a person diagnosed as mentally *ill suffers from a brain disease discovers that the patient was misdiagnosed: the patient did not have a mental illness, he had an undiagnosed bodily illness. The physician's [initial] erroneous diagnosis is not proof that the term 'mental illness' refers to a class of brain diseases."* [10]

But Szasz's conclusion would be true only if the term "mental illness" were mutually exclusive with "brain disease," such that discovery of the latter vitiates diagnosis of the former. But this is by no means either clear or logically necessary. If, by "mental illness", we mean simply "a type of suffering and incapacity expressed in the realm of cognition, affect, or behavior," discovery of "brain disease" as the *proximate cause* of the "mental illness" does not invalidate or vitiate our original designation; i.e., "mental illness." I am grateful to Dr. Muhammad Awais Aftab for making some of these points in an article published in the February 28, 2014, *Psychiatric Times*.

Acknowledgments

My thanks to Prof. Tim Thornton, Prof. Stephen Greenblatt, Prof. Robert Daly, Prof. Joel Kraemer, and Prof. James L. Knoll IV, MD, for their helpful comments on drafts or aspects of this paper; and to Neil Pickering, PhD for his useful book and correspondence. Thanks also to Prof. Amanda Pustilnik for her essays, and to Mr. Jason Kuznicki for his editing of Cato-Unbound. A slightly modified version of this piece appeared in the September 13, 2012, issue of *Psychiatric Times*.

References

[1] Wittgenstein L. The Blue and Brown Books: Preliminary Studies for the Philosophical Investigations. New York: Harper and Row; 1958: 1, 38.
[2] Colton C. Think-exist.com. Charles Caleb Colton quotes [online.]. Available from: http://thinkexist.com/quotation/falsehood_is_never_so_successful_as_when_she/177433.html. Accessed March 1, 2014.
[3] Schaler J, Frances A, Sullum J, Pustilnik AC. Mental Health and the Law [online]. Cato Unbound. Available from: www.cato-unbound.org/issues. Accessed March 1, 2014. (See in particular the numerous postings by Prof. Jeffrey Schaler; also see my letter re: schizophrenia in pathology textbooks.)
[4] Lakoff G, Johnson M. *Metaphors We Live By*. Chicago: University of Chicago Press; 2003.
[5] Ortony A, editor. *Metaphor and Thought*. Cambridge: Cambridge University Press; 1993.
[6] Davidson D. What metaphors mean. *Inquiries Into Truth and Interpretation*. 2nd ed. Gloucestershire, UK: Clarendon Press; 2001.
[7] Pickering N. The Metaphor of Mental Illness. International Perspectives in Philosophy and Psychiatry. New York: Oxford University Press; 2006.
[8] Pies R. Poetry and schizophrenia. In: Graham PW, editor. *Literature and Medicine, Vol 4*. Baltimore: Johns Hopkins University Press; 1985.

[9]   *New Oxford American Dictionary.* 3rd ed. New York: Oxford University Press; 2010.
[10] Szasz T. *Fifty Years After the Myth of Mental Illness.* Available from: http://www.rcpsych.ac.uk/pdf/Szasz%20update.pdf
[11] Goode E, Kovaleski SF, Healy J, Frosch J. Before gunfire, hints of "bad news." *The New York Times.* 2012 August 26. Available from: http://www.nytimes.com/2012/08/27/us/before-gunfire-in-colorado-theater-hints-of-bad-news-about-james-holmes.html?pagewanted=all. Accessed March 1, 2014.
[12] Maimonides. Laws concerning character traits. In: Weiss RL, Butterworth CE, editors. *Ethical Writings of Maimonides.* New York: Dover Publications Inc.; 1983.
[13] Pies R. Maimonides and the origins of cognitive-behavioral therapy. *J Cog Psychother.* 1997;11:21-36.
[14] Pies R. On myths and countermyths: more on Szaszian fallacies. *Arch Gen Psychiatry.* 1979;36:139-144.
[15] Pies R. Moving beyond the "myth" of mental illness. In: Schaler JA, ed. Szasz Under Fire. Chicago: *Open Court Publishing;* 2004:327-353.
[16] Shakespeare W. *The Tragedy of Macbeth.* Available from: http://shakespeare.mit.edu/macbeth/index.html. Accessed March 1, 2014.
[17] Skirry J. Rene Descartes: the mind-body distinction [online]. Internet Encyclopedia of Philosophy. Available from: http://www.iep.utm.edu/descmind/. Accessed March 1, 2014.
[18] The American Century Dictionary. New York: Grand Central Publishing; 1996.
[19] Merriam-Webster [online]. http://www.merriam-webster.com/dictionary/sick. Accessed September 12, 2012.
[20] Isselbacher K, editor. *Harrison's Principles of Internal Medicine.* 8th ed. New York: McGraw-Hill; 1977:1.
[21] Szasz T. Thomas Szasz's summary statement and manifesto [online]. 1998 March. Available from: http://www.szasz.com/manifesto.html. Accessed March 1, 2014.
[22] Malcolm N. Scientific materialism and the identity theory. In: O'Connor J, editor. *Modern Materialism: Readings on Mind-Body Identity.* New York: *Harcourt, Brace, and World:* 1969:72-81.
[23] Daly R. Sanity and the origins of psychiatry. *Assoc Advance Philos Psychiatry Bull.* In press.
[24] Ebdrup BH, Glenthøj B, Rasmussen H, et al. Hippocampal and caudate volume reductions in antipsychotic-naive first-episode schizophrenia. *J Psychiatry Neurosci.* 2010;35:95-104.
[25] Harrison PG, Roberts GW, editors. *The Neuropathology of Schizophrenia: Progress and Interpretation.* New York: Oxford University Press; 2000.
[26] Steen RG, Mull C, McClure R, et al. Brain volume in first-episode schizophrenia: systematic review and meta-analysis of magnetic resonance imaging studies. *Br J Psychiatry.* 2006;188:510-518.
[27] Lyons BG. *Voices of Melancholy.* New York: WW Norton; 1971.
[28] Thornton T. 800 words on Thomas Szasz [online]. In the Space of Reasons blog. 2008 September 18. Available from: http://inthespaceofreasons.blogspot.co.uk/2008/09/800-words-on-thomas-szasz.html. Accessed March 1, 2014.

Addendum

A key claim of Dr. Szasz and his followers was that pathology texts never include psychiatric disorders. I deal with this obvious canard in a letter posted on the Cato Unbound website [1]. There I note the following:

Let's begin with Boyd's *Introduction to the Study of Disease*, Eleventh Edition, published in 1992 [2]. The author, Dr. Huntington Sheldon, was at the time a professor of pathology at McGill University. Dr. Sheldon classifies schizophrenia under the rubric of "functional disorders." He goes on to argue that schizophrenia "…might be regarded as a cancer of the mind, gnawing into the very soul of the patient." Now, those who believe that schizophrenia is only a "metaphorical" disease may dismiss Sheldon's vivid description as mere poetic imagery—not the stuff of hard science. Yet Sheldon goes on to note the beneficial effects of hemodialysis in "a small group of schizophrenics," leading him to hypothesize that there may be "a biochemical substance… that directly affects the ordered functioning of the central nervous system" in schizophrenia. Clearly, for this pathologist, schizophrenia is no mere "metaphorical" illness.

Almost a decade after Dr. Sheldon wrote this, we find another discussion of schizophrenia in the textbook *Biology of Disease*, Second Edition, by Phillips, Murray, and Kirk [3]. Although this is arguably not a "standard" textbook on pathology (it also encompasses elements of clinical medicine), Dr. Murray was then in the department of pathology at the University of Birmingham, United Kingdom. All told, there are seven pages in the text that deal with schizophrenia. Schizophrenia is considered in detail in the chapter entitled "Psychological and social aspects of disease." Phillips et al., observe that "A variety of clinical investigations and imaging techniques… have revealed a number of interesting findings [in schizophrenia], including evidence of cerebral atrophy, left temporal lobe dysfunction, [and] evidence of neuronal loss and disorganization."

The Phillips et al. text goes on to note that the significance of the "inconsistent" pathological findings in schizophrenia are "a matter of current speculation," however there follows a critically important statement: "the biology of *this disease* is as yet poorly understood" (italics added).

Now, critics of psychiatric diagnosis may rush to seize upon the words "poorly understood"—but that would be a serious philosophical error. The biology of many diseases, including some types of cancer, is "poorly understood." The critical words are "this disease." There is simply no question that the authors of the text view schizophrenia as a disease—and that this classification is not dependent on our having a full understanding of schizophrenia's biology.

As Dr. Allen Frances points out, schizophrenia is probably a final common pathway for many different pathophysiological processes; my point here is that psychiatrists are far from alone in using the term "disease" in reference to schizophrenia. Other references to schizophrenia may be found in standard pathology texts, such as the *Oxford Textbook of Pathology* [4]. But the coup de grace for the claim that pathology texts don't recognize schizophrenia is delivered by the 1997 textbook *The Neuropathology of Dementia*, edited by Esiri and Morris [5], in which 20 pages of text discuss the neuropathology of schizophrenia. Moreover, since that text's publication, hundreds of controlled studies of the neuropathology of schizophrenia have appeared in peer-reviewed journals and are converging on several consistent biological abnormalities.

References

[1] Pies, R. Letters: The pathology and reality of schizophrenia [online]. Cato Unbound. Available from: http://www.cato-unbound.org/2012/08/22/editors. Accessed February 18, 2014.

[2] Boyd SH. *Introduction to the Study of Disease*. 11th ed. Philadelphia: Lea & Febiger; 1992.

[3] Phillips J. In: *Biology of Disease*, 2nd Ed. Murray PG, Kirk P, editors. Hoboken, *NJ: Wiley-Blackwell;* 2001.

[4] Talmud PJ, Humphries S. "Molecular genetic analysis of coronary artery disease." In McGee JO, Isaacson PG, Wright NA, Dick HM, editors. *Oxford Textbook of Pathology Volume 1: Principles of Pathology*. New York: Oxford Medical Publications; 1992.

[5] Esri MM, Morris JH, editors. *The Neuropathology of Dementia*. Cambridge: Cambridge University Press; 1997.

~~~~~~~~~~~~~~~~~

OBJECTIVITY IN PSYCHIATRY: IMPLICATIONS FOR DIAGNOSIS AND TREATMENT

Several recent statements from various clinicians and authors in the mental health field have raised serious questions about psychiatry's "objectivity."

But what do *philosophers* mean when they speak of "subjective" and "objective" evidence? According to philosopher and economist Amartya Sen, they often mean something like this. When I say, without having observed your house, "I truly and deeply believe that your house is on fire," I am making a *subjective* claim. In contrast, if two people simultaneously witness what they believe is smoke coming from your house, and say, "We believe your house is on fire," they are making a type of *objective* statement. This does not necessarily mean that your house *is* on fire—after all, someone inside might have been producing a gray-colored vapor of some sort that merely resembles smoke. Thus, the *veridical* nature or "truth value" of objective statements cannot automatically be assumed. But whereas, in theory, we might choose to run that gray-colored vapor through an electronic "vapor analyzer" at some point, we surely would not hesitate to call 911 immediately.

How does all this apply to clinical psychiatry? For philosophers such as Sen, if I say, without having assessed you, "I believe deep in my heart that you have a thought process disorder," I am making an essentially *subjective* claim. On the other hand, if my chief resident and I sit with you for an hour, attending carefully to your speech, and neither of us has a clue as to what you have been saying, we are beginning to develop an "objective" frame of reference. If both the resident and I can point to your use of frequent neologisms and unconventional syntax, as well as to your shifting from idea to idea within the same sentence, we are continuing to develop an "objective" basis for saying that you have a *thought process disorder* of some sort—our agreement being a modest example of "inter-rater reliability." If, upon standardized neurolinguistic testing, we can confirm that, indeed, your use of grammar, syntax, logic, and concept formation are all abnormal, we have further objective evidence of a thought process disorder.

Does all this mean that you have a "mental illness" or a "disease" of any kind? Of course not. To determine that, we need a much broader construct than that of "thought process disorder," and a much wider array of objective data. In philosophical terms, *we need many more observations that can be confirmed by multiple observers.* For example, the resident and I may agree that a thought-disordered patient also has a *blunted* or *flat affect* (based, in part, on our shared experience of "normal" affect). We also observe that he is muttering to himself when sitting alone. We may learn, from a spouse or family member, that the patient has not been showering, feeding himself, or changing his clothes for the past month, and that this represents a dramatic change in his usual behavior. We may learn, from both the patient and the family member, that he is "hearing voices" when nobody is in the room, and that these voices are telling him, *"You deserve to burn in Hell for all eternity!"* We may also learn that, on more than one occasion, the patient has broken into tears and slashed himself with a razor, upon hearing these "voices." At this point, we have built a stronger objective case for saying that the patient has an illness or disease of some sort—perhaps a schizophreniform or psychotic depressive disorder, though other possibilities must be considered (an endocrine disturbance, a brain tumor, a dementing process, etc.).

If, in addition, we can find abnormalities on neurological testing, brain imaging, or laboratory testing, so much the better. (It is clear, on this view, that "objectivity" is not an all-or-none quality, but one that exists along a *continuum* of evidence.) With such testing, we certainly would be strengthening our objective data base—but laboratory studies are not necessary for objectively claiming, in the first place, that the patient has a "disease" of a psychiatric nature.

Historically, the construct of "disease" developed from the notion of *suffering and incapacity* in the absence of an obvious external cause, such as a knife wound. The term *disease* was originally derived from the notion of "*dis*-ease" or discomfort. It is no coincidence that the word *patient* is derived from the Latin *pati,* meaning "to suffer" or "to bear." As physicians, we first recognize *dis*-ease and treat suffering, based on our *clinical* (from Gk. *kline,* "bed") *observations.* In general, it is only *subsequently* that we invoke imaging or laboratory studies to bolster or confirm our diagnosis. As Schwartz and Wiggins have argued, "…we legitimately reason about people's experiences and behaviors in the same manner that we might reason about breathing problems…such reasoning might—or might not—lead us to lesions. But the goal is the relief of suffering, the promotion of health, and the amelioration of the illness…" Of course, a neuropathologist might not offer a diagnosis of "neuroborreliosis" until the organism causing Lyme Disease had been reliably identified. But even a neuropathologist would not deny that a patient who complained, without dissimulation, of profound memory impairment, disorientation, visual hallucinations, and paresthesias had a *disease* of some kind—much less deny that this individual merits our care and treatment.

Indeed, when the average neurologist diagnoses, say, "migraine headaches," he or she rarely uses laboratory or imaging studies, except to rule out *other* disease entities, such as a central nervous system lesion.

Rather, the neurologist relies, in the first place, on the patient's subjective (or *phenomenological*) claims; e.g., "Doc, I get a persistent, throbbing, left-sided pain in my head, along with nausea and sensitivity to light." This claim is then weighed in the context of objective data derived from the medical history and neurological examination. This process is not radically different from the holistic approach a psychiatrist takes in diagnosing schizophrenia or major depression. Nor does it differ from the way most emergency room physicians would make a presumptive diagnosis of *angina pectoris*, even if the patient's EKG were normal.

That some "researchers" may successfully fool clinicians by presenting bogus complaints of hallucinations, headache, or chest pain does not impugn the objective basis of medical diagnosis. Neither does the sad fact that some of our colleagues fail to gather a sufficiently detailed set of phenomenological and objective data, prior to making a diagnosis or offering treatment.

In psychiatry, as in the rest of clinical medicine, it is the patient's unique *experience* of suffering and incapacity—not a blood test or MRI result—that first prompts diagnosis and treatment. Indeed, we would do well to remind ourselves of that famous dictum from Maimonides: "The physician does not cure a disease, he cures a *diseased person*."

Acknowledgements

The author wishes to thank Dr. Scott Lilienfeld and Dr. Michael A. Schwartz for their seminal contributions in the area of psychiatric diagnosis, and expresses appreciation to Dr. Daniel Pistone for his stimulating ideas. A slightly modified version of this piece appeared in the July 1, 2006, issue of *Psychiatric Times*.

For Further Reading

Spitzer RL, Lilienfeld SO, Miller MB. Rosenhan revisited: the scientific credibility of Lauren Slater's pseudopatient diagnosis study. *J Nerv Ment Dis*. 2005;193:734-739.

Slater L. Opening Skinner's Box: Great Psychological Experiments of the Twentieth Century. New York: WW Norton; 2004.

Slater L. Reply to Spitzer and colleagues. *J Nerv Ment Dis*. 2005;193:743-744.

Lilienfeld SO, Spitzer RL, Miller MB. A response to a nonresponse to criticisms of a nonstudy. One humorous and one serious rejoinder to Slater. *J Nerv Ment Dis*. 2005;193:745-746.

Pies R. Psychiatry clearly meets the "objectivity" test. *Psychiatr News*. 2005;40(19):17.

Pies R. Moving beyond the "myth" of mental illness. In: Schaler JA, editor. *Szasz Under Fire*. Chicago: Open Court; 2004: 327-353.

Sen A. Objectivity and position: assessment of health and well-being. In: Chen L, Kleinman A, Ware N. *Health and Social Change in International Perspective*. Boston: Harvard School of Public Health; 1994.

Szasz TS. *The Myth of Mental Illness*. New York: Harper & Row; 1974.

Nagel T. *The View from Nowhere*. New York: Oxford University Press; 1986.

Schwartz MA, Wiggins OP. Psychiatry fraud and force? A commentary on E. Fuller Torrey and Thomas Szasz. *J Humanistic Psychology*. 2005;45:403-415.

PSYCHIATRY AND ANTHROPOLOGY, IN SEARCH OF "SCIENCE"

Have you been following the recent dust-up in the anthropology world? It all started, as Nicholas Wade wrote, "...after a decision by the American Anthropological Association at its recent annual meeting to strip the word 'science' from a statement of its long-range plan" [1]. Commenting on this radical move, Peter Peregrine, president of the Society for Anthropological Sciences,

> "...attributed what he viewed as an attack on science to two influences within anthropology. One is that of so-called critical anthropologists, who see anthropology as an arm of colonialism and therefore something that should be done away with. The other is the postmodernist critique of the authority of science" [1].

There are interesting parallels between the post-modern critique leveled against anthropology, and a similar argument—associated with Michel Foucault—directed against psychiatry, as Dr. Nassir Ghaemi, Sarah Thommai, and I have argued recently [2]. But right now, I'm interested in the other side of the double-edged sword often wielded against psychiatry: not the objections arising from the post-modern tradition, but those arising from *logical positivism*. This was an extreme form of empiricism associated with a group of philosophers known as the "Vienna Circle"—a very high-brow *kaffee klatsch* that met regularly near the University of Vienna. The Circle included luminaries like Moritz Schlick, Rudolf Carnap, Kurt Godel, and Otto Neurath, and did much to promote logical positivism in the early 1920s. (The philosopher Ludwig Wittgenstein sometimes sat in, but never fully embraced the Circle's views—preferring, some say, to read poetry during their meetings!)

Essentially, logical positivism (LP) rejected the "meaningfulness" of any claim that was not based either on a priori *logical necessity* ("All bachelors are unmarried males") or *direct observation*. So, the claim "This rock weighs 0.5 kg" is a meaningful statement to logical positivists. Other kinds of claims, such as "The Mona Lisa is a beautiful painting," or "Stealing is morally wrong," were dismissed as meaningless expressions of emotion. This positivistic view of meaning has infiltrated and colored our modern concept of "science" to a profound degree—notwithstanding the devastating critique of LP from the American philosopher W.V.O. Quine [3] (1908-2000).

Sixty years after Quine's broadside, many in the medical field, in my experience, still take a positivist view of what constitutes "real science." This has left psychiatry open to the charge of not being "scientific"—much as some have said of anthropology. But should all "science" be equated with logical positivism, and held to the rules and paradigms of, say, physical chemistry or molecular biology? And, if we adopt a broader construct of "science," can we maintain that psychiatry is, in fact, very much a science—though it is also far more than that?

A letter in the December 14, 2010, *New York Times* put all these issues in the spotlight. Tom Boellstorff, Editor in Chief of *American Anthropologist,* took the position that "...anthropology helps broaden the definition of science itself." He argued that "...Science takes place not just in laboratories but in field sites..." as one would find in many anthropological studies. So far, so good—I'm with Prof. Boellstorff on that point, and would add, "Science can also take place in the psychiatrist's office!" But the professor goes on to make another claim—perhaps without realizing just how provocative it is. Science, he claims,

"...involves not just experiments but forms of *non-replicable* observation..." Of course, Boellstorff is correct if he means that *no two sets of observations are precisely the same*: it is impossible to recreate exactly the same conditions of the universe at time T2 as at time T1. And, it is widely accepted in the philosophy of science that changing the observer inherently changes the nature of the observation. So up to this point, I have no quarrel with Prof. Boellstorff's statement. However, if he wants to claim that *non-replicable observation is an acceptable and intrinsic design element of science*, I would respectfully disagree—particularly as regards the science of psychiatry.

To be sure: it is difficult, if not impossible, to produce an "essential definition" of either science or the "scientific method" [4, 5]. Nevertheless, Okasha has listed "some of the main features of scientific enquiry" as including *induction, experimental testing, observation, theory construction, [and] inference to the best explanation* [5]. I believe psychiatry partakes of all these elements of science. However, in so far as "observation" is a feature of science, I believe it must entail *replicable* observation. This follows from science's aim to be *objective* (more on this anon). The philosopher Amartya Sen described two essential features of objectivity: *observation dependence* and *impersonality* [6]. "Objectivity demands taking observations seriously," Sen argued [6]. The second term, *impersonality*, implies that in order for an observation to be objective, *the observer's conclusions should be more or less reproducible by other observers*, within the natural limits of human perception. If I write in my mental status exam that "Mr. A. shows marked loosening of associations," I implicitly assert that most English-speaking clinicians are likely to concur with my assessment, assuming that Mr. A's linguistic productions remain relatively constant. The same goes for my notation that "Mr. A. shows markedly flattened affect."

Now—notice that neither notation (loose associations, flat affect) is a straightforward *observation* in the sense that logical positivists probably intended that term: I am not weighing a rock on a scale, after all. First of all, I am implicitly invoking a whole range of *mediating and linking hypotheses*—such as, "There is a direct connection between a person's linguistic expressions and their contemporaneous thought processes;" and, "A tightly-associated train of thought does not contain three or more unrelated ideas within three contiguous sentences." Moreover, I am reaching a clinical *judgment*. Inevitably, a measure of subjectivity inheres in *all* such judgments—including those in general medicine; for example, "This liver cell has borderline atypical morphology." Nonetheless, my mental status exam is both "scientific" and "objective" according to the general criteria I have set forth.

All this goes down the drain, however, if I allow that my observations are "just mine"—that they are, to use Prof. Boellstorff's term, "non-replicable." Indeed, one would be inclined to ask, "Why bother writing them down, if all your notations are non-replicable?" Our entire therapeutic approach to the patient assumes that our observations are largely replicable, both within the circle of our *own* observations—e.g., from session to session—and within the perceptual field of *another competent clinician*. (Of course, the patient's mental status may vary according to mood polarity, course of illness, and many other factors). Without such a general expectation of "replicability", it would make no sense asking another psychiatrist to care for our patients, when we are away!

I have argued previously that psychiatry is a *human science*; specifically, a *science of meaning* [4, 7, 8]. This is not the same as a "physical science", like, say, mineralogy or bacteriology—but it *is* a science nevertheless. However, contrary to the implication I read in Prof. Boellstorff's letter, we cannot maintain our scientific *bona fides* unless we assume that our clinical observations can be replicated, to a large extent, by other clinicians. Finally, I want to be clear that psychiatry is also *more* than mere science: it is also an intense human encounter that defies formula or theorem. The patient is never merely an "It" to be "observed." We must meet the patient empathically, in what Martin Buber called the "I-Thou" relationship. Therein lies the art—and the heart—of what we do as psychiatrists.

Acknowledgment

A slightly modified version of this piece appeared in the December 20, 2010, issue of *Psychiatric Times*.

References

[1] Wade N. Anthropology a science? Statement deepens a rift. *The New York Times*. 2010 December 9. Available from: http://www.nytimes.com/2010/12/10/science/10anthropology.html?_r=1. Accessed March 1, 2014.

[2] Pies R, Ghaemi SN, Thommai S. Getting it from both sides: Foundational and antifoundational critiques of psychiatry. *Psychiatr Times*. 2011 July 1. Available from: psychiatrictimes.com/cultural-psychiatry/getting-it-both-sides-foundational-and-antifoundational-critiques-psychiatry. Accessed March 1, 2014.

[3] Quine WVO. Two dogmas of empiricism. *The Philosophical Review*. 1951;60: 20-43. Reprinted in: *From a Logical Point of View*. Boston: Harvard University Press; 1953.

[4] Pies R. Psychiatry remains a science, whether or not you like DSM5. *Psychiatr Times*. 2010 February 25. Available from http://www.psychiatrictimes.com/bipolar-disorder. Accessed February 27, 2014.

[5] Okasha S. *Philosophy of Science. A Very Short Introduction*. New York: Oxford University Press; 2002.

[6] Sen A. Objectivity and position: assessment of health and well-being. In: Chen L, Kleinman A, Ware N. *Health and Social Change in International Perspective*. Boston: Harvard School of Public Health; 1994.

[7] Ghaemi SN. *The Concepts of Psychiatry*. Baltimore: Johns Hopkins University Press; 2003:90-93.

[8] Wiggins OP, Schwartz MA. Is there a science of meaning? *Integrative Psychiatry*. 1991;7:48-53.

~~~~~~~~~~~~~~~~~~

MISUNDERSTANDING PSYCHIATRY (AND PHILOSOPHY) AT THE HIGHEST LEVEL

Philosophical problems begin when language goes on holiday.—Ludwig Wittgenstein, Philosophical Investigations

Recent book reviews [1] by Dr. Marsha Angell, the former editor-in-chief of the *New England Journal of Medicine,* have stirred great controversy within psychiatric circles, as evidenced by the heated exchange of letters published in the *New York Review of Books* [2-4]. Perhaps—to paraphrase a line from the film *Cool Hand Luke*—"What we got here is a failure to communicate!"

Certainly, when someone of Dr. Angell's presumed sophistication gets psychiatry (mostly) wrong, our profession has a daunting problem on its hands. I do not intend to explore the many erroneous claims proffered in Dr. Angell's reviews and letters, most of which have been rebutted by several prominent psychiatrists [2, 3, 4]. (For a magisterial debunking of the "antidepressants are just expensive placebos" myth, I recommend the splendid monograph by Davis et al., 2011 [5].) Instead, I want to I want to focus on one particularly troubling passage in Dr. Angell's rejoinder to Drs. Richard Friedman and Andrew Nierenberg. She asserts therein that

> "[Drs. Friedman and Nierenberg] are simply wrong in asserting that psychiatry, in using drugs to treat signs and symptoms of illness without understanding the cause of the illness or how the drugs work, is no different from other medical specialties. First, mental illness is diagnosed on the basis of *symptoms* (medically defined as subjective manifestations of disease, such as pain) and *behaviors,* not *signs* (defined as objective manifestations, such as swelling of a joint). Most diseases in other specialties produce physical signs and abnormal lab tests or radiologic findings, in addition to symptoms. Moreover, even if the underlying causes of other diseases are unknown, the mechanisms by which they produce illness usually are, and the treatments usually target those mechanisms…" (italics added) [2].

In my view, Dr. Angell's assertions reflect both a serious misunderstanding of psychiatric diagnosis, and—equally important—a failure to address the core philosophical issues involved in her use of terms like "subjective," "objective," "behaviors," and "signs." The bright lines of separation drawn by Dr. Angell —for example, between "behaviors" and "signs," psychiatry and general medicine—are in fact far fainter than she acknowledges. But this is not surprising. Dr. Angell's analysis is part of a longstanding narrative—alas, sometimes embraced by psychiatrists themselves—that has had the effect, if not the intent, of marginalizing and denigrating psychiatry [6].

Let's focus on the linguistic and philosophical issues that underlie Dr. Angell's claims regarding psychiatric diagnosis. First, let's dispatch the demonstrably erroneous claim that psychiatric diagnosis does not involve "signs." To be sure, most psychiatric diagnoses are made primarily on the basis of the patient's self-expressed reports, experiences, and complaints—in effect, her "symptoms." And, unfortunately, the DSM-IV itself contributes to the confusion by calling *any* feature of psychiatric illness a "symptom." The framers should have been more precise in their terminology!

However, using the definition of "sign" common in general medicine—i.e., "*…Any abnormality indicative of disease, discoverable on examination of the patient; an objective indication of disease, in contrast to a symptom, which is a subjective indication of disease*" [7]—we find that a number of "signs" are indeed part of the criteria sets for several DSM-IV psychiatric disorders:

- Significant weight loss (major depressive episode; anorexia nervosa)
- Psychomotor agitation or retardation "...observable by others, not merely subjective feelings of restlessness or being slowed down" (major depressive episode)
- Increase in goal-directed activity...or psychomotor agitation (manic episode)
- Distractibility (i.e., attention too easily drawn to unimportant or irrelevant external stimuli) (manic episode)
- Motoric immobility as evidenced by catalepsy (including waxy flexibility) or stupor (schizophrenia, catatonic type)
- Stereotyped movements, prominent mannerisms or prominent grimacing (schizophrenia, catatonic type)
- Avoidance of eye-to-eye gaze (autistic disorder)
- Delay in development of spoken language (autistic disorder)

I have deliberately omitted signs of *cognitive disorders* (impaired recent memory, impaired calculation, etc.), such as Alzheimer's Disease, so as to head off the objection that "those are really *neurological* conditions." And I have listed only those findings I believe are unambiguously "signs," according to the definition provided. However, one could make a credible argument that many other determinations made by psychiatrists are in fact observations of "signs"; e.g., pressured speech, loose associations, markedly elevated affect, etc. Then there are the many cognitive functions we assess, such as the patient's ability to perform calculations, recall words, draw a clock face, etc., all of which enter into our diagnosis of delirium, dementia, and the amnestic disorders.

Of course—in addition to data obtained from the mental status exam—psychiatrists routinely assess a variety of external (non-subjective) validators of diagnosis; e.g., the patient's vocational function, prior hospitalizations, substance use, suicide attempts, family psychiatric history, co-morbid medical disorders, etc. Finally, though not yet a part of routine clinical assessment, several biomarkers of psychiatric illness shown considerable consistency across many studies; e.g., enlarged cerebral ventricles and abnormal smooth pursuit eye movements in schizophrenia [8].

Now, I am (painfully!) aware of the kind of argument often marshaled against my list of putative psychiatric "signs." It goes something like this: "Oh, come now, Doctor! With the exception of weight loss, you have really listed *behaviors*, not *signs*—at least, not as that term is understood by other medical specialties. In fact, you are really talking about certain 'disapproved of' behaviors, such as an 'increase in goal directed activity.' Really, now! You are just making value judgments! Who is to say what degree of goal-directed activity is or is not normal? Don't psychiatrists really just mean, 'I don't *like* how much social or sexual activity this guy is carrying out!'? And who is to say that there is anything pathological in maintaining certain postures for long periods? If you watch a group of people performing Tai-chi, you could call them all 'catatonic'! No—in general medicine, a 'sign' is something *objective*, like swelling or pallor or hypoactive reflexes. And, these bona fide signs are usually reflected in abnormalities we can pick up in lab tests, imaging studies, nerve conduction studies, etc."

This essentially "positivist" view of medical diagnosis [6]—and of the distinction between *signs* and *behaviors*—has the ring of superficial plausibility. Indeed, I would guess that a number of psychiatrists would nod (somewhat ambivalently) in general agreement with it. But in my view, this analysis is quite wrong-headed. It creates a spurious distinction which, upon closer examination, is not supported by the way several other medical specialties function in clinical practice. It also employs a sense of the term "objective" that harks back to the largely discredited school of logical empiricism (or logical positivism) that my colleagues and I have addressed elsewhere [6, 9].

Why, for example, does the neurologist's statement, "The patient's hand grip is weak," describe an *objective finding*, whereas the psychiatrist's statement, "The patient's psychomotor activity is abnormally decreased," entails a *subjective judgment*? (Could it be that neurologists simply don't "approve of" certain degrees of muscle weakness? And that in a society that "valued" myasthenia, a weak hand grip would not be deemed pathological?) Why does the claim, "The patient's finger appears swollen," represent an objective finding, whereas the statement, "The patient's speech is pressured," represents merely a subjective judgment? Is there some scientific or epistemological principle that privileges *visual* or *tactile* over *auditory* data, in deciding what counts as "objective"? One philosophically-coherent meaning of "objective" stipulates two main requirements: *careful and repeated observation;* and *concurrence among multiple observers*. On this view, psychiatric diagnosis is, to a considerable degree, an "objective" process [10, 11].

True: a swollen finger might well be correlated with, say, an elevated white cell count, whereas there may be no abnormal lab test associated with pressured speech. But it is not clear why that difference ought to render the determination of pressured speech merely "subjective." (No general physician would dismiss a swollen finger as inconsequential or "merely subjective," *even if all the lab tests came back within normal limits*.)

As for the objection that, "You can *measure* the swelling in a finger, whereas pressured speech is just a judgment call," I would reply thus: if psychiatrists wanted to devise a sophisticated recording device that computed the number and volume of words per minute spoken by the patient, we could easily do so. And, after all, how many general physicians "measure" their arthritic patient's fingers before declaring that they are swollen? Of course, in our pathologizing of both terms—"swelling" and "pressured speech"—there is an irreducibly *non*-objective judgment. This is because each term requires *general agreement on what degree of deviation from the norm constitutes "pathology."* And this is not something that observation alone can tell us: it is ultimately an existential judgment, based on very broad concepts of "health," "disease," "impairment," "suffering," etc.

Furthermore, critics of psychiatric diagnosis need to acknowledge that a number of well-recognized medical and neurological disorders are essentially *symptom-based constructs* that do not necessarily or consistently "…produce physical signs and abnormal lab tests or radiologic findings." Nor are the "mechanisms by which they produce illness" necessarily well understood. Consider the diagnosis of *migraine headaches* by our colleagues in neurology. As one recent review put it,

> "Migraine is a very common disabling brain disorder with unclear pathogenesis…It is now generally accepted that the primary cause of migraine lies in the brain, but *the nature and mechanisms of the primary brain dysfunction that leads to activation of the meningeal trigeminal nociceptors remain incompletely understood and controversial*" (italics added) [12].

Well, it's good to know that the *brain* is involved! The International Headache Society (IHS) criteria are the basis for migraine diagnosis, and these criteria are *entirely symptomatic* and "subjective" in nature; e.g., complaints of unilateral, pulsating headache, often accompanied by nausea or photophobia, etc. [13]. There is no "lab test" or neuroimaging study that is diagnostic of migraine headaches (though such tests may rule out a brain tumor or other pathology). Indeed, unless the physician *witnesses* the patient during an acute migraine attack, one could argue that the migraine diagnosis is made solely on the basis of a normal neurological exam and *the patient's verbal behavior*; i.e., the patient's narrative history of symptoms.

Space limitations prevent discussion of conditions such as *atypical facial pain* or *Meniere's Disease*, but I would contend that these, too, are essentially symptom-based, clinical diagnoses. Even idiopathic *epilepsy* is regarded, to this day, as a *clinical* diagnosis, made primarily on the basis of the patient's history. As neurologist Dr. Anthony Marson puts it, "Epilepsy is a clinical diagnosis....the diagnosis is not based upon the results of tests, but upon an accurate description of the attacks" [14]. Furthermore, even a witnessed tonic-clonic seizure is, arguably, a series of "behaviors": the patient falls to the floor; moves his limbs in a certain manner; bites his tongue, becomes incontinent, etc. In what fundamental sense do these behaviors differ from those of the patient with the catatonic subtype of schizophrenia, who assumes uncomfortable postures for prolonged periods, shows waxy flexibility, stereotypy, automatic obedience, etc.?

If it is argued that the patient with catatonia is "producing" catatonic behaviors, whereas the person with epilepsy is involuntarily "experiencing" epileptic behaviors, I would reply that this amounts to a metaphysical speculation and a certain "theory of mind"—not a scientifically verifiable claim. Indeed, the distinction between "behaviors" and "signs" in both epilepsy and catatonia is largely semantic. *Behaviors are, in effect, a subtype of "sign", and conform to the definition of "...Any abnormality indicative of disease, discoverable on examination of the patient"* [7].

As Dan J. Stein, MD, recently noted, "… both medicine and psychiatry ask about and look for objective signs and subjective symptoms in order to reach a diagnosis" (personal communication, August 17, 2011). I would not go so far as to claim that psychiatry is "no different" than any other medical specialty. And, to be sure, most of the non-psychiatric conditions I have discussed here fall under the rubric of neurology. The data psychiatrists collect often *do* differ from those collected by, say, orthopedists or infectious disease specialists. We are less interested than these specialties in X-rays or urine cultures. We are more interested—as we must be—in the patient's *phenomenology*: the structure and contents of his "inner world" [15]. But the wall of separation implied by Dr. Angell's comments is, in truth, riddled with holes. Indeed, psychiatry bears more similarities to other medical disciplines than many clinicians either understand or acknowledge.

Acknowledgment

I wish to thank Dan J. Stein MD, for his helpful reading of an earlier draft of this paper. A slightly modified version of this piece appeared in the September 8, 2011, issue of *Psychiatric Times*.

References

[1] Angell M. The Illusions of Psychiatry. *The New York Review of Books*. 2011 July 14. Available from: http://www.nybooks.com/articles/archives/2011/jul/14/illusions. Accessed March 1, 2014.

[2] Oldham J, Carlat D, Friedman R, Nierenberg A. "The Illusions of Psychiatry": An Exchange. *The New York Review of Books*. Available from: http://www.nybooks.com/articles/archives/2011/aug/18/illusions-psychiatry-exchange/. Accessed March 1, 2014.

[3] Kramer P. In Defense of Antidepressants. *The New York Times*. 2011 July 9. Available from: http://www.nytimes.com/2011/07/10/opinion/sunday/10antidepressants.html?pagewanted=all. Accessed March 1, 2014.

[4] Ghaemi N. Do antidepressants work? Asking the right questions [online]. Medscape. Free Associations blog. 2011 Aug 3. Available from: http://boards.medscape.com/forums?128@49.4tMIab3F9mH@.2a0c9dc7!comment=1&cat=All&pa=3886333T1313530940564_13135309405641313530940568. Accessed March 1, 2014.

[5] Davis JM, Giakas WJ, Qu J, Prasad P, Leucht S. Should we treat depression with drugs or psychological interventions? A Reply to Ioannidis. *Philos Ethics Humanit Med*. 2011;6:8.

[6] Pies R, Thommi S, Ghaemi N. Getting it from both sides: Foundational and antifoundational critiques of psychiatry. *Psychiatr Times*. 2011 July 1. Available from: psychiatrictimes.com/cultural-psychiatry/getting-it-both-sides-foundational-and-antifoundational-critiques-psychiatry. Accessed March 1, 2014.

[7] MediLexicon [online]. Available from: http://www.medilexicon.com/medical dictionary.php. Accessed March 1, 2014.

[8] Pies R. Beyond reliability: biomarkers and validity in psychiatry. *Psychiatry (Edgmont)*. 2008;5(1):48-52.

[9] Pies R. How "objective" are psychiatric diagnoses? (guess again). *Psychiatry (Edgmont)*. 2007;4(10):18-22.

[10] Pies R. Psychiatry clearly meets the "objectivity" test. *Psychiatr News*. 2005;40(19):17.

[11] Sen A. Objectivity and position: assessment of health and well-being. In: Chen L, Kleinman A, Ware N. *Health and Social Change in International Perspective*. Boston: Harvard School of Public Health; 1994.

[12] Pietrobon D. Insights into migraine mechanisms and CaV2.1 calcium channel function from mouse models of familial hemiplegic migraine. *J Physiol*. 2010;588(Pt 11):1871-1878.

[13] International Headache Society Classification ICHD-II. Migraine without aura. Available from: http://ihs-classification.org/en/02_klassifikation/02_teil1/01.01.00_migraine.html. Accessed February 23, 2014.

[14] Nirza N, Marson A, reviewers. What is epilepsy? [online]. Netdoctor. 2012 March 14. Available from: http://www.netdoctor.co.uk/diseases Accessed March 1, 2014.

[15] Pies R. The anatomy of sorrow: a spiritual, phenomenological, and neurological perspective. *Philos Ethics Humanit Med*. 2008; 3:17.

~~~~~~~~~~~~~~~~~

SENSITIZATION AND ITS DISCONTENTS: ALLERGISTS, PSYCHIATRISTS, AND THE LIMITS OF MEDICAL KNOWLEDGE

It's an embarrassment, no doubt about it. For those of you who have been following the intense debate over the DSM-5, it's high time to ask: how much longer will the public put up with a medical specialty like this?

- A government report finds the field is rife with poorly done studies, misdiagnoses, and tests that give misleading results [1].
- Patients often "shed" the disorder commonly diagnosed by specialists in the field, and no one knows why.
- Specialists can't agree on a definition of the condition they are treating.
- There is good reason to suspect "over-diagnosis," owing to inadequate or inappropriate evaluation.
- One of the most common treatments used by specialists in the field has uncertain benefits, based on published studies.

I know: you are shrugging your shoulders, saying, "So what else is new? People have been saying these things about psychiatry for years!" Well, yes, they have, but—the conclusions above are from the latest report on a subspecialty within the "hard science" of immunology: the field of "food allergies."

A systematic review by Dr. Jennifer J. Schneider Chafen and colleagues, published in *JAMA* found that "...the evidence for the prevalence and management of food allergy is greatly limited by a lack of uniformity for criteria for making a diagnosis" [2]. Indeed, the lead author, Dr. Chafen, is quoted as saying, "Everyone has a different definition" [1] of a food allergy. Apparently, over 80% of the studies reviewed by Chafen and her colleagues used their own definition of "food allergy." Furthermore, the common practice of identifying food allergies by measuring levels of IgE antibodies in the patient's blood proved to be an unreliable test. Prof. Joshuah Boyce, an allergist at Harvard, observed that, "there are plenty of individuals with IgE antibodies to various foods who don't react to those foods at all" [1]. And the *coup de grace*? The common practice among allergists of advising the patient to give up the implicated food—so-called "elimination diets"—is of uncertain and untested benefit [2].

Now, to be clear: my aim is not to cast aspersions on our allergist colleagues; nor is it my intent to give the field of psychiatry a "free pass" on its own shortcomings, which are numerous. Rather, I want to debunk a widespread misconception about psychiatry, as contrasted with other medical specialties. That popular myth goes something like this: *other medical specialties are based on "hard science," known pathophysiology, objective diagnosis, reliable laboratory tests and well-validated biomarkers. Psychiatry,* the myth insists, *lacks each of these characteristics.*

I'll acknowledge the force of the "hard science" argument, if we compare psychiatry to, say, mechanical engineering or physical chemistry. But when we hold psychiatry up to the other medical specialties, we find many more similarities than differences. In each such comparison, we find that the medical specialties in question are struggling with many of the same conceptual and diagnostic conundrums as those besetting psychiatry. To cite just a few examples:

- In oncology, identification of cells and tissues as "cancerous" or "malignant" is by no means straightforward, and many cases of "atypical" cells are notoriously difficult to classify. This is evident, for example, in the notion of "precancer," as one recent review pointed out: "…precancers are associated with a morphological continuum from atypia to dysplasia and invasive neoplasia" [3]. The notion of a "continuum" of pathology should sound eerily familiar to psychiatrists following the DSM-5 controversies.
- In neurology, the classification and diagnosis of headaches has undergone considerable change in the past 20 years. In the most recent international classification of headache disorders (ICHD-II), more than a hundred different kinds of headache are categorized, most of which lack a clearly defined pathophysiology. One expert, commenting on migraine headaches, observed that

"Lacking an external 'gold standard' for headache diagnosis, validity is difficult to judge. Migraine diagnosed according to ICHD criteria responds in 80% to 90% of treatments to injected triptans, drugs that can claim a highly specific mode of action. This proves that clinical diagnosis according to ICHD has been able to identify a group of patients who share a reasonably uniform response to pharmacologic intervention and presumably then share a common pathophysiological pathway" [4].

Well, that word "presumably" is the elephant in the neurologists' examining room. If psychiatrists made the claim, "80% of patients with severe, melancholic major depression respond to ECT [which is true]; therefore, *presumably* these patients share a common pathophysiological pathway," we would be summarily laughed out of the room—particularly if philosophers of science happened to be listening! A more modest assessment of the ICHD-II is provided by neurologist J.W. Swanson :

"The ICHD-II will not be the final word on headache diagnosis and classification. It will undoubtedly be significantly revised as more studies are done to delineate the science of headache. In this regard, the ICHD-II is not unlike the revisions of diagnostic and classification systems that have been developed in multiple areas of medicine such as psychiatry and epilepsy" [5].

1) In rheumatology, the nature and diagnosis of "fibromyalgia" ("chronic fatigue syndrome") remain mired in controversy, even as the condition has been recognized as a medical syndrome by nothing less than the Centers for Disease Control. The underlying pathophysiology and optimal treatment of fibromyalgia remain matters of intense debate. One review by two forensic psychiatrists—published in a rheumatology journal—concluded that "…the only certainty in fibromyalgia is that it is still being diagnosed…" and opined that "…society and medicine have to turn to philosophy rather than to science for the solution of treating and preventing 'syndromes' like fibromyalgia" [6].

But psychiatry and the other medical specialties share more than their struggles with disease demarcation and diagnosis. We also have a practical, everyday clinical issue in common: the high prevalence of psychiatric and mental health problems in many general medical settings. As David Kupfer, MD, and Darrel Regier, MD, MPH, chair and vice chair, respectively, of the *DSM-5* task force, pointed out in a recent editorial, "... in primary care settings, approximately 30% to 50% of patients have prominent mental health symptoms or identifiable mental health disorders, which have significant adverse consequences if left untreated" [7].

In recent years, psychiatry has witnessed impressive growth in its integrated understanding of the biological and psychosocial components of brain-mediated disease, as Nobel laureate Dr. Eric Kandel has shown [8]. This is no time to marginalize or "uncouple" psychiatry from the rest of medicine, as some have suggested. Yes, we have a long way to go, with respect to identifying the genesis, pathophysiology and optimal treatment of the illnesses we confront--but the same may be said of most medical specialties. Psychiatry is, and should remain, well within the fold of general medicine.

Acknowledgment

A slightly modified version of this piece appeared in the May 25, 2010, issue of *Psychiatric Times*.

References

[1] Kolata G. Doubt is cast on many reports of food allergies. *The New York Times*. 2010 May 12. Available from: http://www.nytimes.com/2010/05/12/health. Accessed March 1, 2014.

[2] Chafen JJS, Newberry SJ, Riedl MA et al. Diagnosing and managing common food allergies. *JAMA*. 2010;303:1848-1856.

[3] Cardiff RD, Borowsky AD. Precancer: sequentially acquired or predetermined? *Toxicol Pathol*. 2010;38:171-179.

[4] Oleson J. The International Classification of Headache Disorders. *Headache*. 2008;48:691-693.

[5] Swanson JW. Changes in the international classification of headache disorders. *Current Neurology and Neuroscience Reports*. 2004;4:95-97.

[6] Hazemeijer I, Rasker JJ. Fibromyalgia and the therapeutic domain. A philosophical study on the origins of fibromyalgia in a specific social setting. *Rheumatology*. 2003;42:507-515.

[7] Kupfer DJ, Regier DA. Why all of medicine should care about DSM-5. *JAMA*. 2010;303:1974-1975.

[8] Kandel ER. *Psychiatry, Psychoanalysis, and the New Biology of Mind*. Arlington, VA: American Psychiatric Publishing; 2005.

Psychiatry Remains a Science, Whether or Not You Like DSM5

Quick—which screening test or instrument has greater specificity for the target condition: the PSA (prostate specific antigen) test for prostate cancer, or the BSDS (Bipolar Spectrum Diagnostic Scale), for bipolar disorders?

Wait, one more question: Which physicians are more likely to agree with one another regarding a diagnosis: two radiologists inspecting a renal angiogram for arterial stenosis; or two psychiatrists using a structured interview to assess a patient for possible major depression?

Those of you who are used to "trick questions" on Board exams will probably not be surprised that the answers are, respectively, "the BSDS" (specificity 0.93 vs. 0.33 for PSA); and "the two psychiatrists" (kappa [inter-rater agreement]= 0.73 vs. 0.43 for radiologists) [1-5]. (Disclosure: The BSDS was devised by the present author, then refined and field-tested by Dr. Nassir Ghaemi and colleagues; it is available free of charge on the *Psychiatric Times* website.)

What does this very selective demonstration prove? Not much. Can we conclude that psychiatry is more "scientific" than urology or radiology? Hardly. The exercise was presented mainly to roil the waters surrounding those comfortable cynics who insist that psychiatry is not "scientific" or a "real science." The numerous controversies surrounding the DSM-5—covered at length in *Psychiatric Times*—seem to have brought these critics of psychiatry out in force.

Whatever the failings of the DSM-5, the notion that psychiatry is not a science is profoundly wrong. Proponents of that view persistently confuse science with "logical positivism"—a largely discredited form of scientific fundamentalism [6]—and entirely misunderstand the nature of the scientific enterprise. In fact, my gambit involving PSAs and angiograms was itself a bit misleading. To the extent we can identify the foundational principle of science, it has little to do with lab tests, and a great deal to do with the scientist's *mind-set* and *methodology*.

To be sure, philosophers of science point out that there may be no single, valid definition of "science" or of the "scientific method." As philosopher Samir Okasha puts it, "…science is a heterogeneous activity, encompassing a wide range of different disciplines and theories. It may be that they share some fixed set of features that define what it is to be a science, but it may not" [7].

And so, to assert what science "is" or "is not" with great confidence—or to declare categorically which medical specialties constitute "real science"—is to over-reach in one's epistemology by a considerable stretch.

This doesn't mean that we are left utterly adrift, however, without even a notional definition of science. Recently, the British Science Council spent a full year developing a definition of "science". Their work-product is succinct and yet radically insightful: "Science is the pursuit of knowledge and understanding of the natural and social world following a systematic methodology based on evidence" [8].

Good heavens! No lab tests required for science? No MRIs? No demonstrations of cellular pathology? Why, if this barmy British Science Council has its way, fields as diverse as physics, meteorology, linguistics, and anthropology would qualify as sciences! And, yes, without any question—*so would psychiatry.*

Let's be clear: not all science is *physical* science. Although psychiatry is nowadays associated with "biological psychiatry"—with PET scans, MRIs, neurotransmitters and the like—the domain of psychiatry is broader, deeper, and more pluralistic. As my colleagues Nassir Ghaemi, MD [9], and Michael A. Schwartz, MD [10], have argued, psychiatry may be seen as a *science of meaning*. Wiggins and Schwartz define "meanings" as "...mental processes and their intended objects" [10, p. 49].

We acquire evidence of our patient's mental processes through precisely the "systematic methodology" required by the Science Council's definition: we take a personal and family history; we perform a mental status exam; we observe our patient's facial expression, affect, mannerisms and speech. And we ask countless questions of the patient, aimed at eliciting deeper levels of meaning within the felt experience of the patient's world. In some instances, we supplement these "office based" methods with projective or neuropsychological testing. In selected cases, we ask the patient to complete screening questionnaires or (rarely) to participate in a structured clinical interview. And, consistent with our pluralistic model of "mind," we order appropriate laboratory and somatic tests to rule out underlying medical or neurological disorders.

We then form hypotheses based on these methods, regarding the patient's psychopathology, personality structure, and clinical diagnosis. We test these hypotheses against subsequent observations, and—if we detect inconsistencies—we re-visit our initial formulation. What Okasha identifies as "some of the main features of scientific inquiry" [7, p. 125]—induction, experimental testing, observation, theory construction—are all part of psychiatric methodology. In short, psychiatry is well within the orthodox definition of "science."

Do the methods of the DSM-5 conform to this paradigm? That is a more complicated question, since the DSM-5 work groups do not obtain data in the direct, observational way clinicians do. However, if science is "the pursuit of knowledge and understanding of the natural and social world following a systematic methodology based on evidence," the DSM-5 process is arguably working within the broad framework of science.* Like all such endeavors, the DSM-5 process is buffeted by external forces and pressures that may mar its objectivity and undermine its science. We shall have to wait and see. But whatever the merits or flaws of the DSM-5, psychiatry as a profession remains a science—not a physical, but a *human* science, grounded in a pluralistic understanding of our patients' "meanings."

*For an extended debate on whether DSM-5 is "scientific," please see the essays on the *Psychiatric Times* website, by Dr. Nassir Ghaemi and Prof. Hannah Decker: http://www.physicianspractice.com/couch-crisis/can-validity-pragmatism-go-hand-hand-dsm

Also see my essay, "Science, Psychiatry, and Family Practice: Positivism vs. Pluralism" in this collection.

Acknowledgment

A slightly modified version of this piece appeared in the February 25, 2010, issue of *Psychiatric Times*.

References

[1] Ghaemi S, Miller CJ, Berv DA, et al. Sensitivity and specificity of a new bipolar spectrum diagnostic scale. *J Affect Disord.* 2005;84(2-3):273-277.

[2] Hoffman RM, Gilliland FD, Adams-Cameron M, et al. Prostate-specific antigen testing accuracy in community practice. *BMC Fam Pract.* 2002; 3:19.

[3] Schreij G, de Haan MW, Oei TK, et al. Interpretation of renal angiography by radiologists. *J Hypertens.* 1999;17(12 Pt 1):1737-1741.

[4] Ruskin PE, Reed S, Kumar R, et al. Reliability and acceptability of psychiatric diagnosis via telecommunication and audiovisual technology. *Psychiatr Serv.* 1998;49:1086-1088.

[5] Pies R. How "objective" are psychiatric diagnoses? (guess again). *Psychiatry (Edgmont).* 2007;4(10):18-22.

[6] Hanfling O. Logical positivism. In: Shanker S, editor. Philosophy of Science, Logic, and Mathematics in the Twentieth Century. Routledge History of Philosophy Volume 9. New York: Routledge; 1996:193-213.

[7] Okasha S. *Philosophy of Science.* New York: Oxford University Press; 2002:16-17.

[8] Sample I. What is this thing we call science? [online]. *The Guardian* Notes and Theories blog. 2009 March 3. Available from: http://www.guardian.co.uk/science/blog/2009/mar/03/science-definition-council-francis-bacon. Accessed February 27, 2014.

[9] Ghaemi SN. *The Concepts of Psychiatry.* Baltimore: Johns Hopkins University Press; 2003: 90-93.

[10] Wiggins OP, Schwartz MA. Is there a science of meaning? *Integrative Psychiatry.* 1991;7:48-53.

~~~~~~~~~~~~~~~~

PSYCHIATRY'S NEW BRAIN-MIND AND THE LEGEND OF THE "CHEMICAL IMBALANCE"

Everything should be made as simple as possible, but no simpler.—attributed to Albert Einstein (probably a paraphrase)

Mind and body do not act upon each other, because they are not other, they are one.—Philosopher Will Durant, on Spinoza's monism [1]

I am not one who easily loses his temper, but I confess to experiencing markedly increased limbic activity whenever I hear someone proclaim, "Psychiatrists think all mental disorders are due to a chemical imbalance!" In the past 30 years, I don't believe I have ever heard a knowledgeable, sophisticated, well-trained psychiatrist make such a preposterous claim, except perhaps to mock it. On the other hand, the "chemical imbalance" trope has been tossed around a great deal by opponents of psychiatry, who mendaciously attribute the phrase to psychiatrists themselves [2]. And, yes—the "chemical imbalance" image has been vigorously promoted by some pharmaceutical companies, often to the detriment of our patients' understanding [3]. In truth, the "chemical imbalance" notion was always a kind of urban legend—never a theory seriously propounded by most well informed psychiatrists.

Fortunately, recent advances in cognitive psychology and neuroscience are now converging, with the result that psychiatry may be on the brink of a unified model of so-called mental illness. (The term itself, as we shall see, is belied by the new research.) As described at the APA's 2011 annual meeting by NIMH Director Thomas Insel, MD, neuropsychiatric research is pointing to a complex interplay between factors traditionally dichotomized as "biological" and "psychosocial" [4].

As Insel describes the new model, conditions such as schizophrenia or bipolar disorder are attributable to rare, but highly potent, genetic variations that lead to dysfunction in multiple, complex brain circuits. However, the particular symptomatic manifestation in a given individual—the disease *phenotype*—is partly dependent on the person's experiences and environment. We may hypothesize (and this is my view, not necessarily Dr. Insel's) that given developmentally-based "biases" in various neurocircuits, the young boy or girl may be predisposed to the use of certain dysfunctional cognitive strategies; for example, viewing everyone in the environment as uniformly threatening or "rejecting." These tendencies could easily be exacerbated by, say, childhood traumata or parental neglect.

We can imagine that the "irrational cognitions" so prized by cognitive therapists may develop on this abnormal, biogenetic substrate, and eventually become woven into the very fabric of the individual's personality and world-view. Thus, rather than remain ensnared by the terms "mind" or "brain", we would be better served by what Dr. Dan Stein calls, the "brain-mind". Indeed, "…the two constructs are, in fact, impossible to disentangle" [5]. This is essentially what the philosopher Baruch Spinoza (1632-77) argued more than three centuries ago: "mind" and "brain" are not *two* substances, but *one*—variously understood in "mental" terms for some purposes, and in "physical" terms, for others. And, as Dr. Stein observes, the brain-mind "….is not a computational, apart-from-the-world, passive reflector, but rather a thinking-feeling-actor-in-the-world…" [5].

In short, we cannot afford to view our patients' afflictions in the balkanized terms of "mental" vs. "physical," "mind" vs. "body," "psyche" vs. "soma." Neither can we afford the luxury of supposing that only one type of treatment—medication or psychotherapy—will be effective for the illnesses we treat. On the contrary, the best available evidence suggests that each modality, or their synergistic combination, may be effective—depending on the specific illness. To be sure, as my colleague, Nassir Ghaemi MD, has cautioned, we must not be drawn into a haze of promiscuous eclecticism in our treatment; rather, we must be guided by well-designed studies and the best available evidence [6]. Nonetheless, there is room in our work for both motives and molecules, poetry and pharmacology. The legend of the "chemical imbalance" should be consigned to the dust-bin of ill-informed and malicious caricatures. Psychiatry must now confront the mysteries and miseries of the brain-mind.

Acknowledgment

A slightly modified version of this piece appeared in the July 11, 2011, issue of *Psychiatric Times*.

References

[1] Durant W. *The Story of Philosophy*. New York: Pocket Books; 1953.
[2] See, e.g., Citizens Commission on Human Rights. Blaming the brain: the "chemical imbalance" fraud [online]. Available from: http://www.cchr.org/sites/default/files/Blaming_The_Brain_The_Chemical_Imbalance_Fraud.pdf. Accessed March 1, 2014.
[3] Lacasse JR, Leo J. Serotonin and depression: a disconnect between the advertisements and the scientific literature. *PLoS Med.* 2005;2(12): e392.
[4] Moran M. Brain, gene discoveries drive new concept of mental illness. *Psychiatr News.* 2011 June 17.
[5] Stein DJ. *Philosophy of Psychopharmacology*. Cambridge: Cambridge University Press; 2008:x.
[6] Ghaemi SN. The Rise and Fall of the Biopsychosocial Model: Reconciling Art and Science in Psychiatry. Baltimore: Johns Hopkins University Press; 2009.

Addendum

I have recently posted an updated and expanded essay on the "Chemical Imbalance" canard, in the March 11, 2014 Psychiatric Times. http://www.psychiatrictimes.com/blogs/nuances-narratives-chemical-imbalance-debate/page/0/2

~~~~~~~~~~~~~~~~

DOCTOR, IS MY MOOD DISORDER DUE TO A CHEMICAL IMBALANCE?

Dear Mrs. ──

You have asked me about the cause of your mood disorder, and whether it is due to a "chemical imbalance." The only honest answer I can give you is, "I don't know"—but I'll try to explain what psychiatrists do and don't know about the causes of so-called mental illness, and why the term "chemical imbalance" is simplistic and a bit misleading.

By the way, I don't like the term "mental disorder," because it makes it seem as if there's a huge distinction between the mind and the body—and most psychiatrists don't see it that way. I wrote about this recently, and used the term "brain-mind" to describe the unity of mind and body [1]. So, for lack of a better term, I'll just refer to "psychiatric illnesses."

Now, this notion of the "chemical imbalance" has been much in the news lately, and a lot of misinformation has been written about it—including by some doctors who ought to know better [2]. In the article I referenced, I argued that "…the 'chemical imbalance' notion was always a kind of urban legend—never a theory seriously propounded by well-informed psychiatrists" [1]. Some readers felt I was trying to "re-write history," and I can understand their reaction—but I stand by my statement.

Of course, there certainly are psychiatrists, and other physicians, who have used the term "chemical imbalance" when explaining psychiatric illness to a patient, or when prescribing a medication for depression or anxiety. Why? Many patients who suffer from severe depression or anxiety or psychosis tend to blame themselves for the problem. They have often been told by family members that they are "weak-willed" or "just making excuses" when they get sick, and that they would be fine if they just picked themselves up by those proverbial bootstraps. They are often made to feel guilty for using a medication to help with their mood swings or depressive bouts.

So, some doctors believe that they will help the patient feel less blameworthy by telling them, "You have a chemical imbalance causing your problem." It's easy to think you are doing the patient a favor by providing this kind of "explanation," but often, this isn't the case. Most of the time, the doctor knows that the "chemical balance" business is a vast oversimplification.

My impression is that most psychiatrists who use this expression feel uncomfortable and a little embarrassed when they do so. It's a kind of bumper-sticker phrase that saves time, and allows the physician to write out that prescription while feeling that the patient has been "educated." If you are thinking that this is a little lazy on the doctor's part, you are right. But to be fair, remember that the doctor is often scrambling to see those other twenty depressed patients in her waiting room. To be clear: I'm not offering this as an *excuse*—just an observation.

Ironically, the attempt to reduce the patient's self-blame by blaming his brain chemistry can sometimes backfire. Some patients hear "chemical imbalance" and think, "That means I have no control over this disease!"—which is surely not the case. Other patients may panic and think, "Oh, no—that means I have passed my illness on to my kids!" Both of these reactions are based on misunderstanding, but it's often hard to undo these fears. On the other hand, there are certainly some patients who take comfort in this "chemical imbalance" slogan, and feel more hopeful that their condition can be controlled with the right kind of medication.

They are not wrong in thinking that, either, since we can get most psychiatric illnesses under better control, using medication—but this should never be the whole story. Every patient who receives medication for a psychiatric illness should be offered some form of "talk therapy," counseling, or other kinds of support. Often, though not always, these non-medication approaches should be tried first, before medication is prescribed. But that's another story—and I want to get back to this "chemical imbalance" albatross, and how it got hung around the neck of psychiatry. Then I'd like to explain some of our more modern ideas of what causes serious psychiatric illnesses.

Back in the mid-60s, some brilliant psychiatric researchers—notably, Joseph Schildkraut, Seymour Kety, and Arvid Carlsson—developed what became known as the "biogenic amine hypothesis" of mood disorders. Biogenic amines are brain chemicals like norepinephrine and serotonin. In simplest terms, Schildkraut, Kety, and other researchers posited that too much, or too little, of these brain chemicals was associated with abnormal mood states—for example, with mania or depression, respectively. But note two important terms here: "hypothesis" and "associated." A hypothesis is just a stepping-stone along the path to a fully-developed *theory*—it's not a full-blown conception of how something works. And an "association" is not a "cause." In fact, the initial formulation of Schildkraut and Kety [3] allowed for the possibility that the arrow of causality might travel the other way; that is, that *depression itself might lead to changes in biogenic amines*, and not the other way around. Here is what these two researchers actually had to say back in 1967. It's pretty dense biology-speak, but please do read on:

"Although there does appear to be a fairly consistent relationship between the effects of pharmacological agents on norepinephrine metabolism and on affective state, a rigorous extrapolation from pharmacological studies to pathophysiology cannot be made. Confirmation of this [biogenic amine] hypothesis must ultimately depend upon direct demonstration of the biochemical abnormality in the naturally occurring illness. It should be emphasized, however, that the demonstration of such a biochemical abnormality would not necessarily imply a genetic or constitutional, rather than an environmental or psychological, etiology of depression.

Whereas specific genetic factors may be of importance in the etiology of some, and possibly all, depressions, it is equally conceivable that early experiences of the infant or child may cause enduring biochemical changes and that these may predispose some individuals to depressions in adulthood. It is not likely that changes in the metabolism of the biogenic amines alone will account for the complex phenomena of normal or pathological affect. Whereas the effects of these amines at particular sites in the brain may be of crucial importance in the regulation of affect, **any comprehensive formulation of the physiology of affective state will have to include many other concomitant biochemical, physiological, and psychological factors**" (boldface emphasis added) [3].

Now remember, Mrs. ——, these are the pioneers whose work helped lead to our modern-day medications, such as the "SSRIs" (Prozac, Paxil, Zoloft and others). And they certainly did *not* claim that all psychiatric illnesses—or even all mood disorders—are *caused* by a chemical imbalance! Even after four decades, the "holistic" understanding that Schildkraut and Kety described remains the most accurate model of psychiatric illness. In my experience over the past 30 years, the best trained and most scientifically-informed psychiatrists have always believed in this holistic model, despite claims to the contrary by some anti-psychiatry groups [4].

Unfortunately, the biogenic amine hypothesis got twisted into the "chemical imbalance theory" by some pharmaceutical marketers [5], and even by some misinformed doctors. And, yes, this marketing was sometimes aided by doctors who—even if with good intentions—didn't take the time to give their patients a more holistic understanding of psychiatric illness. To be sure, those of us in academia should have done more to correct these beliefs and practices—and the present writer is no exception. For example, the vast majority of antidepressants are prescribed not by psychiatrists, but by primary care physicians, and we psychiatrists have not always been the best communicators with our colleagues in primary care.

All that said, what have we learned about the causes of serious psychiatric illness in the past 40 years? My answer is, "More than many in the general public, and even in the medical profession, realize." First, though: what we don't know, and shouldn't claim to know, is what the proper "balance" is for any given individual's brain chemistry. Since the late 1960s, we have discovered more than a dozen different brain chemicals that may affect thinking, mood, and behavior. While a few seem particularly important—such as norepineprhine, serotonin, dopamine, GABA, and glutamate—we have no quantitative idea of what the optimal "balance" is for any particular patient. So to speak with great confidence about a specific "chemical imbalance" is to overreach considerably. The most we can say is that, in general, certain psychiatric illnesses probably involve abnormalities in specific brain chemicals; and that by using medications that affect these chemicals, we often find that patients are significantly improved. (It is also true that a minority of patients have significant adverse reactions to psychiatric medications, and we need further study of these medications and their long-term effects [6].)

In the mean time, neuroscience research has moved beyond any simple notion of a "chemical imbalance" as the cause of psychiatric illnesses. The most sophisticated, modern theories posit that psychiatric illness is caused by a complex, often cyclical interaction of genetics, biology, psychology, environment, and social factors [7]. Neuroscience has also moved beyond the notion that psychiatric medications work simply by "revving up" or toning down a few brain chemicals. For example, we have evidence that several antidepressants *foster the growth of connections between brain cells,* and we believe this is related to the beneficial effects of these medications [8]. Lithium—a naturally occurring element found in some mineral springs, and not really a "drug"—may help in bipolar disorder by protecting damaged brain cells and promoting their ability to communicate with each other [9].

Let's take bipolar disorder as an example of how psychiatry views "causation" these days (and we could have a similar discussion of schizophrenia or major depressive disorder). We know that a person's genetic make-up plays a major role in bipolar disorder (BPD). So, if one of two identical twins has BPD, there is better than a 40% chance that the other twin will develop the illness, even if the twins are reared in different homes [10]. But note that the figure is not 100%—so there must be other factors involved in the development of BPD, besides our genes.

Modern theories of BPD hold that abnormal genes lead to abnormal communication between various inter-linked regions of the brain—so-called "neurocircuits"—which in turn increases the likelihood of profound mood swings. There's growing evidence that BPD may involve a sort of top-down "failure to communicate" within the brain. Specifically, the frontal regions of the brain may not adequately dampen over-activity in the "emotional" (limbic) parts of the brain, perhaps contributing to mood swings [11].

So, you ask—is it still all a matter of "biology"? Not at all—the person's environment certainly matters. A major stressor may sometimes trigger a depressive or manic episode. And, if a child with early-onset BPD is raised in an abusive or unloving home, or is exposed to many traumas, this is likely to increase the risk of mood swings in later life [12]—though there is no evidence that "bad parenting" causes BPD. (At the same time, abuse or trauma in childhood may change the "wiring" of the brain permanently, and this in turn may lead to more mood swings—truly, a vicious circle [13].) On the other hand, in my experience, a supportive social and family environment may sometimes improve the outcome of a family member's BPD.

Finally—while the individual's approach to "problem-solving" is not a likely *cause* of BPD—there is evidence that *how the person thinks and reasons* may make a difference in the course of illness. For example, cognitive behavioral therapy and family-focused therapy may reduce the risk of relapse, in BPD [14]. And so, with appropriate support, the person with bipolar disorder can take some control of her illness—and maybe even improve its course—by learning more adaptive ways of thinking.

So, boiling it all down, Mrs.———, I certainly can't tell you the exact cause of your or anybody's psychiatric illness, but it's a lot more complicated than a "chemical imbalance." You are a whole *person*—with hopes, fears, wishes, and dreams—not a brain with a bunch of chemicals sloshing around! The originators of the "biogenic amine" hypothesis understood this over forty years ago—and the best-informed psychiatrists understand it today.

Sincerely,
Ronald Pies, MD

Acknowledgment

A slightly modified version of this piece appeared in the August 11, 2011, issue of *Psychiatric Times*.

References

[1] Pies R. Psychiatry's new brain-mind and the legend of the chemical imbalance. *Psychiatr Times*. 2011 July 11. Available from http://www.psychiatrictimes.com/blogs/couch-crisis/psychiatry%E2%80%99s-new-brain-mind-and-legend-%E2%80%9Cchemical-imbalance%E2%80%9D. Accessed March 6, 2014.

[2] See, for example, Angell M. The epidemic of mental illness: why? *The New York Review of Books*. 2011 June 23. "The shift from "talk therapy" to drugs as the dominant mode of treatment coincides with the emergence over the past four decades of the theory that mental illness is caused primarily by chemical imbalances in the brain that can be corrected by specific drugs..." Available from: http://www.nybooks.com/articles/archives/2011/jun/23/epidemic-mental-illness-why/. Accessed March 1, 2014.

[3] Schildkraut JJ, Kety SS. Biogenic amines and emotion. *Science*. 1967;156:21-37.

[4] See, e.g., Citizens Commission on Human Rights. Blaming the brain: the "chemical imbalance" fraud [online]. Available from: http://www.cchr.org/sites/default/files/Blaming_The_Brain_The_Chemical_Imbalance_Fraud.pdf. Accessed March 1, 2014.

[5] Lacasse JR, Leo J. Serotonin and depression: a disconnect between the advertisements and the scientific literature. *PLoS Med*. 2005;2(12): e392.

[6] El-Mallakh RS, Gao Y, Jeannie Roberts R. Tardive dysphoria: the role of long-term antidepressant use in-inducing chronic depression. *Med Hypotheses*. 2011; 76:769-773.

[7] Moran M. Brain, gene discoveries drive new concept of mental illness. *Psychiatr News*. 2011 June 17.

[8] Castrén E E, Rantamki T. The role of BDNF and its receptors in depression and antidepressant drug action: Reactivation of developmental plasticity. *Dev Neurobiol*. 2010;70:289-297.

[9] Machado-Vieira R, Manji HK, Zarate CA Jr. The role of lithium in the treatment of bipolar disorder: convergent evidence for neurotrophic effects as a unifying hypothesis. *Bipolar Disord*. 2009;11(Suppl 2):92-109.

[10] Kiesepp T, Partonen T, Haukka J et al. High concordance of bipolar I disorder in a nationwide sample of twins. *Am J Psychiatry*. 2004;161:1814-1821.

[11] Lagopoulos J, Malhi G. Impairments in "top-down" processing in bipolar disorder: a simultaneous fMRI-GSR study. *Psychiatry Res*. 2011;192:100-108.

[12] MacKinnon D, Pies R. Affective instability as rapid cycling: Theoretical and clinical implications for borderline personality and bipolar spectrum disorders. *Bipolar Disord*. 2006;8:1-14.

[13] Heim C, Newport DJ, Bonsall R, et al. Altered pituitary-adrenal axis responses to provocative challenge tests in adult survivors of childhood abuse. *Am J Psychiatry.* 2001;158:575-81.

[14] Zaretsky AE, Rizvi S, Parikh SV. How well do psychosocial interventions work in bipolar disorder? *Can J Psychiatry.* 2007;52:14-21.

For Further Reading

Kramer P. In defense of antidepressants. *The New York Times Sunday Review.* 2011, July 9. Available from: http://www.nytimes.com/2011/07/10/opinion/sunday/10antidepressants.html?pagewanted=all. Accessed March 1, 2014.

~~~~~~~~~~~~~~~~~

CAN PSYCHIATRY BE BOTH A MEDICAL SCIENCE AND A HEALING ART? THE CASE FOR POLYTHETIC PLURALISM

Not everything that can be counted counts; and not everything that counts can be counted.—Albert Einstein
The practice of medicine is an art, not a trade; a calling, not a business; a calling in which your heart will be exercised equally with your head.—William Osler

When I was a first-year resident, a revered supervisor of mine made the statement—half-facetiously—that, "In psychiatry, you can do biology in the morning and theology in the afternoon!" That remarkable claim not only intrigued and inspired me—it also became a kind of North Star in my own professional orientation, for the next thirty years. But amidst the intense and sometimes internecine conflicts that rage around and within psychiatry today, I think it is time to re-examine my supervisor's observation. At the very least, it may be useful to use it as a kind of lens, through which recent arguments about psychiatry may be viewed.

The dilemma faced by the psychiatric profession may be epitomized in two emails I recently received, both from very well respected, senior psychiatrists. Senior Clinician #1 is well known in the area of mood disorder classification, and in applying the "medical model" and biological sub-typing to various forms of major depression. He wrote me in reference to my recent essay on "Misunderstanding Psychiatry…" [1] in which I disputed the claim that psychiatric diagnosis does not make use of objective "signs," as in general medicine. He opined that "…psychiatry has rejected the medical model of diagnosis in medical practice" and that the DSM system merely "…looks at the list of symptoms and their duration, rejecting [physical and laboratory] examination, verifying tests and the validation of treatment responses."

Senior Clinician #2 argued nearly the opposite point of view, opining that psychiatric residents these days are "…being inadequately educated, with an emphasis on…[a materialistic] or…so-called medical model." Senior Clinician #2 represents an existential-humanistic approach to psychiatry that seeks to understand the whole person in the context of his or her environment. For him, psychiatry is primarily a "healing art", not a branch of neuroscience. He argued that psychiatry needs to recognize and realize its true nature "…before the field becomes unnecessary and obsolete."

Can both these respected clinicians be right? Has psychiatry really abandoned the "medical model" (whatever that means)? Does the present DSM framework enshrine or ignore this so-called medical model? Has psychiatry become too focused on neuroscience and "materialist" (usually termed "physicalist") models of psychopathology, to the detriment of holistic understanding of the person? Or is the real problem our abandonment of the biomedical model in favor of a kind of promiscuous eclecticism? Can our profession ever hope to overcome all these antinomies, and develop an Einsteinian, "unified field theory" of psychiatric illness? How might such a unified theory partake of both "biology" and "theology", to return to my supervisor's observation? Obviously, this essay can do no more than sketch some very tentative answers to these questions—but here goes.

First of all, what do psychiatrists and other physicians mean by the "medical model"— also called, the "biomedical model"? *Mosby's Medical Dictionary* (8th ed.) defines the "medical model" as

"…the traditional approach to the diagnosis and treatment of illness as practiced by physicians in the Western world since the time of Koch and Pasteur. The physician focuses on the defect, or dysfunction, within the patient, using a problem-solving approach. The medical history, physical examination, and diagnostic tests provide the basis for the identification and treatment of a specific illness. The medical model is thus focused on the physical and biologic aspects of specific diseases and conditions" [2].

In this sense, the last two DSMs can hardly be seen as exemplars or instantiations of "the medical model." As McHugh & Slavney point out, the DSM-III was primarily interested in *enhancing diagnostic reliability*—essentially, agreement on diagnosis among observers—and *not* in establishing the biological validity of any condition [3]. Nor have biological factors been a central (or even a peripheral) part of the DSM diagnostic criteria, from DSM-III to the DSM-5 (though there are some neurobiological data in the text sections of the new manual).

So, it would be wrong to characterize the DSMs as exemplars of "the medical model" or of "biological psychiatry," as many commentators often claim. Notice, by the way, that there is nothing inherent in this dictionary definition of the medical model that precludes careful attention to the patient's *verbal account* of what is wrong; or that "encourages a view of the patient as a machine" [4]. These misattributions become important when we consider Dr. Nicolas Kontos's argument, below, concerning the "biomedical Straw Man" [5].

Rather remarkably, Mosby's Dictionary goes on to note that,

"Nursing differs from the medical model in that the patient is perceived primarily as a person relating to the environment holistically; nursing care is formulated on the basis of a holistic nursing assessment of all dimensions of the person (physical, emotional, mental, and spiritual) that assumes multiple causes for the problems experienced by the patient. Nursing care then focuses on all dimensions, not just physical" [2].

This is actually an extraordinary statement, and I'll come back to it when I introduce the concept of "polythetic pluralism"—but on its face, this description of the "nursing model" ought to give every physician pause, particularly psychiatric physicians. Another reason to reconsider the "medical model" is the politico-rhetorical "baggage" this term has acquired in recent decades, as public disenchantment with medical diagnosis—and particularly, psychiatric diagnosis—has grown. Consider this claim from a U.K. website, advocating for the disabled:

> "Under the medical model, disabled people are defined by their illness or medical condition. They are disempowered: medical diagnoses are used to regulate and control access to social benefits, housing, education, leisure and employment" [6].

"Straw man" or not, similar claims about the medical model have been voiced by various advocacy groups—and many psychiatrists—highly critical of psychiatric diagnosis and practice. These critics usually use the term "reductionistic" in speaking of the medical model, with the implication that ordinary emotions and "problems in living" are being increasingly and inappropriately "medicalized" [7]. Yet it was a *physician*, Dr. George Engel—a professor of medicine and psychiatry—who most prominently called attention to the reductionist nature of the traditional medical model, and who called for a new approach—one that would "...include the psychosocial without sacrificing the enormous advantages of the biomedical approach" [8].

It should also be noted that "reductionism" in psychiatry is not confined to those who advocate either a *DSM-* categorical approach or a strictly biomedical approach. As Dr. Glen Gabbard has observed, "Both [psychoanalysts] and their patients secretly are drawn to simple formulations that eschew complexity" [9]. Reductionism, in short, is an equal-opportunity habit of mind.

To be sure, Engel's biopsychosocial model (BPSM) has come in for pointed criticism in recent years. Some, like Nassir Ghaemi MD, have argued that the BPSM has led to a sort of mishmash of treatment approaches, in which the psychiatrist adds "a little of this and a little of that" (my phrase, not Ghaemi's) to the treatment mix, without basing the decision on rigorous evidence [10]. And, in a thoughtful critique, Nicolas Kontos MD has argued that Engel himself created a kind of "Straw Man", by mischaracterizing the biomedical model; e.g., as one that effectively discourages dialogue with the patient, and "encourages a view of the patient as a machine". Kontos persuasively argues that promulgation of this "Straw Man" model has led to the misperception that "...most physicians are purposefully complicit in efforts to promote inadequate patient care" [5]. Indeed, this is a charge often leveled against psychiatrists who supposedly adhere to this bowdlerized version of the medical model.

A complete discussion of the BPSM is beyond the scope of this essay. Nevertheless—while acknowledging both deficiencies in and misrepresentations of the model—the BPSM at least represented a conscientious attempt to move psychiatry toward a humane and holistic approach to the patient. It seems to me that Engel must be given substantial credit for this, regardless of his own possible mischaracterizations of biomedicine or the misapplication of the BPSM by some clinicians.

I have already noted that the DSM framework does not exemplify the "medical model" as defined above. Ironically—and with all due respect to the conscientious efforts of its framers—the present DSM approach manages to achieve the "worst of both worlds": it does not adhere to a robust form of the biomedical model, but *neither does it provide a rich, coherent existential-phenomenological basis for understanding the patient's psychology.* There are very few diagnostic criteria in the DSM that help explain anything important about the *inner world* of the emotionally disturbed individual. (For a sense of what I mean, I recommend Silvano Arieti's magisterial description of the inner world of the patient with schizophrenia [11].)

This "worst of both worlds" quality of the DSM has a curious analogy in psychiatry's present predicament. As many critics have observed—reference Senior Clinician #1—he typical psychiatric practice today puts little emphasis on such traditional biomedical concerns as the physical and neurological exam, neuroendocrine measures, or the use of validated assessment instruments. (How many psychiatrists, these days, perform even a rudimentary neurological exam on a new patient? How many check the patient's pulse or blood pressure when monitoring medication side effects? Yet these are basic components of careful medical practice.) On the other hand, the inexorable pressure to constrict the therapeutic "hour" and eschew psychotherapy means that we have been less able to pursue the more subjective and humanistic elements of our calling.

Underlying this predicament is the continued ideological divide that has bedeviled psychiatry for decades, eloquently described in Tanya Luhrmann's classic book, *Of Two Minds* [12]. Very roughly put, Lurhmann described the dueling models of biomedical science and pharmacotherapy, on the one hand; and psychodynamics and psychotherapy, on the other. Thus, psychiatry seems to be trapped in a conceptual dilemma—in part, of its own making—akin to what the philosopher Ludwig Wittgenstein termed, "the fly bottle". If so, how does psychiatry escape "the fly bottle"? Put another way: *how does psychiatry maintain itself as a science-based, medical discipline, while also remaining a humanistic, healing art?*

Polythetic Pluralism

In an important essay brought to my attention by Dr. Sara Hartley, the psychoanalyst Harry Guntrip explores the concept of a "psychodynamic science" [13]. In the process, Guntrip goes on to anatomize a number of terms, such as "physical science," "natural science," "material science," and "mental science." He also alludes to a "science of human experience." All these terms, of course, share the designation "science", and it seems we must pause to offer at least a rough, notional definition of what that term may mean. Unfortunately, this turns out to be a complicated and controversial enterprise, perhaps best left to philosophers! [14] For purposes of this essay, however, I will define a "science" as *any discipline that studies some aspect of the world by means of repeated, systematic observations and investigations by multiple observers; constantly attempts to validate and invalidate its own hypotheses and theories; and which accords a high value to the replicability, reliability, and validity of its findings* [15].

The term "scientific" is thus closely related to the term "objective." In so far as a discipline carries out such systematic, empirical investigations, and demonstrates that its findings have good "inter-rater agreement," the discipline is engaging in an "objective" activity [16]. Paradoxically, this claim holds, even when the discipline's "object of investigation" is the *patient's subjectivity*. This, indeed, is a tenet of some types of *phenomenological psychiatry*, such as that of Karl Jaspers. Jaspers regarded phenomenological psychiatry as an "empirical" and descriptive process [17]*. Neurology and psychiatry share this dual, "objective/subjective" dimension; for example, the sensory exam in neurology "..,relies on a patient's subjective report and is therefore prone to additional variability" [18].

Now, Guntrip makes the following critical points. First, he warns us of the "false antithesis between a scientific and a human approach" to the patient. Thus, Guntrip observes that, "A surgeon can be capable of sympathy with his patient, however objectively and impersonally scientific he is in his medical theory and practice" [13].

Just so! How, then, can psychiatry be both medical science and healing art? I believe the way forward is via what I call "polythetic pluralism." "Polythetic" refers to several *shared characteristics*, none of which is essential for membership in a particular class. "Pluralism" refers to the use of several *different models*, approaches, or methods, not all of which may be appropriate in any given situation—the best model or method being dependent on the evidence supporting it and the facts at hand. Thus, the model of psychiatry I have in mind is characterized by *the use of several different approaches to diagnosis and treatment, sharing some features in common, no one of which defines the "essence" of psychiatry*. In this sense, I fully agree with Kontos's conclusion that "...the complexity of contemporary medicine is such that it cannot be served by just one model at either the macro (i.e., scientific and clinical) or micro (i.e., within clinical) levels." So much for airy abstraction—how might polythetic pluralism work in clinical practice?

> *Consider Ms. Thumos, a 34-year-old single woman who complains of "terrible, life-long, depression" which has worsened in the past six months. The patient's mother died when she was only four years old, and she was raised "an only child" by her father, an emotionally-detached man who spent little time with his daughter. The patient describes herself as "severely shy," with few friends or social contacts. She describes herself as "lonely, most of the time." Her family history is positive for a maternal grandmother and two uncles with severe major depression. The patient recently lost her job as a computer programmer, and has experienced increasing fatigue, weight gain, constipation and lethargy over the past four months. She also complains of "feeling cold all the time," despite adequate heat in her apartment. A physical exam showed slightly delayed ankle jerk (Achilles reflex), but was otherwise normal. However, lab studies revealed a TSH of 15 (normal <10 milli-international* units *per liter), with normal T3 and T4.*

In my estimation, no single "model" of medical or psychiatric diagnosis adequately "explains" Ms. Thumos's depression. Her family history suggests a strong genetic diathesis for major depressive disorder (MDD); the loss of her mother at an early age is also a risk factor for subsequent development of MDD. From an object relational standpoint, the patient's emotionally distant father may have further impaired her ability to form a positive sense of self, which in turn may have led to her pathological shyness and social avoidance. Her lack of close friends may have contributed to her life-long depression, which may now be exacerbated by recent unemployment, and subclinical hypothyroidism. *Comprehensive psychiatric treatment of Ms. Thumos must consider all these psychodynamic, interpersonal, and biological factors.* Our treatments, however, must reflect the *best available evidence for the particular disorder (or disorders) in question*—and that's quite different than throwing "a little of this, and a little of that" at the patient, thereby misapplying George Engel's teachings.

Psychotherapy, perhaps of the interpersonal type, could be very helpful to Ms. Thumos. But the best available evidence would suggest that correction of her thyroid problem should be the first step in caring for the patient, in that depression is not likely to respond optimally until underlying hypothyroidism is adequately treated [19]. If the patient's depression persists despite euthyroid status and psychotherapy, then antidepressant treatment may be warranted.

(Incidentally, in my own practice, I would typically prescribe the thyroid hormone in cases such as that of Ms. Thumos, usually in consultation with an endocrinologist.) So, in a sense, the holistic psychiatrist must indeed be prepared to do biology in the morning and theology in the afternoon!

Conclusion

In my view, psychiatry should not aim to be a "physical science" or a "natural science"—but neither should it confine itself, in Cartesian fashion, to being a "mental science." Psychiatry ought to be both a *medical science* and a *healing art*—and must find a way to embrace and meld elements of both. Psychiatry should be a medical science in so far as it studies conditions of health and disease; adheres to the best available controlled evidence; and uses the tools of "objective" medical practice, such as laboratory studies and brain imaging. At the same time, psychiatry should be a healing art, in so far as it concerns itself with the intimate subjectivity and "inner world" of the patient. There is no incompatibility or conflict between these complementary realms: "molecules" and "motives" are simply two lenses through which we view one and the same human condition.

What I am describing is akin to what Ghaemi describes as the "biological existentialism" of Karl Jaspers [20]. And—though some physicians may chafe at this—the model I am proposing is also close in spirit to the "nursing model" described above: i.e., "a holistic....assessment of all dimensions of the person (physical, emotional, mental, and spiritual) that assumes multiple causes for the problems experienced by the patient." (However, as Dr. Kontos commented to me (personal communication, October 12, 2011), this putative "nursing" model really represents the qualities found in all good *physicians*, independent of any theoretical "model" of medical care and treatment.)

Albert Einstein once observed, "The intuitive mind is a sacred gift and the rational mind is a faithful servant. We have created a society that honors the servant and has forgotten the gift." In order for psychiatry to escape the "fly bottle" in which it now finds itself, we must bring together the intuitive and the rational mind. And we must do this not in service of a theory or ideology, but in the service of reducing suffering and enhancing the quality of life for our patients.

Acknowledgments

I would like to thank Nicolas Kontos, MD, for his helpful comments on an early draft of this paper; and Sara Hartley, MD, for referring me to the paper by Guntrip. I also wish to thank Max Fink, MD, and Melvin Gray, MD, for their important insights into psychiatric diagnosis and practice. A slightly modified version of this piece appeared in the October 19, 2011, issue of *Psychiatric Times*.

References

[1] Pies R. Misunderstanding psychiatry (and philosophy) at the highest level. *Psychiatr Times*. 2011 September 8. Available from: http://www.psychiatrictimes.com/articles/misunderstanding-psychiatry-and-philosophy-highest-level. Accessed March 1, 2014.

[2] *Mosby's Medical Dictionary*. 8th ed. 2009. Available from: http://medical-dictionary.thefreedictionary.com/medical+model. Accessed March 6, 2014.

[3] McHugh PR, Slavney PR. *The Perspectives of Psychiatry*. Baltimore: Johns Hopkins University Press; 1986.

[4] Engel GL. The clinical application of the biopsychosocial model. *Am J Psychiatry*. 1980;137:535-544.

[5] Kontos N. Biomedicine—menace or straw man? Reexamining the biopsychosocial argument. *Academic Medicine*. 2011;86:509-515.

[6] Anonymous. Models of disability. Available from: http://www.forwardmid.org.uk/2012_directory/directory_disability_models.html

[7] Frances A. Good grief. *The New York Times*. 2010 August 14. Available from: http://www.nytimes.com/2010/08/15/opinion/15frances.html. Accessed March 1, 2014.

[8] Engel GL. The need for a new medical model: a challenge for biomedicine. *Science*. 1977;196:129-136.

[9] Gabbard GO. "Bound in a nutshell": thoughts on complexity, reductionism, and "infinite space." *Int J Psychoanal*. 2007:88(Pt 3):559-574.

[10] Ghaemi SN. The rise and fall of the biopsychosocial model. *Br J Psychiatry*. 2009;195(1):3-4.

[11] Arieti S. *Interpretation of Schizophrenia*. New York: Basic Books; 1974.

[12] Luhrmann T. Of Two Minds: The Growing Disorder in American Psychiatry. New York: Knopf; 2000.

[13] Guntrip H. The concept of psychodynamic science. *Int J Psychoanal*. 1967;48:32-43.

[14] Okasha S. *Philosophy of Science. A Very Short Introduction*. New York: Oxford University Press; 2002.

[15] Carroll BJ. Diagnostic validity and laboratory studies: rules of the game. In: Robins LN, Barret JEW, editors. *The Validity of Psychiatric Diagnosis*. New York: Raven Press, Ltd; 1989: 229-244.

[16] Sen A. Objectivity and position: assessment of health and well-being. In: Chen L, Kleinman A, Ware N. *Health and Social Change in International Perspective*. Boston: Harvard School of Public Health; 1994.

[17] Wiggins OP, Schwartz MA. Karl Jaspers. In: Embree L, Behnke EA, Carr D et al., editors. *Encyclopedia of Phenomenology*. Kluwer Academic Publishers; 1997. Available from: Karl Jaspers Forum, note 90: www.kjf.ca/N90-SCH.rtf. Accessed March 1, 2014.

[18] *In his text, *General Psychopathology*, Jaspers states, in a footnote, that "Phenomenology is for us purely an *empirical method of enquiry*..." though these investigations "...are quite different from those in the natural sciences." (italics in original). Hoenig JMW, Hamilton MW, translators. Baltimore: Johns Hopkins University Press; 1997: vol 1 p. 55.

[19] Rosenfeld J, Martin RA, Bauer D. Numbness: a practical guide for family physicians. Available from: https://www.aan.com/uploadedfiles/website_library_assets/documents/9.careers/1.job_seekers/family%20practice%20curriculum.pdf
[20] Pies RW. The diagnosis and treatment of subclinical hypothyroid states in depressed patients. *Gen Hosp Psych.* 1997;19:344-354.
[21] Ghaemi SN. Existence and pluralism: the rediscovery of Karl Jaspers. *Psychopathology.* 2007;40:75-82.

~~~~~~~~~~~~~~~~~

HUME'S FORK AND PSYCHIATRY'S EXPLANATIONS: DETERMINISM AND THE DIMENSIONS OF FREEDOM

An item that appeared in the Boston Globe recently caught my eye. Apparently, a man who was fired by a large corporation for visiting an adult "chat room" while at work is suing the company. The man is claiming he is an "Internet addict" who "…deserves treatment and sympathy rather than dismissal" [1].

Another item reported recently concerned a lawyer who argued that her client was not responsible for a rampage he had committed because "…he had been obsessed with comic book superheroes as a kid" [2].

These items piqued my interest not merely because they play into the public's worst stereotypes, concerning psychiatric diagnosis—"You shrinks think every kind of bad behavior is a *disease!*"—but also because they raise the most fundamental questions concerning freedom, responsibility, and mental illness. Since the vexing question of "free will" has been debated by theologians and philosophers for centuries—more recently, the neuroscientists have weighed in—I do not propose to resolve this matter in the space of one column (even medical editors are not that grandiose). I do hope to present an overview of the philosophical issues as they impinge upon psychiatric theory and practice; and to put forward a conceptual schema for understanding how individuals may be both "mentally ill" *and yet responsible in some measure for their actions.* But to accomplish the latter, I first need to put forth a somewhat unfamiliar, if not unwelcome concept, of what it means to act with "free will." In formulating my position, I am indebted to the work of philosophers Moritz Schlick (1882-1936), Thomas W. Clark [3], Owen Flanagan [4], and Daniel C. Dennett [5], among many others.

Stuck by Hume's Fork

Let's begin by considering a paradox known in philosophical circles as "Hume's Fork" [6], ostensibly derived from the work of the great Scottish philosopher, David Hume. The paradox goes something like this: Either all our actions are determined, in which case we are not responsible for them; or, our actions are the result of random events—in which case we are *still* not responsible for them! To understand the first part of this dilemma, we need briefly to consider the concept of *determinism.* In its most basic formulation, determinism simply asserts that *everything that happens is caused*; and that when an event occurs, *nothing other than that event could have occurred at that particular moment, given precisely the same conditions immediately preceding the event.* Determinism is not to be confused with *fatalism* or *predestination,* both of which imply that no matter what we do, the future will turn out in one and only one way. Determinism asserts, on the contrary, that our actions are crucial in shaping the future.

Now, with this in mind, we can see that the first part of Hume's dilemma might imply nothing less than this: if all our wishes, desires and actions are merely the inevitable result of innumerable causal factors coalescing since the beginning of time, we cannot possibly have "free will", or reasonably be held *morally accountable* for our actions. (Thomas Aquinas appreciated these implications more than seven centuries ago.) You can easily imagine how this argument, applied to the subset of individuals with serious *psychiatric disorders*, becomes even more destructive of our commonly-held notions regarding freedom and responsibility: if *everyone's* actions are merely the result of a chain of causation extending back ad infinitum, how much *less* "free will" must someone suffering with schizophrenia have? He or she, after all, carries the added "causal burden" of *brain pathology*, based on the best available science. And how could we possibly argue that such brain-impaired individuals should be held accountable in any way for their actions? On this view, surely, our "internet addict" (whatever that means) might just have a case, in denying any culpability for his on-the-job behavior.

And, alas, the other "tine" in Hume's Fork doesn't help us much, either, if we are intent on salvaging our *ordinary* concept of personal responsibility. For if our actions do *not* proceed from an unbroken chain of causal events; if, on the contrary, our behavior is the product of random factors operating *beyond the realm of causality*, then we are clearly not the authors of our actions in any meaningful sense. By the way, the "quantum mechanics loophole"—the hypothesis that strict determinism may not hold at the level of subatomic particles—does not do us much good, since the molecular and electrochemical events in the brain occur on a scale many magnitudes larger than that of Heisenberg's wave-particle "uncertainty principle."

Bending Hume's Fork

Philosophers, ethicists, and theologians have proposed several ways out of Hume's dilemma, and it is beyond the scope of this brief piece to review them [4, 6, 7]. However, I would like to defend the position—taken prominently by the German philosopher Moritz Schlick—that determinism and causal law do not vitiate "free will" or moral responsibility. On the contrary, Schlick argued, our ability to act with genuine freedom *depends upon causality and determinism* [7]. Schlick pointed out that causal laws are not *proscriptive*, in the way that civil laws are; rather, they are *descriptive*, and merely tell us how the physical world actually functions. The view that determinism and free will are compatible is sometimes termed "compatibilism" or, in more recent versions, "neo-compatibilism" [4]. Of course, Schlick's position rests on the admittedly controversial hypothesis that determinism invariably operates throughout the universe—and thus, in the sphere of our own thoughts, feelings, and actions.

Essentially, the compatibilist argument is that we cannot be free or responsible beings, if our actions are mysteriously "chosen" by some entity that somehow slips the surly bonds of causal law and acts independently of our goals, values, and wishes. On the contrary: whether we call that volitional entity "will," "soul," "psyche," or "I," it must be *causally linked* with our core values, in order to effect morally responsible actions. That is, in order to *preserve free will*, "…the state of my will (itself determined by prior and contemporaneous causes) must be a sufficient cause of any choice I make" [4, p. 126]. Indeed, I want to suggest that the "tighter" the causal links between our decision-making capacity and our innermost values, the "freer" and more responsible our decisions.

Degrees of Freedom

Notwithstanding the compatibility of freedom and determinism (in my view), freedom is not an "either/or" condition. Rather, actions may be *more or less free*, and more or less "responsible", depending on a number of contingent factors. There are, in short, *degrees of freedom*. Psychiatrists can be most helpful, in my view, in so far as we can describe, study, and categorize these degrees of freedom, and the psychopathological conditions that so tragically undermine them.

And yet, while I do not believe that the notion of an "autonomous self" *free of causal law* (contra-causal free will) can be scientifically defended, I do not want to jettison the concept of the autonomous self. Indeed, with proper conceptual rehabilitation, the concept still has what philosopher William James might have called, "cash value": it can still do useful philosophical "work" for us, if understood properly. (As the pragmatic James famously put it, "*Theories thus become instruments, not answers to enigmas…*" [8].)

To appreciate all this, let's begin with a thought experiment. Imagine that some nefarious inventor has contrived an evil device I shall call the *assault machine*. This dastardly machine is attached to the arm, rather like a blood pressure cuff, and has an electrode that penetrates the substance of the brain. The assault machine (or AM) has a visual recognition component that activates its motor apparatus—the purpose of which is to "whack" the nearest person within one's reach! The AM has the ability to override the person's higher brain centers, such that he or she is *absolutely powerless* to resist carrying out the assault. Let's now suppose that Jones is hooked up to the AM, quite against his will. Smith happens to walk by Jones and, as expected, Jones—well, his *arm* at least!—whacks Smith in the head. Now, in my view, the AM provides what my Cornell philosophy professor, Max Black [9], used to call "a perfectly clear case" in which freedom of will and agential action are essentially *inoperative*, as understood in what Black would call our "ordinary language." That is, Jones's assault on Smith is *not causally related to the hopes, wishes, goals, and rational purposes unique to Jones*; rather, the proximal cause of the assault is the action of the nefarious device. And how is this thought experiment related to the concept of the "autonomous self"? Essentially, the AM vitiates our ordinary language understanding of the autonomous self. To appreciate this, let's consider another vignette on the opposite side of the continuum I am developing here.

Our friend Jones—having been acquitted of any criminal charges in the Smith assault incident—now returns to his home where he is enjoying his hobby of painting. He stands, brush in hand, deliberating as to what he will now paint; in what style (abstract expressionism? realism? Etc.) and with what colors. Jones has not been externally constrained, so far as we know, in any way: he has not been commissioned to produce one kind of painting or another; he has no limits as to available art supplies, choice of paint, etc. Again, I would argue that this is a "perfectly clear case" in which the autonomous self and agential action—action taken by a rational and deliberative person—are essentially *preserved*. Now this is surely not to argue that any of Jones's artistic decisions are somehow *uncaused*, or supernaturally liberated from the laws of physics and neurochemistry! Jones's actions are, to be sure, mediated by his brain—and his brain is a physical entity constrained by physical laws. Yet, in our ordinary language, I believe we would consider Jones to be acting freely—indeed, *with free will*. We would also say, in my view, that Jones, as artist, is now *responsible* for his actions, in a very robust sense.

Before relating all this to psychiatric disorders, let's consider, finally, a middle case. Let's suppose it is the year 2025, and neuroscientists have isolated a neuropeptide dubbed, "assaultin." Assaultin, it turns out, is coded for by the gene BAD2U. Behavioral scientists have established, in 32 randomized, controlled studies, that when this neuropeptide is injected into the cerebrospinal fluid of human subjects, fully 65% of them become immediately and dramatically assaultive. Ah—but 35% of subjects *do not* become assaultive. Indeed, psychological studies of these non-assaultive subjects reveal that nearly all employ a certain cognitive strategy to overcome the powerful impulse to become assaultive—they repeat a sort of mantra that helps them retain self-control. Moreover, when the 65% of subjects who *do* become assaultive are *taught* this marvelous mantra, 50% are able to *resist* the effects of subsequent assaultin injections. Now the key question: where, on the "degrees of freedom" continuum, would we place the *brain state* (or states) associated with "assaultin injection", in relation to (a) the condition of being strapped to the assault machine [Jones case 1]; and (b) the condition of being left alone with one's paints and canvass [Jones case 2]? I would argue that we would place the neuropeptide-induced brain state(s) somewhere in between the other two instances—probably closer to Jones case 1 than to Jones case 2.**

Now, if this heuristic model has any utility in psychiatry, we ought to be able to place a variety of brain states and psychiatric disorders somewhere along the "degrees of freedom" continuum. (I am assuming here that psychiatric disorders are essentially highly complex, aberrant brain states). I have suggested a few purely speculative placements in Figure 1. The actual placement of brain states and putative disorders would depend crucially on the empirical evidence gathered in understanding these conditions: for example, to what degree does an individual with schizophrenia have the ability to resist obeying so-called "command hallucinations" to harm someone? The answer undoubtedly differs from patient to patient—depending on a multitude of genetic, biochemical, and psychological factors. (The term "psychological" is not intended to imply something *non-material*; rather, it is a short-hand term for brain processes that we experience and express in terms of *motivations, wishes, understandings, fears*, etc.). In part II of this essay, I will elaborate on the "naturalistic" model of freedom and autonomy, and suggest how it may be applied to psychiatric disorders and medico-legal determinations of culpability.

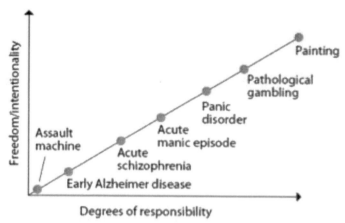

Source: Ronald Pies, MD (with permission from Psychiatric Times)

Figure 1. Degrees of Freedom Continuum.

Notes

**I believe the example holds up whether or not we can isolate or discover a single, invariable neuroanatomical or neurochemical brain state associated with this drug. The degree of freedom I am positing is still intermediate, with respect to the other two cases.

Acknowledgments

I wish to thank Thomas Clarke and Robert Daly MD for their helpful comments on this essay. Excellent discussions of free will and determinism may be found at the website http://www.naturalism.org/freewill.htm. I also highly recommend Thomas W. Clark's book, *Encountering Naturalism*, published by the Center for Naturalism. A slightly modified version of this piece appeared in the August 1, 2007, issue of *Psychiatric Times*.

References

[1] Man fired for visiting chat room sues IBM. *The Boston Globe*. 2007 February 19.
[2] "Q & A." *The Boston Globe*. 2007 March 4.
[3] Clark TW. Applied ethics: science and freedom. Free Inquiry. 22(2). Available from: http://www.secularhumanism.org/index.php?section=library&page=clark_22_2. Accessed March 6, 2014.
[4] Flanagan O. *The Problem of the Soul*. New York: Basic Books; 2002.
[5] Dennett DC. *Freedom Evolves*. New York: Viking; 2003.
[6] Blackburn S, editor. *Oxford Dictionary of Philosophy*. New York: Oxford University Press; 1994.
[7] Berofsky B. Free will and determinism. In: Weiner PP, editor. *Dictionary of the History of Ideas*. Vol 2. 1974: 236-242. Available from http://xtf.lib.virginia.edu/xtf/view?

docId=DicHist/uvaGenText/tei/DicHist2.xml;chunk.id=dv2-28;toc.depth=1;toc.id=dv2-28;brand=default. Accessed March 6, 2014.

[8] James W. *What Pragmatism Means.* (1907) Available from: http://iws.collin.edu/amiller/William%20James%20-%20Pragmatism.pdf

[9] Black M. Definition, presupposition, and assertion. *The Philosophical Review.* 1952;61(4):532-550.

~~~~~~~~~~~~~~~~~

PSYCHIATRIC NATURALISM AND THE DIMENSIONS OF FREEDOM: PART II

Implications for Psychiatry and Law

In the first part of this essay, I argued that individual freedom is not only compatible with determinism, but also dependent upon it. I also argued that "freedom" is not an "either/or" condition. Rather, actions may be *more or less free*, and therefore more or less "responsible," depending on a number of contingent factors, yielding various *degrees of freedom*. Psychiatrists, I suggested, can be most helpful in so far as we can describe, study, and categorize these degrees of freedom, and the psychopathological conditions that undermine them. Now, in this concluding portion, I want to elaborate on the "naturalistic" model of freedom and autonomy, and suggest how it may be applied to psychiatric disorders and medico-legal determinations of culpability.

By "naturalistic," I mean simply that we need not posit *non-material* or metaphysical entities—though these might exist—in order to explain ourselves or the world. As the Center for Naturalism puts it, "Nothing about us escapes being included in the physical universe, or escapes being shaped by the various processes—physical, biological, psychological, and social—that science describes. On a scientific understanding of ourselves, there's no evidence for immaterial souls, spirits, mental essences, or disembodied selves which stand apart from the physical world" [1].

And yet—in the face of all this, I maintain that we *do* experience and possess a very real kind of freedom. In what, then, might this freedom consist? And how might such freedom be vitiated in the presence of certain kinds of brain dysfunction? Finally, how does such a view square with our everyday understanding of moral responsibility and societal punishment for "evil-doing"?

I believe that the ancient Stoics had it about right when they construed freedom in essentially "negative" terms; that is, in terms of what is *not present* when we say that we act "freely." At the very least, the Stoic formulation may help us toward a first approximation of what we mean by "freedom."

In his *Discourses*, the Stoic philosopher Epictetus described the free individual as being *free from* certain inhibiting conditions; specifically, he or she is (a) free from distress (*alupos*); (b) free from fear (*aphobos*); (c) free from violent emotions (*apathes*); and (d) free from hindrance (*akolutos*) [2]. In our ordinary linguistic use of the term "free," I believe these components are usually understood or intended. That is, we say that "Jones acted freely" if (among other criteria yet to be specified), *Jones acted at a time when, with respect to the act in question, he was not under great duress; not being coerced; not experiencing some overwhelming emotional turmoil, and was not hindered from pursuing his wishes at the time.* I believe that these "negative aspects" of freedom bring us to what I would call the first threshold of a free act. These "non-constraint" features, in my view, are generally necessary, but not sufficient, to constitute what, in ordinary language, we mean by a "free act." (I am again appealing to what our *ordinary language* tells us about words such as "freedom"; and, as the philosopher Ludwig Wittgenstein reminded us, "...ordinary language is all right" [3].)

The second threshold, in my view, involves the presence of *intentionality*. The philosopher Keith Seddon defines intentionality as follows: "In order for any action to be intentional, we have to understand the background of the situation against which we intend to act; what we hope to accomplish, and why it is *reasonable* to suppose that this action will produce that result" (italics added) [2 p. 42].

Note that Seddon's concept of intentionality entails more than simply acting *consciously* or with a *purpose* in mind—it entails a kind of *rationality* as well. On this admittedly stringent view of intentionality, someone who decided, say, that the KGB had implanted an electrode in his brain; that the only way to correct this situation was to remove the electrode with an ice pick; and that this could be accomplished only by kidnapping the Russian ambassador would not be acting "intentionally." Nor, in my view, would that individual be acting "freely" in the sense I wish to develop. It may also be seen that this unfortunate individual would not meet most ordinary-language definitions of "sane". Indeed, Prof. Robert Daly has developed the concept of *sanity* in a way that is readily transferable to the concept of *freedom* I am developing. Daly writes: "A person is judged to be "sane" when the behavioral and experiential foundations of his capacity for action (his personality) are so integrated with his knowledge and capacity to choose that he is...able to secure his prudential interests" (personal communication, March 21, 2007). If we substitute the word "free" for "sane" in this passage, we will arrive at something like what I mean by this "second threshold" of freedom.

The third threshold for a truly free act, in my view, is quite straightforward and intuitively obvious: the act undertaken must be *subjectively experienced as consistent with the individual's wishes*. Simply put, we feel "free" when (in addition to the aforementioned conditions) we feel that we are acting in accordance with our own wishes—what Thomas Clark calls the *authorship criterion* of free action. In part I of this essay, I described a hypothetical "assault machine" which—when strapped to the person's arm and connected to the brain—overrides the individual's intentions and wishes, and causes him or her to strike the nearest person. Assuming the individual does not wish to be assaultive, it is evident that the act of assault cannot be "free", in this hypothetical scenario.

Note that this third threshold involves an *experiential* or *phenomenological* element of freedom: very simply, we *feel free* as we are carrying out most of our everyday actions, regardless of how a deterministic science might explain these actions. (Dr. Nassir Ghaemi has pointed to psychiatrist and philosopher Karl Jaspers* as one who understood the importance of this transcendent "world of personal freedom" [4].) Some proponents of determinism argue that this feeling of freedom is nothing more than a kind of "trick" played on us by our brains—a comforting delusion that belies the causal mechanisms that determine our actions. I strongly disagree: nothing in the nature of determinism or causality vitiates or renders illusory our conscious *experience* of being free. That feeling is as "real" as rocks or trees or atoms. It is as real as experiencing sugar as sweet. Indeed, none of the three main threshold criteria I have described is vitiated by the operation of physical law, neurochemical processes, causality, or determinism.

To summarize, in Clark's term: a free act is *unconstrained, rational, and experienced as self-authored* [6]. These criteria do not require us to posit some contra-causal "autonomous self" that rises up, sundered from physical laws, and magically "chooses" a course of action. Indeed, the "capacity to choose" I cited in Robert Daly's work need not be understood as a faculty disconnected from determined, causal events. Rather, the individual's *capacity to choose* may be understood as *the repertoire of contemplated acts and behaviors that the individual perceives, evaluates, and, in principle, is capable of performing, immediately prior to acting.*

This repertoire is akin to what computer scientist Marvin Minsky refers to as the "resources" available to the human brain at the moment an action is contemplated [5]. These might include, for example, neuronal circuits or brain regions dedicated to aggression, passivity, avoidance, etc. In the case of highly creative and abstract actions, such as painting a portrait (see Part 1), this repertoire of available acts ("resources") might include neuronal pathways representing, say, "impressionist techniques" or "classic style." Note that I said, capable of performing *in principle*. There are always sufficient reasons why, at a given moment, all *potentially* available actions are not *in fact* carried out by the individual. Indeed, that is why determinists argue that, for any action that we have performed, we could not have done otherwise, at that particular moment. This, however, does not mean that our actions are easily predictable, or that we can't *modify our behavior* when contemplating similar actions in the future. On the contrary, the entire foundation of psychotherapy requires the presupposition that we can help many of our patients acquire an ever more flexible, adaptive, and existentially fulfilling repertoire of behaviors.

Thus, psychotherapy is not threatened by determinism; rather, psychotherapy of any type *relies upon causality* as the underlying basis for favorably modifying thought, emotion, and behavior. It is simply that the "causes" we ordinarily attend to in psychotherapy are those proximately linked to the patient's behavior : those we ordinarily understand as the patient's enduring *wishes, beliefs, impulses, fantasies, and goals*. In short, we understand that the proximate cause of the patient's behavior is his or her *personality,* or *personhood*—essentially what the Stoics called "the ruling principle" (*hegemonikon*).

So: how does all this theorizing apply to individuals with psychiatric disorders? And how does a model of "psychiatric naturalism" help us achieve a humane and rational system of justice and rehabilitation?

In this brief space, I can only sketch some answers to these questions. (A much richer and more elegant exposition is provided in Thomas Clark's book, *Encountering Naturalism* [6].) Let's start with a hypothetical patient, Mr. A., who carries a diagnosis of chronic paranoid schizophrenia. Let's posit that, in the midst of an acute psychotic decompensation, Mr. A. is attending to command auditory hallucinations telling him, "Drive your car into the nearest pedestrian." Let's also posit that Mr. A. is terrified that, if he does not comply with the "voice"—which he takes to be that of "Satan"—he will be thrown into a pit of fire. In fact, Mr. A. sees no viable alternatives to complying with these diabolical voices. As a consequence of this psychopathology (or "brain state", to use an alternative framework), Mr. A. appears to be highly agitated, according to several witnesses; for example, he is perspiring heavily, and hyperventilating, as he steps into his car. Tragically, Mr. A proceeds to drive his car into a pedestrian; is subsequently arrested, and charged with "vehicular homicide" [7].

Subsequent investigation reveals that Mr. A. had made a decision, two weeks earlier, to discontinue his antipsychotic medication—despite having been warned repeatedly against doing so, by both his psychiatrist and his wife. Mr. A., at that time, was not showing any evidence of acute psychosis. He convinced his physician that he understood the risks of stopping his medication, including the potential for violent acts, but elected to stop the medication anyway because, "I don't like the side effects."

Based on the model we have constructed, what can we say about Mr. A's actions? First, it seems clear that his act of driving into the pedestrian—terrible as it was—cannot be considered a *free* act. Assuming we have our facts right (and, in principle, this is a matter of empirical investigation). Mr. A. was acting under just the kind of *internal coercion* the Stoics viewed as inconsistent with a free act. He was also in a state of *marked emotional turmoil*, judging from the reports of witnesses. Furthermore, Mr. A's act was evidently not *intentional*, in the strict sense we have defined it. Recalling Seddon's requirement that an intentional act entails our rationally understanding "...the background of the situation against which we intend to act..." it seems clear that Mr. A. did not have such a rational understanding (though he may well have *believed* himself to be rational at the time). Mr. A. did not, for example, appear to realize that the "Satanic voices" were causally related to his having stopped taking his antipsychotic medication. Finally, from the posited facts of the case, Mr. A. *felt compelled* to act as he did, rather than experiencing his actions as *self-motivated expressions of his own wishes*. In sum, with respect to his mowing down the pedestrian, Mr. A. met none of the three threshold criteria for acting freely.

On the other hand, Mr. A's earlier decision to stop taking his medication—though no less determined than any other action by any individual—appears to have been undertaken with a *greater degree of freedom,* as we have defined it. That is, from what we have posited, Mr. A. elected to stop his medications while in a relatively non-coerced, and rationally informed, mental state. In ethical terms, therefore, we might plausibly argue that whereas Mr. A. was not fully responsible for his running down the pedestrian, he was at least *largely responsible* for (unwisely) discontinuing his medication. I am positing, in other words, a *direct relationship between degrees of freedom and degrees of responsibility.* Indeed, I would define "responsibility" as essentially *the ethical dimension of freedom*. Responsibility, as Clark notes, is also "...the dimension which legitimizes social sanctions and rewards as a way to change behavior..." (personal communication, April 12, 2007). And though I am not putting forward an explicitly *legal* claim, I believe that our legal system can draw on such philosophical reasoning, in so far as society applies various "remedies" to acts such as those of Mr. A.

In our present legal system, based on the Model Penal Code (MPC) promulgated by the American Law Institute, it seems likely that Mr. A. would be found guilty of either manslaughter or negligent homicide. As Prof. Daniel W. Shuman informs me (personal communication April 23, 2007), "Under MPC, a person with a mental disability who is aware of a potential for violence when unmedicated may be liable for reckless or negligent homicide if he fails to remain on medication and then kills [someone—even if at the time of the crime he would meet the test for not guilty by reason of insanity." Mr. A. could be found guilty of manslaughter because "...he consciously disregarded his physician's warning and subsequently killed someone; or for negligent homicide, because he failed to be aware of the reasonable risk that driving after he discontinued his medication would result in physical injury to others."

All this is more or less consistent with our naturalistic model of freedom. That is, a jury might implicitly understand that whereas Mr. A's mowing down the pedestrian was not *in itself* a free act for which he should be held responsible, his refusal to take appropriate medication *was* a free act, for which he *should* be held responsible.

However, our current system of justice would most likely diverge from our model of psychiatric naturalism at this point. As Prof. Shuman notes, criminal law as we know it still has "retributive goals"—psychiatric naturalism does not. (For a rebuttal of Prof. Michael Moore's contention that retribution is "intrinsically good," see Clark [8].) Under our present system, Mr. A. might very well be sentenced to prison, in most states.

In contrast, our model (and perhaps some judges in specialized "mental health courts") might prompt another course of action; e.g., involuntary inpatient commitment or partial hospitalization; mandatory (court-enforced) depot antipsychotic medication; and immediate suspension of Mr. A's driver's license. (This last sanction might remain in force until such time as Mr. A's compliance with, and positive response to, medical treatment are unambiguously established). Mr. A. might also be ordered to compensate the family of the pedestrian he killed, and to perform some type of long-term community service. Under our model of psychiatric naturalism, this outcome would be deemed more rational (and less retributive) than putting Mr. A. in prison.

We can apply this same sort of reasoning to a wide spectrum of psychiatric disorders, ranging from schizophrenia to so-called "internet addiction." Psychiatrists can contribute to legal decision-making by providing general empirical evidence regarding specific brain states and disorders; and the degree to which they may undermine free and responsible action. Indeed, the Chinese have actually developed a "diminished criminal responsibility rating scale" (DCRRS) that has been used to distinguish varying degrees of culpability in patients with schizophrenia [9].

In the end, it must be left to the legal system to determine "criminal responsibility," and to apply the most useful and humane remedies or sanctions. Psychiatric naturalism does not compel us, either logically or morally, to abandon our feelings of outrage or revulsion in the face of, say, terrorism, homicide or genocide; nor does it require us to jettison our belief that such acts are profoundly wrong. Rather, psychiatric naturalism compels us to re-examine the belief that *retribution for retribution's sake* is based on sound reasoning or wise public policy [8]. Finally, psychiatric naturalism permits us to retain those elements of the criminal justice system that promote such valid objectives as "...public safety, deterrence, rehabilitation, community restoration, and victim restitution" [10].

Acknowledgments

I wish to thank Dr. Robert Daly and Thomas W. Clark for their helpful comments on both parts I and II of this essay. I also wish to acknowledge the assistance of the late Prof. Daniel Shuman; and of Prof. Alan Stone MD, for their helpful comments on portions of this essay. A slightly modified version of this piece appeared in the August 1, 2007, issue of *Psychiatric Times*.

References

[1] Tenets of naturalism. Available from: http://www.naturalism.org/tenetsof.htm. Accessed February 23, 2014.
[2] Seddon K. Epictetus' Handbook and the Tablet of Cebes. London: Routledge; 2005.
[3] Wittgenstein L. The Blue and Brown Books: Preliminary Studies for the Philosophical Investigations. New York: Harper and Row; 1958: 28.
[4] Ghaemi SN. Existence and pluralism: the rediscovery of Karl Jaspers. *Psychopathology*. 2007;40:75-82.
[5] Minsky M. The Emotion Machine: Commonsense Thinking, Artificial Intelligence, and the Future of the Human Mind. New York: Simon & Schuster; 2006.
[6] Clark TW. *Encountering Naturalism*. Somerville, MA: Center for Naturalism; 2007.
[7] Vehicular Homicide (no author listed). Accessed at: http://definitions.uslegal.com/v/vehicular-homicide/
[8] Clark TW. Against retribution. Available from: http://www.naturalism.org/criminal.htm#AgainstRetribution. Accessed February 23, 2014.
[9] Huang FY, Cai WX, Zhang QT et al. The application of diminished criminal responsibility rating scale to schizophrenia offenders. *Fa Yi Xue Za Zhi*. 2006; 22: 288-90.
[10] Clark TW. Naturalism and punishment: real world implications for criminal justice. Available from: http://www.naturalism.org/stanko.htm. Accessed February 23, 2014.

*For more on Jaspers, see: OP Wiggins, MA Schwartz. Edmund Husserl;s influence on Karl Jaspers's phenomenology. *Philosophy, Psychiatry, & Psychology*. 1997;4.1;15-36.

~~~~~~~~~~~~~~~~~

SCIENCE, PSYCHIATRY, AND FAMILY PRACTICE: POSITIVISM VS. PLURALISM

For now we see through a glass, darkly...—1 Corinthians 13: 12-13

When I was growing up in the late 1950s, "science" was all the rage among my young classmates. The manned space program was in its infancy, and most of my friends had fashioned "space helmets" out of 5-gallon ice-cream tubs and collected picture cards showing the seven Mercury astronauts. Fifty years later, I am amazed at how the cachet of "science" has dominated the recent debate over psychiatric diagnosis, the DSM-5, and the issue of psychiatry's supposed "medicalization" of normality [1]. Ironically, both friends and foes of psychiatry invoke the prestige of "science" in asserting their views. Critics of the DSM-5 insist that the new manual's modifications are not "scientific," while the DSM-5 itself informs us that it has incorporated "scientific findings from the latest research" [2]. Meanwhile, the National Institute of Mental health promotes its "RDoC" (Research Domain Criteria) project—emphasizing neurocircuits—as the new "scientific agenda" for psychiatry [3].

But for the philosophically inclined, these confident pronouncements on "science" present more questions than answers. For example: what, exactly, does the word "science" mean? What is denoted by the term "scientific"? Is "scientific" a *binary* term—for example, is a particular claim, or diagnostic category, either "scientific" or "not scientific"? Or can claims and categories be *more or less* "scientific"? Similarly, is there a continuum of scientific *validity*? Are biological "tests" and observable neuropathology necessary to validate a psychiatric diagnosis? Does diagnosis in general medicine and psychiatry typically involve the identification of a well-defined lesion or pathoanatomical "entity"? The remainder of this essay will offer some very provisional answers to these questions.

What Is Science and the Scientific Method?

The nature of "science" and the meaning of "scientific" are far from settled matters—even among scientists. Prof. Sean Carroll, a theoretical physicist at the California Institute of Technology, writes that, "Defining the concept of "science" is a notoriously tricky business. In particular, there is long-running debate over the demarcation problem, which asks where we should draw the line between science and non-science" [4].

Nevertheless, Carroll makes clear that science is *not* a particular set of facts or lab tests, but a three-part *process*: (1) Developing several hypotheses about some aspect of the world. (2) Carefully examining that aspect of the world and collecting relevant data; and 3. Choosing the hypothesis that best "fits" or explains the data, whenever possible. This, essentially, is what Western science calls, "the hypothetico-deductive method." But Sean Carroll notes that "every one of these three steps is highly problematic in its own way" [4], particularly the third step. That's because any set of data may yield several quite reasonable hypotheses, any one of which may "explain" the phenomenon in question—what philosophers refer to as the *underdetermination* of the data.

To take a recent example from the DSM-5, consider "Jimmy," a 7-year-old boy who is nearly always irritable or angry, most of the day, nearly every day. Let's say Jimmy also shows severe, recurrent, and sometimes violent temper outbursts three times per week, which are felt to be inconsistent with his developmental level. Let's say Jimmy has shown these features for the past 18 months, and has never met criteria for a manic or hypomanic episode. We might offer two quite different hypotheses to account for this child's presentation.

The first says, "Jimmy is a normal, 7-year-old child who, like many children his age, often has bad moods and temper tantrums. He's probably upset by problems within his family, feels ignored, and hasn't learned appropriate ways of expressing anger." The second hypothesis says, "Jimmy has a pathological condition called Disruptive Mood Dysregulation Disorder (DMDD), which can be distinguished from both 'normal' moodiness and bipolar disorder. DMDD is often a precursor of a depressive or anxiety disorder, and is associated with specific attentional problems not seen in normal children or those with bipolar disorder." The second hypothesis is roughly the basis for the controversial new DSM-5 category of DMDD [5].

Now, we can certainly question whether the DSM-5 work group was justified in positing DMDD as a specific disorder, despite their review of the available epidemiological, clinical, and neuropsychological data. And, it might turn out that, indeed, Jimmy is just a normal but temperamental child. But, as Prof. Carroll construes the scientific method, it would be unfair to say that the DSM-5 work group has been "unscientific" in its deliberations on DMDD.

Indeed, the British Science Council (BSC) has defined science as, quite simply, "...the pursuit of knowledge and understanding of the natural and social world following a systematic methodology based on evidence." In my view, the most serious and debilitating psychiatric disorders encountered in clinical practice—*schizophrenia, bipolar disorder*, and *melancholic major depressive disorder*—are, without a doubt, scientifically-based, using the BSC definition. While the specific DSM criteria have changed somewhat from DSM-III to DSM-5, our basic clinical descriptions of these conditions are grounded in many decades of careful observations, as well as thousands of systematic research studies.

This doesn't mean that the DSM work groups are never swayed by political, economic or social pressures [6]. Other medical specialties, too, are sometimes motivated by "extra-scientific" considerations and values. For example, the recent recommendation by the American Medical Association to declare obesity a "disease" appears to have been driven primarily by the wish to encourage better treatment of this condition—a laudable goal, surely, but *not* a purely "scientific" decision, if by that term, we mean "value-free" [7].

Finally, it's important to note that *use of the scientific method* doesn't guarantee that our diagnostic categories are *valid* or clinically useful. After all, many careful scientific observations led to the hypothesis that a small planet—*Vulcan*, no less!—existed somewhere between Mercury and the Sun. Yet ultimately, this claim was *invalidated*. It is certainly possible that DMDD and other DSM-5 categories will suffer the same fate—but this is all part of the scientific process. **

What Properties Confer Validity on a Diagnosis?

Clinicians want their diagnostic categories to be both *reliable* and *valid*. *Reliability* refers to the degree of inter-rater agreement that can be achieved with a particular set of diagnostic criteria, represented by the designation "kappa." So, let's say two people viewing a picture of a horse-like creature with a horn in the middle of its forehead agree that the picture represents a unicorn, and agreement occurs 100% of the time with all other observer pairs. This picture elicits perfect inter-rater agreement, and would have a *kappa* of 1.0. But this tells us nothing about the existence of unicorns!

Validity is quite another matter. Very broadly, validity describes the "*is*-ness" of a diagnosis or set of criteria; i.e., the degree to which a diagnostic category actually identifies something "real"—or at least, a clinically useful and meaningful diagnostic entity. How is validity established in clinical medicine and psychiatry?

Dr. Bernard Carroll's description of "convergent validity" helps answer this question. He explains that our disease constructs take shape through a process of "convergent validation." This entails "...iterative attention to signs, symptoms, course of illness, response to treatments, family history, and laboratory data" [8].

Like the term "scientific," validity is not a binary term. Diagnostic categories may have *varying degrees* of validity. As I wrote several years ago, in order for a diagnostic category to gain a least a modicum of validity,

> "...the criteria for "Disease X" must be "sharp" enough to distinguish its sufferers from those with Disease Y or Z. Its "elements" must cohere, in the way we would expect the pieces of a jigsaw puzzle to fit together. For example, if Disease X is defined by the presence of auditory hallucinations, dry skin, elevated blood pressure, and tremor, one would expect high degrees of concordance and overlap among these features. One would also expect a good correlation between this symptom picture and the course, outcome, and response to treatment of Disease X..." [9].

How many DSM-5 diagnostic categories will meet these fairly stringent tests of "validity"? No one knows—maybe a handful, maybe a few dozen. I believe that, at a minimum, schizophrenia, bipolar disorder, panic disorder, obsessive-compulsive disorder, and the melancholic subtype of major depressive disorder will make the grade. (My colleague, Nassir Ghaemi, MD, estimates that, among DSM-III categories, "about two dozen" were based on "decent scientific evidence" [6] (see footnote).

But even by these harsh lights, there is no foundation for the claim that *all* psychiatric diagnoses, across the board, lack validity. Even DSM categories not yet fully validated are not necessarily *in*valid. Indeed, it is seldom understood that the same kinds of rigorous studies that would *validate* a DSM category would be required to *invalidate* it. Furthermore, diagnostic validity is always *provisional* and probabilistic. Thus, our level of confidence in a set of disease criteria may increase or decrease, as new data or discoveries emerge. (I believe the "DSM-5.1"—i.e., expected updates of the DSM-5—must provide ongoing validity data that support its newer categories, or the credibility of the manual will continue to be questioned).

Nevertheless, even if some of DSM-5's *categorical distinctions* prove invalid, this in no way invalidates the construct of *psychiatric disease*, understood in neuropathological terms. For example: the most recent investigations of schizophrenia and psychotic bipolar disorder suggest that there is substantial neurobiological overlap of these conditions, with respect to white matter abnormalities [10]. If these preliminary findings are replicated, we might reasonably infer that—in the case of these afflictions—Nature is not "carved at its joints" so much as shaded at its borders. But such "fuzziness" at the schizophrenia-bipolar border does not render the aforementioned white matter abnormalities—much less, the patient's suffering and incapacity!—any less "real." As the philosopher Ludwig Wittgenstein observed, a fuzzy beam of light is just as real as a sharply focused one [11].

Are Biomarkers or Lab Tests Necessary for a Diagnostic Category to Be Valid?

Once again, Dr. Bernard Carroll hits the mark:

> "We need to be clear that the existence of disease is not predicated on having a biological test. It's nice when we do have one, but there are many areas in medicine where there is no conclusive diagnostic test. Think migraine. Think multiple sclerosis. Think chronic pain. Indeed, clinical science correctly recognized many diseases long before lab tests came along for confirmatory diagnostic application. Think Parkinson's disease, Huntington's disease, epilepsy... it's a long list" [8].

Indeed, Dr. Kurt Kroenke points out that physicians can easily overestimate the value of lab and imaging tests, noting that *the patient's history* "...typically accounts for 75% or more of the diagnostic yield when evaluating common symptoms" [12]. The physical examination accounts for 10-15%, and diagnostic testing, generally less than 10% of the diagnostic yield.

Moreover, lab tests and biomarkers can never be any better than the *clinical criteria* that define the disorder under investigation—and useful "lab tests" or biomarkers for a disorder must always *follow* the development of reliable and valid clinical criteria. As Bernard Carroll succinctly puts it, "Laboratory measures are the servants of clinical science, not the other way around" [8].

Diagnosis in Psychiatry and Family Practice: Lumps vs. Patients

Critics of psychiatric diagnosis often argue that our disease categories do not identify or name any "ontological entity"—a real "thing" like an abscess or tumor. These critics point to medical specialties like microbiology, in which one can see a pathogenic organism under the microscope, and even isolate it from the patient's infection site. For the critics, this makes microbiology a "real" science that treats "real" diseases, in contrast to psychiatry, which allegedly treats only "metaphorical" disease [13]. I believe this "lumps and bumps" concept of disease is deeply misinformed and represents the regressive legacy of *logical positivism*—an early 20th century school of thought now largely discredited by most philosophers of science [14].

In his Skinner Lecture of 1942 [15], professor of radiology Dr. Henry Cohen described "two main trends...in our conception of disease." The first was that of the *Hippocratic school*, which, in Cohen's words, "...stressed *the patient*--his complaints, his appearance, his habits, his work, his environment, his relatives, his sputum, urine...and the like" (italics added) [15]. The contrasting trend—which Cohen saw as a late outgrowth of Platonic philosophy—is close kin to the positivist, "lumps and bumps" school of thought. It conceived of a disease in terms of a specific *ontological entity*—what family physician Kirsti Malterud MD, PhD defines as, "...a solid fact representing the actual pathology..." [16].

One might have thought that a radiologist would be in sympathy with this positivist outlook, but Cohen clearly was not. Rather, he tartly observed that,

> "Our textbooks describe 'entities'—model and composite pictures of such diseases as typhoid fever...cancer and the like...[and] our goal has been a diagnostic penny-in-the-slot machine; for then, treatment and prognosis too follow automatically. Not a few physicians act as if, by a combination of X rays with clinical pathological reports, that goal has been achieved. From time to time, voices have been raised stressing the importance of the patient; of his environment, of the mental reaction to, and the mental components of his illness, but they have gone unheeded..." [15]. ^^

Dr. Malterud observes that it is rare, in family practice, that the physician can link specific observable signs to a specific localized lesion or pathological process. On the contrary, "The professional norm that objective signs are supposed to confirm subjective symptoms and thereby reveal monocausal disease processes falls apart in the sea of medical complexities encountered by the family physician" [16].

Nevertheless, Dr. Malterud notes that, "...the solution of the patient's problem can often be achieved despite the impossibility of reaching an established medical diagnosis" [16]. Indeed, in psychiatry, as in family practice, we can still be of great help to the patient, even when we have not identified a specific lesion, pathophysiological process, or other "ontological entity" as the culprit. Thus, the patient may present with a puzzling mix of anxiety, depression, obsessive features, rejection sensitivity, and mild ideas of reference. No specific diagnostic "entity," lesion, or pathophysiological process may be discernible—yet the patient is suffering and unable to function. The psychiatrist, proceeding from a Hippocratic and "holistic" perspective [17], may understand the genesis of the patient's problem in biological, psychosocial, environmental, and even spiritual [18] terms. Most important: *the psychiatrist may find effective ways of helping the patient feel and function better*. This, arguably, is a type of Hippocratic medicine [16,17] and there is nothing "unscientific" about it—so long as the physician's approach is grounded in careful and repeated observation; frequent testing of one's hypotheses; and the use of well-founded somatic and psychosocial treatments.

As for those vaunted lab and imaging findings psychiatry's critics are always demanding, Dr. Malterud notes that "test results...are only interesting if they can support or refute a first-class *clinical* question" (italics added) [16].

When we elevate lab tests to the level of Supreme and Ultimate Standard, we are engaging not in science, but in *scientism*—"an exaggerated trust in the efficacy of the methods of natural science applied to all areas of investigation (as in philosophy, the social sciences, and the humanities)" [19].

Sometimes, of course, a pathophysiological approach is necessary; for example, in ensuring that a patient's panic attacks are not a complication of a pheochromocytoma; or his auditory hallucinations, the result of a temporal lobe tumor. But these examples are atypical, in both family medicine and psychiatry. Usually, our patients' complaints are more subtle, complex, and overdetermined [16]. I believe they are best addressed by maintaining a dynamic tension between what Karl Jaspers proposed as two basic methods of discernment in psychiatry: *Erklären* (causal explanation) and *Verstehen* (meaningful understanding) [20]. Very roughly, these modes of discernment correspond, respectively, to the pathoanatomical and patient-centered perspectives.

Conclusion

Neither family practice nor psychiatry is a "natural science", like biophysics. Rather, they are *medical sciences*—hybrid constructs, compounded of observation and interpretation; molecules and motives; nanograms and narratives. Indeed, the core values of clinical psychiatry have always been Hippocratic, pluralistic and holistic. Even the dean of neuropsychiatry in the U.K.—Prof. William Alwyn Lishman—had this to say:

> "The study and treatment of those psychiatric disorders deriving from brain malfunction must capitalize on all that psychiatry has to offer. There are psychodynamic, social and cultural aspects of neuropsychiatry to be considered; exploration of conflict must take its place alongside the physical examination in differential diagnosis; psychotherapy alongside pharmacotherapy in treatment" [21, p. xiii-xiv].

Such rich pluralism does not undermine psychiatry's status as a medical science. But psychiatry is also an art [22], grounded in deeply personal human relationships. The danger to our profession comes from those who insist on stark dichotomies, as Dr. Malterud explains:

> "Dichotomous thinking is dangerous because it encourages the practitioner to choose one alternative and dismiss the other. Instead...physicians must be ready to merge paradoxes and opposing perspectives...the narrative structure of medical knowledge is gaining increasing recognition. Yet, an ongoing simultaneous attention to biomedical processes should never be neglected" [16].

Yes, the physician's knowledge is almost always fragmentary and incomplete—and often, "we see through a glass, darkly." But we must not allow these limitations to deter us from diagnosing and treating our patients to the best of our ability.

Notes

** My colleague, Dr. Nassir Ghaemi, has suggested that "in clinical diagnosis, the specific scientific criteria are the five [Robins and Guze] criteria of validity"; and that one cannot justifiably "separate science from validity when discussing nosology" (personal communication, August 29, 2013). (The Robins & Guze criteria [Am J Psychiatry. 1970 Jan;126(7):983-7] comprise *clinical description, laboratory study, exclusion of other disorders, follow-up study, and family study*—often considered the fundamental elements of "construct validity"). To be sure: "science" is intimately related to construct validity—but they are distinct concepts. "Construct validity" is essentially an outgrowth and subset of the long-established *scientific method*, which dates from Roger Bacon's work in the 13th century. An empirical claim may be proved "invalid" yet be eminently "scientific." For example, the "steady-state" theory of the universe was unquestionably grounded in the scientific method, but was eventually *invalidated* and replaced by the "Big Bang Theory." By the same token, the DSM-5's decision to eliminate the subtypes of schizophrenia (paranoid, disorganized, etc.) might someday be invalidated, based on new data—but it would be unfair, retrospectively, to call the DSM-5's decision "unscientific." (See Highlights of Changes from DSM-IV-TR to DSM-5, American Psychiatric Association, 2013).

^^These different aspects of the patient's condition have been discussed in terms of "disease" (pathoanatomical entity) and "illness" (the patient's subjective reaction) by Dr. Arthur Kleinman.

Acknowledgments

My deep appreciation to Dr. S. Nassir Ghaemi and Dr. Bernard J. Carroll, for their helpful comments on this article. The views presented here, however, are my own. A slightly modified version of this piece appeared in the October 14, 2013, issue of *Psychiatric Times*.

References

[1] Pies R. Psychiatry and the myth of medicalization. *Psychiatr Times*. 2013 April 18. Available from: http://www.psychiatrictimes.com/depression. Accessed March 6, 2014.

[2] American Psychiatric Association. *Diagnostic and Statistical Manual of Mental Disorders*, 5th ed. Washington, DC: American Psychiatric Association; 2013: xlii.

[3] Cuthbert B. First-generation RDoC standard data elements. National Advisory Mental Health Council. *NAMHC Concept Clearance*. 2013 May 30. Available from: http://www.nimh.nih.gov/funding. Accessed March 6, 2014.

[4] Carroll S. What is science? [online]. Sean Carrol blog. 2013 July 3. Available from: http://www.preposterousuniverse.com/blog/2013/07/03/what-is-science/.

[5] Accessed March 9, 2014.

[6] Leibenluft E. Severe mood dysregulation, irritability, and the diagnostic boundaries of bipolar disorder in youths. *Am J Psychiatry*. 2011;168:129-142.

[7] Ghaemi SN. Requiem for DSM. *Psychiatr Times*. 2013 July 17. Available from: http://www.psychiatrictimes.com/dsm-5-0/requiem-dsm. Accessed March 9, 2014.

[8] Pies R. With obesity, a new disease is born: its profound implications for psychiatry [online]. Psych Central. World of Psychology blog. Available from: http://psychcentral.com/blog/archives/2013/06/22/with-obesity-a-new-disease-is-born-its-profound-implications-for-psychiatry/. Accessed February 27, 2014.

[9] Carroll BJ. Comment on Medscape Psychiatry [online]. Available from: http://www.medscape.com/viewarticle/804408?nlid=31347_421&src=wnl_edit_medp_psyc&spon=1

[10] Pies R. What should count as a mental disorder in DSM-V? *Psychiatr Times*. 2009 April 14. Available from: http://www.psychiatrictimes.com/dsm-5-0/what-should-count-mental-disorder. Accessed March 9, 2014.

[11] Skudlarski P, Schretlen DJ, Thaker GK, et al. Diffusion tensor imaging white matter endophenotypes in patients with schizophrenia or psychotic bipolar disorder and their relatives. *Am J Psychiatry*. 2013;170:886-898.

[12] Wittgenstein L. The Blue and Brown Books: Preliminary Studies for the Philosophical Investigations. New York: Harper Torchbooks; 1965.

[13] Kroenke K. Diagnostic testing and the illusory reassurance of normal results. *JAMA Intern Med*. 2013;173:416-417.

[14] Pies R. Mental illness is no metaphor: five uneasy pieces. *Psychiatr Times*. 2012 September 13. Available from: http://www.psychiatrictimes.com/articles/mental-illness-no-metaphor-five-uneasy-pieces?iframe=true&width=90%25&height. Accessed March 8, 2014.

[15] Pies R, Thommi S, Ghaemi SN. Getting it from both sides: Foundational and antifoundational critiques of psychiatry. *Psychiatr Times*. 2011 July 1. Available from: psychiatrictimes.com/cultural-psychiatry/getting-it-both-sides-foundational-and-antifoundational-critiques-psychiatry. Accessed March 1, 2014.

[16] Cohen H. The nature, methods and purpose of diagnosis. *The Lancet*. 1943;241:23-25.

[17] Malterud K. Diagnosis—A tool for rational action? A critical view from family medicine. *Atrium*. 2013; Winter:26-35.

[18] Ventegodt S, Kandel I, Merrick J. A short history of clinical holistic medicine. *The Scientific World Journal*. 2007;7:1622-1630.

[19] Pies RW, Geppert C. Ethical issues in the psychiatric treatment of the religious "fundamentalist" patient [online]. Medscape Psychiatry. 2013 March 19. Available from: http://www.medscape.com/viewarticle/780839. Accessed March 8, 2014.
[20] Merriam-Webster [online]. Available from: http://www.merriam-webster.com/dictionary/scientism. Accessed March 8, 2014.
[21] Ghaemi SN. Paradigms of psychiatry: eclecticism and its discontents. *Curr Opin Psychiatry*. 2006;19:619-624.
[22] Lishman WA. Organic Psychiatry: the Psychological Consequences of Cerebral Disorder. 3rd edition. Hoboken, NJ: Wiley-Blackwell; 1998.
[23] Ghaemi SN. The Rise and Fall of the Biopsychosocial Model: Reconciling Art and Science in Psychiatry. Baltimore: Johns Hopkins University Press, 2012.

For Further Reading

Pies R. DSM-5's Validity: *Non Sumus Angeli!* [online]. Medscape Psychiatry. 2013 June 12. Available from: http://www.medscape.com/viewarticle/805365. Accessed March 8, 2014.
Markova IS, Berrios GE. Epistemology of psychiatry. *Psychopathology*. 2012;45:220-227. (This paper discusses the concept that psychiatry is a "hybrid discipline" whose objects of inquiry are themselves "hybrid" constructs.)

~~~~~~~~~~~~~~~~

THE 5-MINUTE PHENOMENOLOGIST: A PRIMER FOR PSYCHIATRISTS

In 5 minutes, so much can be accomplished.— Rabbi Menachem Mendel Schneerson [1]

Let's imagine that you, Dr. Jones, are sitting in your office on a warm day in June, waiting for your next patient, and staring out the window that overlooks the street, one story below. Suddenly, a woman strolling on the sidewalk catches your attention. She has long, blond hair; a look of keen intelligence, and a smile on her face. All at once, you feel overwhelmed with emotion. Your eyes brim with unexpected tears; your heart flutters; your face flushes, then quickly blanches.

How would we explain your psychophysiological reaction in response to seeing this woman? How would we understand it? These 2 terms—explanation and understanding—turn out to be conceptual windows into 2 different yet complementary approaches to human psychology. Thus, a neurophysiologist might offer (very roughly) the following explanation of your reaction:

> *Dr. Jones's retinal photoreceptors registered the image of the woman and sent electrical impulses to his/her optic nerve. The impulses passed through the optic chiasm to the lateral geniculate bodies of the thalamus, and eventually to Dr. Jones's occipital lobe. At the same time, a second visual pathway allowed nerve impulses to activate*

primitive limbic system structures, including the amygdala. Activation of the amygdala resulted in Dr. Jones's strong emotional reaction to the woman.

Now, allowing for considerable oversimplification, this is a perfectly reasonable causal explanation for your emotional reaction. But few of us would argue that it provides us with much *rational understanding* of why this particular woman seemed to have such a dramatic effect on you. Enter our friend, the phenomenologist, who—for purposes of our discussion—has a detailed understanding of your mental state, personal history, and relationships. She gives the following account:

Dr. Jones did not actually know the particular woman who passed by on the sidewalk. The two had never met. But the woman reminded Dr. Jones of a dear friend from college, who had died over 20 years ago. Dr. Jones had long harbored guilt feelings about failing to stay in touch with this friend, and felt particular regret over not having visited her when the woman was gravely ill. When Dr. Jones saw the woman outside, he initially experienced a mixture of joy and sorrow, followed almost instantaneously by deep remorse and anxiety.

Ah—a much more satisfying narrative, but no more "correct" than our neurophysiologist's explanation. The 2 narratives are complementary, and represent 2 different modes of knowledge. The philosopher of history, Wilhelm Dilthey—and later, the psychiatrist Karl Jaspers—used the terms *erklaren* (causal explanation) and *verstehen* (meaning-based understanding) to describe these two modes of knowing [2]. In all the sciences—but particularly in the human science of psychiatry [3]—we often experience a dialectical tension between *erklaren* and *verstehen*. For example, the psychiatrist who is seeing a severely depressed patient may view the patient's condition using two basic schemas, sometimes oscillating from one frame of reference to the other: (1) This individual's brain function—her serotonergic system, neurocircuits, nerve growth factors, etc—may be aberrant in some way that is causally contributing to her depression (*erklaren*); (2) In addition, and equally important, this person's recent job loss has led to a profound loss of meaning and self-esteem in her life, which is clearly relevant to her current depression (*verstehen*). We can analogize this dialectic to viewing that famous "perceptual ambiguity" picture, which may be seen either as a young or an old woman, depending on what elements of the picture you are attending to—there is only one picture, but two ways of perceiving it.

Phenomenology may be understood as a *subtype of meaning-based understanding*: it is concerned with the meaning a particular perception has for a subject. For the phenomenologist, a perception is not merely the passive reception of data. Rather, perception is always about something—it is *intentional*. Perception is always accompanied by interpretation, and has a particular intrapsychic structure. For example, Dr. Jones's perception of the woman strolling on the sidewalk was structured by Dr. Jones's chronological recollection of events and their associated feelings. Phenomenology thus aims at a structural understanding of the person's felt experience [4].

It should be evident that this approach is quite different than that of either the neuroscientist, or of the external observer using a largely descriptive method, such as we find in the DSM-5. Phenomenology is not hostile to neurobiological or descriptive approaches; nor does it take sides in the perennial controversies over mind versus brain, psychological versus neurological causation, etc. Phenomenology simply "brackets" such controversies—

i.e., suspends judgment on these issues—and returns to "the things themselves," to use philosopher Edmund Husserl's famous saying [4]. That is, phenomenology is concerned with how the person actually experiences the world, not with theories that try to account for that experience.

By now, the busy psychiatrist-reader is entitled to ask, "OK, so how does all this phenomenology help me in my day-to-day work with patients?" Or, in the pragmatic terms of philosopher William James, what is the "cash value" of phenomenology, as it relates to clinical practice? Well, to begin with, phenomenology has a clear connection to the *sine qua non* of nearly all successful therapy; namely, *empathy*. After all, if the psychiatrist hasn't a clue regarding the contents and structure of the patient's felt experience—the way the patient interacts with and interprets her world—how can he or she possibly have empathy for the patient?

Furthermore, by understanding the contents and structure of the patient's felt experience, the psychiatrist may be guided toward one or another diagnostic conclusion. The distinction between ordinary grief and clinical depression provides a case in point. To be sure, there is no bright line between intense, prolonged grief and clinical depression, and the two states have several features in common. As Dr. Sidney Zisook and I pointed out [5], both grief and major depression often involve intense sadness, problems sleeping, concentrating, eating, and interacting with others. But the underlying *experiential structure* of normal, productive, or uncomplicated grief differs in important ways from the psychic structure of major depression. For example, in the grief that follows the loss of a loved one, the bereaved person often experiences pleasant memories of the deceased; believes that the grief will eventually pass; and has a sense that better times are ahead. These positive features are rarely present in a bout of severe, major depression. Moreover, unlike the person with major depression, the person with ordinary grief does not typically have the sense of being a worthless or unlovable person, nor is he usually suicidal. Note that none of the features could be gleaned simply by observing the patient, or by obtaining DSM-type data (e.g., by noting the patient's affect, psychomotor activity, weight, sleep pattern, etc). Rather, the phenomenological features are part of the patient's experience. It often requires persistent and empathic exploration to elicit these contents of consciousness.

Even psychotic conditions lend themselves to a phenomenological analysis. For example, the psychiatrist Silvano Arieti [6], in his classic work, *Interpretation of Schizophrenia*, provides a rich and detailed analysis of the phenomenology of schizophrenia—in effect, deconstructing the world-view of many individuals suffering with schizophrenia. Consider Arieti's description of the patient in the advanced stages of schizophrenia:

> "A certain equilibrium seems to have been reached; the patient seems to have accepted, at least to some extent, his illness; and anxiety seems decreased or even absent . . . typical of this stage, however, is the effort to stop the decline, to retain whatever grasp is possible on the escaping reality . . . in some patients the delusions and the hallucinations have lost a great many of their unpleasant qualities . . . some [patients] hear voices that bring them comfort. In some of these cases, the delusions of persecution have been replaced by delusions of grandeur."

How much richer these phenomenological descriptions are than the symptom check-lists of the DSM framework—and how much more, they explain [7]! Moreover, an understanding of the inner world of our patients may have important implications for the therapeutic alliance. After all, if you do not understand that your patient finds comfort in his auditory hallucinations [8], how will you understand his deep-seated reluctance to take antipsychotic medication?

Psychiatry nowadays is often tarred with the label of being "overly biological" or "reductionistic." To be sure, psychiatrists struggling to understand their patients during 15- or 20-minute "med checks" are well aware of the limitations under which they work. In-depth understanding and phenomenological analysis take time. Nonetheless, many of us remain interested in the contents and structure of our patients' inner world [9]—and if we ask the right kinds of questions, more can be accomplished in five minutes than you might think.

Acknowledgments

I would like to thank Michael A. Schwartz, MD, for his helpful comments and references. This essay is dedicated to the memory of two fine "phenomenological" psychiatrists: Paul Genova, MD, and Vic Himber, MD. A slightly modified version of this piece appeared in the April 29, 2010, issue of *Psychiatric Times*.

References

[1] Schneerson MM. *Toward A Meaningful Life*. New York: William Morrow; 1995:143.
[2] Ghaemi SN. The Concepts of Psychiatry: A Pluralistic Approach to the Mind and Mental Illness. Baltimore: Johns Hopkins; 2003.
[3] Pies R. Psychiatry remains a science, whether or not you like DSM5. *Psychiatr Times*. 2010 February 25. Available from http://www.psychiatrictimes.com/bipolar-disorder. Accessed February 27, 2014.
[4] Gallagher S, Zahavi D. The Phenomenological Mind: An Introduction to Philosophy of Mind and Cognitive Science. London: Routledge; 2008.
[5] Pies R, Zisook S. DSM5 criteria won't "medicalize" grief, if clinicians understand grief. *Psychiatr Times*. 2010 February 16. Available from: http://www.psychiatrictimes.com/home/content/article/10168/1523978.
[6] Accessed March 8, 2014.
[7] Arieti S. *Interpretation of Schizophrenia*. New York: Basic Books; 1974: 398-399.
[8] Genova P. Dump the DSM! *Psychiatr Times*. 2003 April 1. Available from: http://www.psychiatrictimes.com/display/article/10168/47316?pageNumber=3. Accessed March 8, 2014.
[9] Waters F. Auditory hallucinations in psychiatric illness. *Psychiatr Times*. 2010 March 10. Available from: http://www.psychiatrictimes.com/cme/display/article /10168 /1534546. Accessed March 8, 2014.
[10] Wiggins OP, Schwartz MA. Is there a science of meaning? *Integrative Psychiatry*. 1991;7:48-53.

For Further Reading

Uhlhass PJ, Mishara AL. Perceptual anomalies in schizophrenia: integrating phenomenology and cognitive neuroscience. *Schizophr Bull*. 2007;33:142-156.

Chapter 2

PSYCHIATRIC DIAGNOSIS AND THE DSM DEBATES

WHAT SHOULD COUNT AS A MENTAL DISORDER IN DSM-5?

If sick men fared just as well eating and drinking and living exactly as healthy men do...there would be little need for the science [of medicine].—attributed to Hippocrates

Well, while I'm here, I'll do the work—and what's the work? To ease the pain of living...—Allen Ginsberg

What exactly is a "mental disorder"? For that matter, what criteria should determine whether *any* condition is a "disease" or a "disorder"? Is "disease" something like an oak tree—a physical object you can bump into or put your arms around? Or are terms like "disease" and "disorder" merely abstract, value-laden constructs, akin to "injustice" and "immorality"? Are categories of disease and disorder fundamentally different in psychiatry, compared with other medical specialties? And—by the way—how do the terms "disease," "disorder," "syndrome," "malady," "sickness," and "illness" differ?

Anyone who believes there are easy or certain answers to these questions is either in touch with the Divine Mind, or out of touch with reality. To appreciate the complexity and ambiguity in this conceptual arena, consider this quote from the venerable *Oxford Textbook of Philosophy and Psychiatry*: "The term 'mental illness' is probably best used for those disorders that are intuitively most like bodily illness (or disease) and, yet, mental rather than bodily. This of course implies everything that is built into the mind-brain problem!" [1, p.11].

In a single sentence, we are already grappling with the terms "illness" "disorder" and "disease", not to mention Cartesian psychology! And yet—daunting though these issues are, they are central to the practical task now before the DSM-5 committees: *figuring out what conditions ought to be included as psychiatric disorders.*

To prefigure one element of my own position, I again quote from the *Oxford Textbook*'s chapter 20, entitled, "Values in Psychiatric Diagnosis":

"Our conclusion...[is] that the traditional medical model, and the claim to value-free diagnosis on which it rests, is unsupportable; and that, to the contrary, diagnosis, although properly grounded on facts, is also, and essentially, grounded on values...[this] is consistent with late twentieth century work in the philosophy of science...showing the extent to which the scientific process, from observation and classification to explanation and theory construction, does not depend on merely passively recording data, but is instead actively shaped in complex judgments…" [1, p. 565].

The Oxford authors wisely observe that "adding values" does not entail "subtracting facts." Thus, when we assert that someone with paraplegia has a *pathological* (from Gk. *pathos*, "suffering") condition, we are making a claim grounded in a certain kind of *value judgment*; namely, that the inability to move one's legs is in some sense "not a good thing." In a society that greatly valued paralysis and devalued walking, paraplegia would not constitute "pathology." On the other hand, we also "add facts" in reaching the conclusion that Mr. Jones—who cannot move his legs—has suffered a fracture-dislocation of the lumbar vertebrae. In short, medical diagnosis is a matter of "facts *plus* values" [1]. (Incidentally, we do not escape this evaluative dimension by appealing to some putative "evolutionary standard" based on notions of how we humans were "designed" [2]. As clinicians, we must still make value judgments as to *what degrees of departure* from supposed evolutionarily-designed responses should—or should not—count as "disease").

Similarly, when psychiatrists adduce evidence of *suffering and incapacity* in diagnosing a psychiatric disorder, we implicitly invoke certain broad values; for example, that it is generally "not a good thing" when a human being is unable to eat, sleep, think, and work. At the same time, we "add facts": we note that the patient has lost 20 lbs in the last month; that she gets only 3 hours of sleep each night; that she cannot subtract serial 7s accurately; and perhaps, in some cases, that she shows marked elevation of her serum cortisol [3]. That the facts we adduce as psychiatrists often differ from the kind cited by, say, orthopedists, does not render our data less "factual!" Indeed, some of the most important facts about the suffering and incapacitated psychiatric patient are facts *intrinsic to the person's experience*—the phenomenology or "life world" of the patient [4, 5, 6]. Thus, when the depressed patient tells us, "I feel like I'm being suffocated by my depression;" and "I feel like an empty shell about to be crushed," we justifiably regard these as *facts*—i.e., as facts of the patient's felt experience.

The prejudicial notion that only conditions associated with anatomical lesions or abnormal physiology count as "real" diseases—the "lumps and labs" model of disease [7]—denigrates the phenomenological realm. It arbitrarily declares as "facts" only those data obtained through the lens of a microscope or in a CT scan, and relegates to mere metaphor the facts of the patient's experience. This is bad science, bad history, and bad clinical practice. Sadly, such misplaced positivism—based on a crude understanding of pathologist Rudolph Virchow's views—has been used to whack psychiatry over the head for nearly fifty years [8, 9]. That said, in the model I shall develop, the search for abnormal neuroanatomy, physiology, and biomarkers does play an important role in the *later stages* of disease classification.

****

Deciding what should "count" as a mental disorder is not the same as *offering an essential definition* of "mental disorder." An essential definition is one that specifies necessary and sufficient conditions; for example, "a closed figure consisting of three line segments linked end-to-end" constitutes the necessary and sufficient conditions for ascribing the term "triangle." The philosopher Ludwig Wittgenstein (1889-1951) taught us that—with the possible exception of mathematical terms—commonly-used words *do not have essential definitions* [10, 11]. For example, it is almost impossible to specify the necessary and sufficient conditions that define the term "game." On the other hand, Wittgenstein argued, we *can* identify certain "resemblances" among members of a particular "family." These family resemblances—blond hair, blue eyes, etc.—help us recognize the family, even though no single feature is present in every family member. Wittgenstein likens a family resemblance to the long, overlapping fibers of a rope: no single fiber runs the entire length of the rope, but the rope is still held together by these fibers.

Following the lead of the late Dr. Robert E. Kendall [12], I believe that *suffering* and *incapacity* are the main "fibers" making up the disease concept. When prolonged and severe suffering and incapacity are present in the *affective, cognitive, or interpersonal-behavioral realms*, we are then entitled to speak generically of "psychiatric disease." (For many reasons, I believe this term preferable to "mental disorder" or "mental illness," but I will retain the term "mental disorder" because it is used in the DSMs).

The failure to recognize the distinction between *disease* in its primordial, conceptual sense (in German, *die Krankheit*) and *specific diseases* (*die Krankheiten*) has led to much confusion, in my view [8, 9]. What we humans ordinarily "count" as disease (*die Krankheit*) represents a pragmatic existential decision. It is not a determination akin to observing a bacterium under a microscope. Indeed, the concept of disease (etymologically, *dis-ease*) does not originate in the realm of "expert" determination; rather, *ordinary human beings decide that someone is "dis-eased" based on everyday observations and reports of suffering and incapacity*. It does not take a microbiologist or pathologist to know that someone "has disease" or "is diseased"—though both specialists may ultimately contribute to determining the *particular type* of disease.

In the words of Maurice Natanson, a philosopher who helped introduce the work of Jean-Paul Sartre and Edmund Husserl in the United States, "*Disease [is originally recognized] not by experts, but by ordinary men*" (italics added) [13]. Similarly, with respect to cognitive and emotional derangement, we do not require biological validators to identify the presence of psychiatric disease per se. Thus, my teacher, Dr. Robert W. Daly, has written that "To affirm that someone is mad is to make a practical judgment based on immediate and reflective knowledge of the activities, experiences, and circumstances of the person in question...as a particular human agent" [14].

The Evolution of a Specific Mental Disorder

So how do we develop a practical model for determining whether a condition represents, in the first place, *dis-ease*; and, secondarily, whether it constitutes a *specific* disease, on a par with, say, Bipolar I Disorder? For example, how do we decide whether to consider "pathological bigotry" or "internet addiction" specific mental disorders? I have developed a pyramidal model (see Figure 2) that illustrates the evolution of a condition from primordial *dis-ease* to a *fully-realized disease entity*.

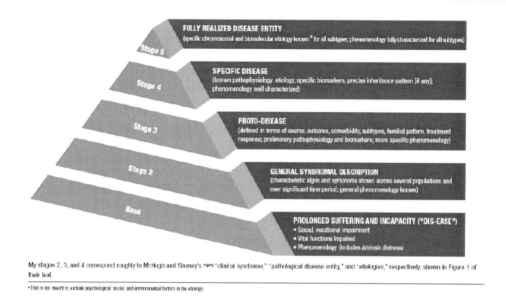

Source: Ronald Pies MD, with permission of Psychiatric Times.

Figure 2. Evolution of a Disease Entity.

At the base of the pyramid is the everyday recognition of substantial and prolonged suffering and incapacity. In my view, at least some of the "suffering" must be an *intrinsic element of having the condition*—not simply a consequence of society's punitive responses to the person's behaviors (e.g., putting someone in jail because of certain sexual behaviors). We can specify "suffering and incapacity" in terms, for example, of *social and vocational impairment, impaired vital functions*, and *distortions in the phenomenological realm* (e.g., feeling "totally worthless," "like I'm nothing," etc.). The next level of the pyramid comprises the *general syndromal description* of the condition; e.g., people with (hypothetical) Syndrome X typically experience olfactory hallucinations, memory loss, impaired calculation, and loss of taste. At the syndromal level, we usually have evidence that these signs and symptoms reliably "hang together" over long periods of time, and in geographically-distant populations. The next level (stage 3) comprises what I call the *proto-disease*. By now, we have characterized the syndrome in terms of usual course, outcome, comorbidity, familial pattern, and response to treatment. We may also have preliminary data on pathophysiology and biomarkers, and a more specific understanding of the afflicted person's phenomenology. By stage 4, the condition has moved from proto-disease to *specific disease*, for which there is a known pathophysiology, etiology, specific set of biomarkers, and (in some cases) inheritance pattern. Phenomenology is well characterized at this stage. Finally, in stage 5 ("Fully-realized disease entity") we are able to specify the precise chromosomal and biomolecular etiology, and the phenomenology, for all disease subtypes. (The term "biomolecular etiology" should not be construed as precluding a role for social and psychological factors, however). Clearly, stage 5 is theoretically possible, but rarely achieved, even in most areas of general medicine. Note that a syndrome (at stage 2) may ultimately yield two or more specific disease entities, at stages 4 and 5; e.g., "anemia" ultimately resolves into B-12 deficiency anemia, iron-deficiency anemia, etc.**

Also note that "phenomenology"—the patient's felt experience—enters into *all* stages of the evolution of the disease entity (hardly a feature of the present DSM framework). There is *no contradiction between biological and phenomenological data*, in this pluralistic model. Rather, these are complementary modes of analysis and observation, each enhancing our understanding of a disease entity. Indeed, in principle, *nothing in this model would preclude a purely phenomenological set of criteria for a given disease*; however, I believe the pluralistic approach taken here strengthens the evidentiary foundations of our nosology. (I am grateful to Dr. Nassir Ghaemi for pointing out affinities between my approach and the "biological existentialist" approach of Karl Jaspers).

Validating Our Disease Categories

While the designation "disease" may involve both subjectivity and "values", there are, nevertheless, empirically-based parameters that help us gauge the soundness of our judgment. As pathologist L.S. King observed over 50 years ago, "A [disease] pattern has reasonable stability only when its criteria are sharp, its elements cohere, and its utility in clarifying experience remains high" [15].

The key here is the phrase "clarifying experience." King is pointing to the *instrumental* function of disease classification—what the pragmatist philosopher and psychologist William James would have termed the "cash value" of the concept. If, in the long run, a particular disease category fails in its instrumental function, then it ceases to be a useful category—*even if it is grounded in molecular biology of the most sophisticated sort*. And what instrumental functions should a disease category serve? First, the criteria for "Disease X" must be "sharp" enough to distinguish its sufferers from those with Disease Y or Z. Its "elements" must cohere, in the way we would expect the pieces of a jigsaw puzzle to fit together. For example, if Disease X is defined by the presence of auditory hallucinations, dry skin, elevated blood pressure, and tremor, one would expect high degrees of concordance and overlap among these features. One would also expect a good correlation between this symptom picture and the course, outcome, and response to treatment of Disease X. Finally, the overall construct of Disease X should allow us to *understand the life experience* of those who suffer with it: not only *what* these patients suffer, but *how* and *why*.

Readers may understandably protest that very few current psychiatric disorders meet these idealized tests of utility—and I would agree! Taylor and Fink have argued that their construct of melancholia amounts to a "definable syndrome" [3], but their data on pathophysiology suggest that melancholia may already be at the level of a "proto-disease" (Stage 3). This is roughly where I would place schizophrenia and bipolar disorder, though some would argue that they are still at the syndromal level [16].

That few current DSM diagnoses would qualify for Stage 4 (much less stage 5) of my schema does not render them "myths"—it means that we have our work cut out for us, as we try to "elevate" each diagnostic category toward the top of the evidentiary pyramid. Based on this pyramidal model, I have argued that two diagnoses proposed for DSM-5—"Pathological Bigotry" [17] and "Internet Addiction" [18]—fall well short of the threshold for specific disease or disorder, in our present state of knowledge. (I am pleased that neither made it into the new diagnostic manual, though "Internet Gaming Disorder" is included as a condition requiring "further study.")

We shall see how the framers of DSM-5 judge these matters. My hope is that the model described here will at least serve as a rough guide to what should and should not "count" as specific psychiatric disease entities.

Notes

^^The DSM-5 states, "A mental disorder is a syndrome characterized by clinically significant disturbance in an individual's cognition, emotion regulation, or behavior that reflects a dysfunction in the psychological, biological, or developmental processes underlying mental functioning. Mental disorders are usually associated with significant distress or disability in social, occupational, or other important activities...socially deviant behavior...and conflicts that are primarily between the individual and society are not mental disorders unless the deviance or conflict results from a dysfunction in the individual..." [19, p. 20]. Note that this definition does not define "dysfunction" or what normal mental functioning denotes—philosophical problems, no doubt, but probably not clinical problems. For more on normal mental functioning and "sanity," see the paper by Dr. Robert Daly [14].

**My stages 2, 3, and 4 correspond roughly to McHugh and Slavney's "clinical syndrome," "pathological disease entity," and "etiologies," respectively, shown in Figure 1 of their text [16, p. 36].

Acknowledgments

I wish to thank Robert Daly, MD, Nassir Ghaemi, MD, and Derek Bolton, PhD, for their helpful comments. A slightly modified version of this piece appeared in the April 14, 2009, issue of *Psychiatric Times*.

References

[1] Fulford KWM, Thornton T, Graham G. *Oxford Textbook of Philosophy and Psychiatry*. New York: Oxford University Press; 2006.
[2] Horwitz AV, Wakefield JC. *The Loss of Sadness*. New York: Oxford University Press; 2007.
[3] Taylor MA, Fink M. Melancholia. *The Diagnosis, Pathophysiology and Treatment of Depressive Illness*. Cambridge: Cambridge University Press; 2006.
[4] Gallagher S, Zahavi D. *The Phenomenological Mind*. London: Routledge; 2008.
[5] Schwartz MA, Wiggins O. Science, humanism, and the nature of medical practice: a phenomenological view. *Perspect Biol Med*. 1985;28:231-261
[6] Ghaemi SN. Feeling and time: the phenomenology of mood disorders, depressive realism, and existential psychotherapy. *Schizophr Bull*. 2007;33:122-130
[7] Szasz TS. *The Myth of Mental Illness*. New York: Harper & Row; 1974.
[8] Pies R. On myths and countermyths: more on Szaszian fallacies. *Arch Gen Psychiatry*. 1979; 36:139-144.

[9] Pies R. Moving beyond the "myth" of mental illness. In: Schaler JA, editor. *Szasz Under Fire.* Chicago: Open Court; 2004: 327-353.
[10] Schulte J. *Wittgenstein: An Introduction.* Brenner WH, JF Holley JF, translators. Albany, NY: State University of New York Press; 1992.
[11] Wittgenstein L. The Blue and Brown Books: Preliminary Studies for the Philosophical Investigations. New York: Harper and Row; 1958.
[12] Kendell RE. The concept of disease and its implications for psychiatry. *Br J Psychiatry.* 1975;127:305-315.
[13] Natanson M, Strauss EW, Ey H. Philosophy and psychiatry. In: Natanson M, editor. *Psychiatry and Philosophy.* New York: Springer-Verlag; 1969: 85-100.
[14] Daly RW. A theory of madness. *Psychiatry.* 1991;54:368-385.
[15] King LS. What is disease? *Philos Sci.* 1954;21:193-203.
[16] McHugh PR, Slavney PR. *The Perspectives of Psychiatry.* Baltimore: Johns Hopkins University Press; 1983.
[17] Pies R. Is bigotry a mental illness? *Psychiatr Times.* 2007 May 1. Available from: http://www.psychiatrictimes.com/display/article/10168/55226. Accessed March 8, 2014.
[18] Pies R. Should DSM-V designate "internet addiction" a mental disorder? *Psychiatry (Edgemont).* 2009;6:31-37.
[19] American Psychiatric Association. *The Diagnostic and Statistical Manual of Mental Disorders, 5th ed.* Washington, DC: American Psychiatric Association; 2013.

For Further Reading

Ghaemi SN. *The Concepts of Psychiatry.* Baltimore: Johns Hopkins University Press; 2003. (See especially Dr. Ghaemi's discussion of "The Essentialist Fallacy" and the work of psychologist Peter Zachar and philosopher Daniel Dennett).
Ghaemi SN. On the nature of mental disease: the psychiatric humanism of Karl Jaspers. *Existenz.* 2008;3:1-9.
Lloyd GE. *Hippocratic Writings.* New York: Penguin Books; 1978: 71.

~~~~~~~~~~~~~~~~~

BEYOND DSM-5, PSYCHIATRY NEEDS A "THIRD WAY"

The recent spate of Op-Eds in the *New York Times* says it all: both the psychiatric profession and the general public have strong feelings about the pending DSM-5—what many in the media like to call "Psychiatry's Bible." These emotions are certainly understandable. Apart from the many ethical and philosophical problems raised by changes in psychiatric diagnosis, there are millions of dollars at stake: depending on how the DSM-5 evolves, individuals with major depression, Asperger's syndrome, ADHD, and a number of other diagnoses may or may not be eligible for coverage by third-party payers.

Most of the controversy over the DSM-5 has focused on "boundary" issues: where do we draw the line between the introspective and the autistic individual, or between the bereaved widow experiencing ordinary grief and the one with a major depressive episode? But most of the vociferous critics of the DSM-5 have been nibbling around the edges of the diagnostic system as a whole. Few have argued that the entire DSM approach is in need of a drastic overhaul.

The DSMs over the past 30 years have attempted to "carve Nature at its joints"—a metaphor first used by Plato in his *Phaedrus*. By requiring certain necessary and sufficient conditions for diagnosing a disorder, the DSMs have provided researchers with a means of ensuring "inter-rater reliability"—in effect, making sure that those investigating schizophrenia or bipolar disorder have identified subjects with the same condition. Implicit in this categorical approach is the notion that there is an "essence of schizophrenia" or an "essence of panic disorder," much like the Platonic "forms" that defined the nature of triangles or spheres. Critics of this approach have argued that "Nature" may not have "joints" and that human disease states are too varied and complex to conform to essentialist definitions. Call this the "anti-pigeonhole" critique of the DSMs.^^

Some of these critics have argued for a "dimensional" approach to diagnosis, in which patients are rated on a number of different measures of psychopathology; for example, Mr. Jones might be categorized as having high anxiety, moderate depression, and minimal cognitive disorganization. Proponents of the dimensional approach believe it allows clinicians to address the patient's problems in a more targeted and fine-grained way, without reifying the patient's condition as a specific disease entity. But a dimensional approach makes it much harder to group patients together for research purposes, and nearly impossible to exchange "shorthand" information between clinicians. After all, it's much easier to tell a colleague, "I saw an elderly man with bipolar I disorder" than to break down the patient's problem into 4 or 5 symptom dimensions.

One thing we know for sure: many clinicians routinely ignore the present DSM system. For example, a study by Dr. Mark Zimmerman and colleagues found that nearly 25% of psychiatrists used the DSM-IV criteria to diagnose major depression less than half the time—and this was true of more than two-thirds of the non-psychiatrist physicians studied. Many clinicians find the cut-and-dried DSM criteria too superficial to capture the nuances of the patient's condition. Others (this writer among them) complain that the DSM embodies the worst of both worlds: it lacks validated biochemical "markers" for the major disorders, while also ignoring the kind of *depth-psychology* emphasized by psychoanalysts and existential therapists. Furthermore, the convoluted "exclusion rules" demanded by the DSM criteria—for example, the recently removed "bereavement exclusion" for major depression—are often too confusing for most clinicians.

The DSM-5 has now been published, warts and all, and will be with us for at least another decade or two. But we *can* begin to think beyond the DSM-5, and beyond "categorical" versus "dimensional" models: we can begin to consider a "third way."

Decades ago, the psychiatrist Karl Jaspers (1883-1969) advocated the use of so-called *ideal types* in psychiatric diagnosis. Similarly, in recent years, other clinicians have argued for the use of "prototypes"—basically, narrative descriptions of typical disease presentations, sometimes in the language patients themselves use to describe their experience (i.e., *phenomenological* prototypes). Prototypes—unlike the rigid DSM categories—have "fuzzy" boundaries. They try to capture the core features of an illness like schizophrenia without specifying an "essence," or a list of necessary and sufficient criteria. In this sense, they reflect developments in the philosophy of language best epitomized in the work of Ludwig Wittgenstein (1889-1951).

Rather than proffering a Platonic "essence" to define a category, Wittgenstein referred to "family resemblances"—like, say, blue eyes and blond hair in three of five members of the Jones family, and tallness in four of the five. No single feature invariably identifies a Jones family member, but the "blue eyes, blond hair, and tall" prototype helps us do so. My colleague, Dr. Nassir Ghaemi, and I used a modified prototype approach in developing a screening tool—the Bipolar Spectrum Diagnostic Scale (BSDS)—for identifying bipolar spectrum disorders. Rather than relying on a fixed set of criteria, the BSDS presents a kind of narrative "story" to the patient, who is then asked how closely the bipolar prototype fits his or her condition. The BSDS has proved useful in identifying patients on the "softer" end of the bipolar spectrum. Similarly, I have recently used the prototype method to develop a potential screening tool—the *Post-Bereavement Phenomenology Inventory* (PBPI)—for distinguishing ordinary grief from clinical depression. (The ICD diagnostic system also uses a modified prototype approach to diagnostic entities.)

Of course, insurance companies are bound to oppose the use of prototype diagnoses—after all, it's much easier to deny (or approve) a claim based on a hard-and-fast set of "essential" criteria. Indeed, we can always retain such strict criteria in a separate manual, designed for researchers, or as an appendix to a prototype-based manual. But psychiatry needs to move beyond the DSM system, and beyond the perennial categorical versus dimensional debate. I believe that work-a-day clinicians will welcome a "third way"—one that allows us to appreciate the fluidity, complexity, and depth of our patients' problems.

Notes

^^ I do not mean to imply that the framers of DSM-IV and DSM-5 are naïve about categorical diagnosis and its limitations, or that they overtly embrace an "essentialist" perspective on psychiatric diagnosis. The DSM-5, for example, acknowledges that, "...the boundaries between many disorder "categories" are more fluid over the life course than DSM-IV recognized, and many symptoms assigned to a single disorder may occur...in many other disorders" (DSM-5, p. 5).

Acknowledgment

A slightly modified version of this piece appeared in the February 8, 2012, issue of Psychiatric Times.

For Further Reading

Ghaemi, SN, Miller CJ, Berv DA, et al. Sensitivity and specificity of a new bipolar spectrum diagnostic scale. *J Affect Disord.* 2005;84:273-277.

Pies R. Why psychiatry needs to scrap the DSM System [online]. Psych Central. World of Psychology blog. Available from: http://psychcentral.com/blog/archives /2012/01/07 /why-psychiatry-needs-to-scrap-the-dsm-system-an-immodest-proposal.
Accessed February 27, 2014.
Schwartz MA, Wiggins OP, Norko MA. Prototypes, ideal types, and personality disorders: the return to classical psychiatry. *J Pers Disord.* 1989;3:1-9.
Vázquez GH, Romero E, Fabregues F, et al. Screening for bipolar disorders in Spanish-speaking populations: sensitivity and specificity of the Bipolar Spectrum Diagnostic Scale-Spanish Version. *Compr Psychiatry.* 2010;51:552-556.
Wittgenstein L. The Blue and Brown Books: Preliminary Studies for the Philosophical Investigations. New York: Harper Torchbooks; 1965.
Zimmerman M, Galione JN, Ruggero CJ, et al. A different approach toward screening for bipolar disorder: the prototype matching method. *Compr Psychiatry.* 2010;51:340-346.
Zimmerman M, Galione J. Psychiatrists' and nonpsychiatrist physicians' reported use of the DSM-IV criteria for major depressive disorder. *J Clin Psychiatry.* 2010;71:235-238.

~~~~~~~~~~~~~~~~~

PSYCHIATRY AND THE MYTH OF "MEDICALIZATION"

Whatever happened to common sense? You know what I mean— these psychiatrists "medicalize" every ordinary feeling and behavior, every normal stress and strain of living. Why, the way they want to call ordinary shyness "Social Anxiety Disorder," or call ordinary grief "Major depressive disorder"—it's ridiculous! These so-called diagnoses are just "false positives"—not cases of disease or disorder. These self-appointed "experts" keep invading the territory of normal human experience like conquistadors! Then they prescribe all kinds of harmful medications for non-existent diseases. And now, they are expanding their diagnostic system, to the point where nobody is normal anymore!

Are any of these claims even controversial these days? Even for some readers of *Psychiatric Times*, I suspect not. After all, we have heard this line of argument from respected academics; many patients or "consumers;" some of psychiatry's own luminaries; and from many sincere and conscientious clinicians. Recently, one particularly renowned critic pointed to the DSM-5's "diagnostic imperialism." [1]. Indeed, before the final text of the DSM-5 had even appeared, several books criticizing the new manual were already out or in press.

But does this narrative of psychiatry's "medicalization of normality" really represent *common sense*—or is it mostly common nonsense? In my view, the "medicalization" narrative contains some kernels of truth, and many defenders of the term proceed from honorable and well-intentioned motives; for example, the wish to reduce unnecessary use of psychotropic medication--and who could be opposed to *that*? But on the whole, I believe the medicalization narrative is philosophically naïve and clinically unhelpful. Upon close examination, the term "medicalization" proves to be largely a rhetorical device, aimed at ginning up popular opposition to psychiatric diagnosis. It not only stigmatizes the field of psychiatry and those who practice in it; it also undermines our ability to provide the best care to our patients, by spuriously "normalizing" their suffering and incapacity [2].

I am not claiming that *careless diagnosis* and *over-diagnosis* never occur in psychiatry. Alas, as in all of medicine, sometimes they do—particularly when insufficient time is allowed for the initial evaluation of the patient, and when no validated scales or screening instruments are used [3]. (*Under*-diagnosis also occurs, as in the failure to recognize major depressive disorder in some settings—but that's another story [4].) Neither am I voicing a full-throated defense of the new DSM-5 manual. Indeed, while I respect the good-faith efforts of the DSM-5's framers, I have serious concerns regarding some of DSM-5's decisions, such as lowering the threshold for the diagnosis of somatoform disorders [1] (now called "Somatic Symptom Disorders").

What I do want to claim is that when a psychiatric diagnosis is *accurately and carefully made*, according to generally accepted (e.g., DSM or ICD) criteria, it should not be "normalized" or declared "non-disordered" because its manifestation is "understandable" or "explained" by the psychosocial context in which it occurs—or because it is deemed "proportionate" to some hypothetical "evolved mechanism" [5].

The Normality Fallacy

For the proposition, "Psychiatry is medicalizing normality" to be true, we would need, first; adequate definitions of the terms "medicalizing" and "normality"; and second, convincing evidence that psychiatry is actually *doing* what the proposition asserts. Yet all three elements of "truth" turn out to be complex and problematic. For one thing, psychiatry's critics almost never bother to define the terms "medicalizing" or "normality." (Does "medicalization" refer to application of the "medical model", or to the use of medication? And what is the "medical model," exactly? Is "normality" a purely statistical term? Is it used in relation to a particular cultural subgroup; to the human species as a whole; or in relation to the particular patient's usual state of affairs?)

Moreover, those who argue that psychiatry "medicalizes" normality while simultaneously asserting that there is no clear demarcation between "normality" and "abnormality" [6] effectively refute their own argument. For if there are no absolute, categorical and universally agreed upon boundaries separating "normal" from "abnormal", then the claim, "Psychiatry is medicalizing normality" cannot logically be sustained: *the argument is devoured by its own premise.* That is: if "normality" has no precise boundary in the realm of disease—including psychiatric disease—then *there can be no verifiable "medicalization" of normality*. Neither can there be a veridical demonstration of psychiatry's alleged diagnostic "imperialism" or its supposed creation of diagnostic "false positives." Such claims are no more verifiable than a landowner's complaint that someone has impermissibly planted a tree on his property, when there are no clearly established property lines. But let's be clear: this doesn't mean that we can't make reasoned, empirically-grounded judgments as to *what conditions merit medical evaluation or treatment,* as I'll explain below.

Psychiatry's Ethical Aim Is the Relief of Suffering and Incapacity

So long as the patient is experiencing a substantial or enduring state of suffering and incapacity, *the patient has disease* (dis-ease) [5]. (Unlike the DSMs, which emphasize distress *or* impairment, I prefer to include both suffering *and* incapacity as core features of disease, though there are undoubtedly exceptions to this). To assert this is not to "medicalize" normality, but to affirm what physicians have recognized as an ethical imperative, for millennia: the need to relieve the misery and dysfunction of the patient. Indeed, as Prof. H. C. Erik Midelfort, professor of history at the University of Virginia, author of the book, *A History of Madness in Sixteenth-Century*, comments:

> ". . . for ancient and early modern physicians, there was no clear, bright line between disease and health. They did not, generally, decide that someone was suffering an understandable and proportionate sadness and was not therefore 'ill.' They generally decided that if one were suffering, for whatever reason and whether proportionate or disproportionate, they would do what they could to help . . . [and their remedies] did not depend upon a strict decision that so-and-so was fundamentally 'ill' while someone else was merely sad for good, sufficient, and proportionate reasons" (personal communications, October 2008 and March 2012).

Indeed, as historian and *Psychiatric Times* blogger, Prof. Greg Eghigian has commented:

> "...Midelfort get[s] at something important that many commentators on the history of psychiatry often either ignore or consider unimportant: the fact that the overwhelming majority of patients treated by psychiatrists, 'mad-doctors,' mental healers, etc. over the centuries have presented symptoms clearly crossing the 'threshold of chronicity or severity.' And indeed, this is one of the reasons why I have problems with the way in which self-identifying critics of psychiatry invoke the term 'medicalization'—they more often than not neglect the extraordinary and painful nature of the maladies...[patients] were/are facing" [7].

Prof. Eghigian leads us toward a critical insight: the obsessive debate about what is or is not "normal" is largely a distraction from the two practical issues facing all physicians: first; what is the threshold for considering a condition a "disease" or "disorder"; and second, how can we best help the patient? As a practical matter, internists do not consider an upset stomach as crossing the threshold of disease; nor do psychiatrists of any wisdom consider a mildly "fidgety," bored and inattentive child to have a disease or disorder called "ADHD." But in both instances, these threshold decisions are based primarily on *the absence of pronounced or enduring suffering and incapacity*—not on an obsessive fixation on what is "normal." (If every-day, "upset stomach" suddenly became vanishingly rare, it still would not qualify as "disease." Michael Moore makes a similar point re: a "cubical" stomach [8]. Physicians, fundamentally, are not philosophers or evolutionary biologists. We do not, as a matter of daily routine, entertain metaphysical and semantic questions, such as "What is truly normal for the human species?" Rather, physicians have a general concept of what constitutes "health", and a general concept of enduring and significant departures from health. We find ourselves faced with a waiting room full of distressed and often incapacitated human beings who, in ordinary circumstances, are voluntarily seeking our help. We do our best to respond to them not as specimens of "abnormality," but as suffering individuals--and as fellow human beings.

Acknowledgment

A modified version of this article appears in *Philosophy Now*, Nov-Dec 2013. My thanks to the editors of that piece.

References

[1] Frances A. Yet another way the medically ill will be misdiagnosed as mentally disordered. *Psychiatr Times*. 2013 February 28. Available from: http://www.psychiatrictimes.com/blog/frances/content/article/10168/2130515. Accessed March 8, 2014.

[2] Zisook S, Corruble E, Duan N, et al. The bereavement exclusion and DSM-5. *Depress Anxiety*. 2012; 29(5):425-443.

[3] Aboraya A, France C, Young J, Curci K, Lepage J. The validity of psychiatric diagnosis revisited: the clinician's guide to improve the validity of psychiatric diagnosis. *Psychiatry (Edgmont)*. 2005;2(9):48-55. Available from: http://www.ncbi.nlm.nih.gov/pmc/articles/PMC2993536/. Accessed March 8, 2014.

[4] Egede LE. Failure to recognize depression in primary care: issues and challenges. *J Gen Intern Med*. 2007;22:701-703.

[5] Pies R. Context does not determine "disorderness" or normality. *Psychiatr Times*. 2013 January 15. Avaiable from: http://www.psychiatrictimes.com/blog/pies/content/article/10168/2122512. Accessed March 8, 2014.

[6] Frances A. What's normal? What's not? *Psychiatr Times*. 2013 April 1. Available from: http://www.psychiatrictimes.com/blog/frances/content/article/10168/2135602. Accessed March 8, 2014.

[7] Eghigian G. The medicalization of grief: what we can learn from 19th-century nervousness. *Psychiatr Times*. 2013 March 1. Available from: http://www.psychiatrictimes.com/blog/eghigian/content/article/10168/2130801. Accessed March 8, 2014.

[8] Moore MS. Some myths about "mental illness." *Arch Gen Psychiatry*. 1975;32:1485-1490.

~~~~~~~~~~~~~~~~~

DIAGNOSIS AND ITS DISCONTENTS: THE DSM

As to diseases, make a habit of two things—to help, or at least to do no harm.— Hippocrates, *Epidemics*, in Hippocrates, trans. W. H. S. Jones (1923), Vol. I, 165 (emphasis added)

An agnostic is someone who doesn't know, and di- is a Greek prefix meaning "two." So "diagnostic" means someone who doesn't know twice as much as an agnostic doesn't know.—Walt Kelly, Pogo

A funny thing happened to me on the way to the New York Times "Sunday Dialogue"—I made myself unclear [1]. This is not supposed to happen to careful writers, or to those of us who flatter ourselves with that honorific. So what went wrong?

In brief, I greatly underestimated the public's strong identification of psychiatric diagnosis with the *categorical approach* of the recent DSMs. But whereas my letter to the *Times* was indeed *occasioned* by the DSM-5's release in May 2013, my argument in defense of psychiatric diagnosis was not a testimonial in favor of any one *type* of diagnostic scheme—categorical, dimensional, prototypical [2] or otherwise. Each of these diagnostic schemes has its advantages and disadvantages. My personal preference is for a *prototype-based* schema, for everyday clinical use; and a DSM-type categorical schema for purposes of psychiatric research [2]. The categorical approach is usually preferable for most research studies, because it provides precise "cut-points" for entry criteria. But we should not suppose that our diagnostic categories necessarily "carve Nature at its joints," in Plato's famous phrase. Indeed, as philosopher Alexander Bird quipped, "The classifications of botanists do not carve nature at its joints any more than the classifications of cooks" [3]. The DSM-IV itself understood this, and explicitly recognized its own limitations. In the often-ignored introduction, the DSM-IV stated,

> "Making a DSM-IV diagnosis is only the first step in a comprehensive evaluation. To formulate an adequate treatment plan, the clinician will invariably require considerable additional information about the person being evaluated beyond that required to make a DSM-IV diagnosis" [4, p. xxv].

The DSM-5 is equally cautious in its remarks on diagnosis. But I would add that our diagnostic methods need more than symptom check-lists. In order to gain a full and deep understanding of the patient, psychiatrists must also delve into the patient's "world view"—her way of "being in the world." The phenomenologists therefore focus on the *structure and contents of the patient's conscious experience* [5, 6]. For example, does he or she invariably experience the world as a hostile and threatening place? Are all her relationships perceived as threats to her autonomy? And how do the patient's spiritual concerns and beliefs shape his world-view [7]? From the psychodynamic perspective, as Dr. James Knoll observes (personal communication, March 26, 2013), what are the wishes, fantasies, experiences, fears, and desires that shape the patient's conscious and unconscious life? Such depth-psychology is unlikely to be captured in either a categorical or a dimensional "diagnosis" of the patient. Deeper understanding demands that we enter into the patient's way of "being in the world."

Physicians, of course, have been reaching diagnostic conclusions since the time of Hippocrates—quite without the help of diagnostic manuals. The word "diagnostic"—notwithstanding Walt Kelly's sardonic jab—may be understood as "knowing (*gnosis*) the difference between (*dia-*)" one condition and another. So, when we recognize that a patient's auditory hallucinations are related to complex partial seizures and not a psychosis, we are engaging in diagnosis.

A diagnosis, however, need not name a "disorder" or disease. Our diagnosis of Mr. Smith may be, "Perfectly happy chap—nothing to treat here!" Sometimes, in my consultative practice, a patient would ask me for my diagnosis, and I might reply, "Well, I think you have a serious problem with regulation of your mood and your anger. I can give you a formal name for your condition, but I'd rather hear what kind of information you would find most helpful."

That, too, is a "diagnosis"—though not necessarily the "CPT code" an insurance company would accept.

Kudos and Brickbats

Reaction to my letter was decidedly mixed. While most colleagues were very supportive, many comments in the blogosphere ranged from the dismissive to the abusive. Predictably, some critics trotted out the old war-horses of anti-psychiatry (were these not led out to pasture decades ago?): psychiatry is not "scientific," because it doesn't have verifiable laboratory tests or biomarkers for its disorders; psychiatric diagnoses are just the "subjective impressions" of the clinician; psychiatry amounts to "totalitarian oppression," etc.

These canards and slurs have been addressed in many other contexts [8, 9, 10] and I won't belabor their fallacious assumptions here. Yet psychiatrists should not underestimate the deep currents of public anger and resentment toward our profession, and we must acknowledge that sometimes, we have not served our patients well. Psychiatric diagnosis—like diagnosis in other fields of medicine—is sometimes premature. Psychiatric treatments—like many treatments in general medicine—are sometimes ineffective or injurious, despite our best intentions. Patients who have been hospitalized against their will—even when justified on the basis of imminent "dangerousness" and ordered through due process of law—may still have bitter memories of that experience. I truly believe that psychiatry is a force for genuine good—and sometimes quite literally a lifesaver [11]—but I am also aware of the many challenges we face in building trust with the general public.

The Public's Misconception of "Science"

One thing was abundantly clear from responses to my letter: the general public still does not understand that "science" is fundamentally *a habit of mind and method*—not a microbe in a dish, or a shadow on a CT scan. Recently, the British Science Council spent a full year developing a definition of "science." Their conclusion was radically insightful and succinct: "Science is the pursuit of knowledge and understanding of the natural and social world following a systematic methodology based on evidence" [12]. Specifically, science entails *careful and systematic observation; hypothesis-formation; and repeated testing of one's hypothesis, using empirical methods.* In this sense, there is no question that psychiatry and psychology are sciences—though they are also more than that.

t the concept of science is so badly muddled—even by some health care professionals—is testament to the baneful legacy of *logical positivism*, and its close cousin, *scientism* [13]. These ideologies have led to the public's abiding confusion between the *physical sciences*, like biology and biochemistry; and the *sciences of human emotion and behavior*—the domain of psychiatry, psychology, and related disciplines. Psychiatry, as a medical discipline, partakes of *both* the physical and human sciences. *But psychiatry is not physics!* As Schwartz and Wiggins have observed, "Medicine is a science, insofar as its concepts, methods, and techniques are based on evidence, but it is a practical and not a pure science. Medicine is a practical science because its goals—the promotion of health and the amelioration of illness—are practical ones" [14].

Of course, good clinicians know that there is also "art" in what we do, and that some subjective elements of the patient-doctor dyad are not easily expressed in the terms of science. Therein lies the art—and poetry—of our work with patients [15].

Are Psychiatric Diagnoses Inherently "Stigmatizing"?

Other arguments put forth by my critics were more troubling [1]. Many readers bristled at my claim that a psychiatric diagnosis is not *inherently*—that's the key word—"stigmatizing" or "dehumanizing." (The diagnosis, of course, may simply be incorrect.) These critics pointed with understandable outrage to personal experiences of prejudice, discrimination, and mistreatment at the hands of people who learned of their psychiatric "label." (It is interesting that nobody calls a diagnosis of *migraine headache* or *epilepsy* a "label." The reasons for this discrepancy, however, would take us far afield—suffice to say that neither condition is diagnosed on the basis of a "lab test" or demonstrable pathophysiology). More subtly and poignantly, some readers described how *internalizing* their psychiatric diagnosis adversely affected their self-esteem and identity—stunting their emotional growth and depriving them of purpose, dignity, and worth. On one level, this should not surprise us. After all, hearing from an orthopedist that your ankle is broken is existentially different than hearing from a psychiatrist that your very *self* is broken.

And yet, I stand squarely behind my claim: there is nothing *inherently* stigmatizing or dehumanizing in the psychiatric diagnosis itself. If the patient feels diminished or dehumanized, it is largely owing to one or more of these factors: (1) the patient has been subjected to bigotry, insults, or discrimination at the hands of ignorant and insensitive people; (2) the psychiatrist or clinician has (unconscionably!) presented the diagnosis in an overly pessimistic or depreciating way—one that leaves the patient feeling hopeless, disrespected or demeaned; or (3) the patient himself has engaged in a process of *self-deprecation*.

This last point needs clarification. I am not trying to "blame" the patient for feeling bad. However, I am suggesting that the patient who receives a psychiatric diagnosis *need not* feel diminished, dehumanized, or demoralized. So much depends on how the diagnosis is framed, both by the clinician and the patient. A patient may say to herself, "Well, the doctor says I'm a schizophrenic. That must mean I'm crazy, and no good to anybody! I'm nothing, a nobody. My life is over—I might as well pack it in." Of course, this patient will feel dehumanized and demoralized! But another patient, given the same diagnosis, may think, "OK, this schizophrenia thing is very upsetting and scary—but it's not the end of the world. I can still be a creative, loving, and productive person. I'm still me, and I'm still a good person." This patient is far less likely to be bludgeoned by the diagnosis.

Indeed, such cognitive reframing is a critical part of the growing "recovery movement," which emphasizes the patient's *possibilities* rather than his limitations. For example, Bellack has noted that as many as 50% of people with schizophrenia actually have good outcomes [16]. Ironically, when critics of psychiatry claim that a diagnosis is *inherently* "stigmatizing," they undermine the goal of recovery in psychiatric patients. They implicitly deny that patients can "re-envision" the *meaning* of their diagnosis—surely a disparaging notion! Furthermore, *when critics of psychiatric diagnosis insist that terms like "schizophrenia" or "bipolar disorder" are inherently stigmatizing, they are unwittingly perpetuating the very prejudice they wish to end.* It is time to shine a bright light on this self-fulfilling prophecy. As blogger and journalist Sandy Naiman has put it: "There is no stigma. Just prejudice and discrimination. When you say the word 'stigma' you actually incite stigma." [17]. Precisely!

That said, it must be admitted that some psychiatrists have been slow to accept the "recovery" paradigm, which often has been advanced by "consumer" activists outside the medical community [16]. We need to do better in this respect. When we provide a diagnosis, we must also provide hope, comfort, and realistic optimism. But let us be clear: psychiatrists must never cease the activity of diagnosis, or be intimidated by unreasoning critics. To abandon diagnosis is to violate our most fundamental Hippocratic duty: *to help our patients.*

Or, as the poet, Allen Ginsberg, put it, in a different context: "Well, while I'm here I'll do the work—and what's the work? To ease the pain of living" [18].

Acknowledgments

I would like to thank James L. Knoll IV, MD, and Michael A. Schwartz MD, for their helpful comments on an earlier draft of this article. Dr. Sidney Zisook has been extremely helpful in developing my views on diagnosis. I also appreciate the many colleagues and readers who commented on my letter, and the careful editing of Sue Mermelstein at *The New York Times*. Thanks also to the American Psychiatric Association for taking note of my letter. A slightly modified version of this piece appeared in the March 29, 2013, issue of *Psychiatric Times*.

Disclosure

Dr. Pies has had no official relationship with the committees or work groups responsible for the DSM-5. He is a member of the American Psychiatric Association.

References

[1] Pies R, and others. Sunday dialogue: defining mental illness [letters to the editor]. *The New York Times*. 2013 March 24. Available from: http://www.nytimes.com/2013/03/24/opinion/sunday/sunday-dialogue-defining-mental-illness.html?_r=0. Accessed March 8, 2014.

[2] Phillips J, Frances A, Cerullo MA, et al. The six most essential questions in psychiatric diagnosis: a pluralogue part 1: conceptual and definitional issues in psychiatric diagnosis. *Philos Ethics Humanit Med*. 2012;13;7:3.

[3] Bird A. Natural kinds [online]. The Stanford Encyclopedia of Philosophy. 2008 September 17. Available from: http://plato.stanford.edu/entries/natural-kinds/. Accessed March 8, 2014.

[4] American Psychiatric Association. *Diagnostic and Statistical Manual of Mental Disorders, 4th ed*. Washington, DC: American Psychiatric Association; 1994.

[5] Wiggins OP, Schwartz MA. Is there a science of meaning? *Integrative Psychiatry*. 1991;7:48-53.

[6] Pies R. The 5-Minute phenomenologist: A primer for psychiatrists. *Psychiatr Times.* 2010 April 29. Available from: http://www.psychiatrictimes.com/articles/5-minute-phenomenologist-primer-psychiatrists. Accessed February 27, 2014.

[7] Pies RW, Geppert C. Ethical issues in the psychiatric treatment of the religious "fundamentalist" patient [online]. Medscape. 2013 March 19. Available from: http://www.medscape.com/viewarticle/780839. Accessed February 23, 2014.

[8] Pies R. Moving beyond the "myth" of mental illness. In: Schaler JA, editor. *Szasz Under Fire.* Chicago: Open Court; 2004: 327-353.

[9] Pies R. Psychiatric diagnosis and the pathologist's view of schizophrenia. *Psychiatry (Edgmont).* 2008;5:62-65. Available from: http://www.ncbi.nlm.nih.gov/pmc/articles/PMC2695726/. Accessed February 27, 2014.

[10] Pustilnik A. Calling mental illness "myth" leads to state coercion [online]. Cato Institute. Cato Unbound 2012 August 13. Available from: http://www.cato-unbound.org/2012/08/13/amanda-pustilnik/calling-mental-illness-myth-leads-state-coercion. Accessed February 27, 2014.

[11] Pies R. The good psychiatry does: A brief review. *Psychiatr Times.* 2010 February 2. Available from: http://www.psychiatrictimes.com/articles/good-psychiatry-does-brief-review. Accessed February 27, 2014.

[12] Sample I. What is this thing we call science? [online]. *The Guardian.* Notes and Theories blog. 2009 March 3. Available from: http://www.guardian. Accessed February 27, 2014.

[13] Pies R. Psychiatry remains a science, whether or not you like DSM5. *Psychiatr Times.* 2010 February 25. Available from http://www.psychiatrictimes.com/bipolar-disorder. Accessed February 27, 2014.

[14] Schwartz MA, Wiggins OP. Psychiatry fraud and force? A commentary on E. Fuller Torrey and Thomas Szasz. *Journal of Humanistic Psychology* 2005;45:1-13.

[15] Halpern J, Lewis B. Introduction: why does psychiatry need the humanities? *Psychiatr Times.* 2013 March 12. Available from: http://www.psychiatrictimes.com/display/article/10168/2132712. Accessed February 27, 2014.

[16] Bellack AS. Scientific and consumer models of recovery in schizophrenia: concordance, contrasts, and implications. *Schizophr Bull.* 2006;32:432-442.

[17] Naiman S. Comments on day two: the toxic word ~ "stigma" ~ ban it! [online]. Psych Central. Coming Out Crazy blog. Available from: http://blogs. Accessed February 27, 2014.

[18] Ginsberg A. "Memory Gardens." In: Hyde L. *On the Poetry of Allen Ginsberg.* Ann Arbor: University of Michigan Press; 1985: 212.

For Further Reading

Frances A. Giftedness should not be confused with mental disorder. *Psychiatr Times.* 2010 March 13. Available from: http://www.psychiatrictimes.com/adhd/content/article/10168/2132869. Accessed February 27, 2014.

Lothane Z. Dramatology: a new paradigm for psychiatry and psychotherapy. *Psychiatr Times.* 2010 June 4. Available from: http://www.psychiatrictimes.com/articles/dramatology-new-paradigm-psychiatry-and-psychotherapy. Accessed February 27, 2014.

PANIC ON THE PRECIPICE: DOES "CONTEXT" DETERMINE DISORDER IN PSYCHIATRY?

Part 1: Why Panic Attacks Are Nearly Always Pathological

When...you see someone pale with worry...this man is disordered in his desires and aversions.—Epictetus, Discourses

Let's say a patient comes to you with a recent history of a single florid panic attack, in the context of giving a speech before an audience of 2,000 colleagues. I don't mean a case of the "jitters"—I mean a 10-minute episode of palpitations, shaking, sweating, choking, dizziness, derealization, and the belief that he was dying. Since you are remarkably empathic, and have had some public speaking anxiety yourself, you think, "I can understand how someone could have an attack like that, under those circumstances."

Let's hold off on suggesting any formal diagnoses (a panic attack is not a formal DSM diagnosis—only a "building block" for one). Was this episode "normal" and "non-disordered" anxiety, because it is "understandable" to you? What about a patient with the identical set of symptoms, in the context of, say, hanging by his fingers over the edge of a cliff? If you can "understand" the occurrence of a panic attack in this context, was it therefore "normal"? These may sound like very theoretical questions, but they go to the heart of what we think of as "normal" or "disordered", both in psychiatry and general medicine. How we answer these questions also has important implications for what we mean by the term "false positive" in psychiatry, and what categories we create for the DSM-5.

At the last annual meeting of the APA—where I had just spoken on the experiential differences between grief and major depression—a very well-respected, senior researcher in the audience rose to comment, evidently quite perturbed. He expressed great surprise at my claim that an "explanatory context" shouldn't determine our clinical assessment of "disorder" or "abnormality." My critic gave the example of someone who has a full-blown panic attack while hanging by his fingers, over a steep cliff. Surely, he insisted, "context" is critically important in such a case! After all, the context *explains* the person's panic attack, and thus renders the attack *non-pathological.*

This is a perfectly plausible position, and probably represents the prevailing opinion among the general public. Indeed, many clinicians may be inclined to say, "Hey, *I'd* have a panic attack, too, if I were hanging by my fingers, over a cliff!" So calling such a panic attack "normal" is just "common sense." Maybe so—but as Einstein once reminded us, "Common sense is the collection of prejudices acquired by age eighteen." *Science* is the systematic testing of "common sense" assumptions against the range of alternative theories.

In my view, the hypothetical panic attack on the precipice is inherently *pathological* and *disordered*. And this "disorderness"—i.e., that state in which healthy and adaptive organismic function is disrupted--*is not negated by any explanatory context*. Furthermore, I want to suggest that "explanatory context" is usually a misleading guidepost, in so far as the determination of disorderness is concerned. It leads us to erroneous conclusions in other areas of psychiatry, besides panic attacks, such as whether to regard bereavement-related major depressive syndromes as instances of "normal sadness" or of bona fide Major Depressive Disorder [1].

And so, I want to suggest that the general concept of *disorderness* in psychiatry ought to be—with very few exceptions—*non-contextual*. But before my psychodynamically-oriented colleagues recoil in horror, I hasten to add that context is critically important in working *psychotherapeutically* with patients. After all, there is a world of difference, psychotherapeutically speaking, between a severely depressed patient who has just lost a loved one; and an equally depressed patient who is being investigated for bank fraud—though, in my view, *both are in a disordered state* and deserve professional treatment.

The Background Story: Panic on the Precipice

Recently, I came across an article that may have been the genesis of my distinguished colleague's "hanging off the edge of a cliff" scenario. In his 2007 review of the book, *The Loss of Sadness* [2], by Jerome C. Wakefield and Allan V. Horwitz, the eminent researcher and scholar, Dr. Kenneth Kendler wrote as follows:

> "If an individual experience[s] a full-blown panic attack when…he loses his grip and falls 40 feet before a rope catches him…no psychiatrist I know would consider this to be a psychopathological phenomenon. A panic attack is not—in and of itself—psychopathological. It only becomes pathology when it occurs in certain contexts—at times and in places when it should not. Thus the diagnostic status of panic disorder is inherently contextual. It is not a disorder in and of itself but only in certain contexts…" [3].

Later in his review, Dr. Kendler alludes to what he takes to be a unanimous consensus among psychiatrists, regarding "…our all agreeing that the climber dangling from the rope has a clearly 'understandable' and hence non-pathological panic attack" [3]. He then contrasts panic attacks with, for example, a bizarre delusion, such as, "A hard drive has been installed in my head by aliens..." He regards the latter as *inherently pathological*. But, regarding the panic attack, is Dr. Kendler correct?

On a purely *pragmatic* view of "psychopathology", I believe Dr. Kendler is—mostly—correct. Undoubtedly, no psychiatrist would say to our mountain-climber, after his cliff-hanger panic attack, "You need psychiatric treatment. Please set up an appointment with me right away!" Nor would many competent psychiatrists say, "You are likely to need psychotherapy and perhaps medication, given that you experienced this panic attack."

So, in terms of clinical *praxis*, Dr. Kendler is right to claim that the panic-on-the-precipice scenario would probably not be interpreted as *psychopathology*—at least in the sense that the term "psychopathology" is typically used in the psychoanalytic literature; i.e., as a disturbance of internalized objects, unresolved unconscious conflicts, use of primitive ego defenses, etc. Dr. Kendler is also technically correct in noting that Panic Disorder (like its building-block, the panic attack) is "inherently contextual," in the limited sense that the DSM-IV and DSM-5 criteria require that PD be characterized by recurrent and *unexpected* ("spontaneous") panic attacks. "Unexpected" attacks are, in essence, "contextless" attacks—ones that come "out of the blue." The clear implication is that there is such a thing as "expected" panic attacks. In DSM-IV and DSM-5, "expected" implies that the attack is associated with a *situational trigger*, such as a "cue" or reminder of a previous trauma; i.e., the attack occurs in an understandable "context."

It's not clear how the framers of DSM-IV or DSM-5 would classify the panic attack in our "cliff-hanger" scenario. But while such an attack may not represent *psychopathology*, there are no compelling clinical reasons for viewing such a context-based panic attack as "normal" or "*non-pathological.*" After all, anxiety related to a pheochromocytoma may not be associated with *psychopathology* in the sense described, yet the resultant anxiety may be *pathological* in its intensity and incapacity. Thus, I believe Dr. Kendler erred in suggesting that the mountain climber's panic attack was, "…'understandable' and hence [a] non-pathological panic attack." The problem is with the use of the word, "hence." That an event is "understandable" does not, by itself, render the event *non-pathological*. (Dr. Kendler, of course, is well aware of this with respect to major depressive symptoms in the context of recent bereavement, and has so argued on the DSM-5 website [4]). Similarly, I believe Prof. Jerome C. Wakefield errs when he comments on the Kendler scenario, arguing that the mountain climber's panic attack "…was *normal* because that is precisely the *context* in which such intense anxiety experiences were biologically designed to occur" (italics added) [5].

I know of no empirical evidence whatsoever that human beings are "biologically designed" (whatever that expression means) to experience panic attacks in *any* circumstance or context—precipice or no precipice! Nor am I aware of any evidence that "such intense anxiety" in objectively dangerous situations is in any way *advantageous* to the human organism, as Wakefield's quasi-evolutionary claim implies. In my view, panic attacks do not demonstrate "biological design," but *biology gone awry*. Here, I believe, Wakefield confuses *anxiety* with *fear*. The latter is a *realistic* and *adaptive* emotion in the face of some objective, external threat—like, say, a Mack truck heading straight for your car. Unlike ordinary fear, panic attacks *do not* prepare the endangered person for appropriate defensive action—rather, if anything, panic usually *incapacitates* the person experiencing it.**

Furthermore, it is misleading to claim that labeling a panic attack as "pathological" or "disordered" represents a "false positive," if the attack occurs in an "understandable" context [5]. Indeed, the entire notion of a "false positive" in psychiatry rests on an unproved ontological assumption; i.e., that there exist "natural types" of disease entities ("taxons") defined by *necessary and sufficient criteria*, against which diagnostic claims may be judged "false" [6].

As Lilienfeld notes, "Such terms as 'false positives' and 'overdiagnosis' carry no ontological meaning in the absence of a taxon [a genuine category that exists in nature], as they presume the existence of at least some true breaking point in nature" [7].

One possible reason for confusion among "contextualist" writers—particularly those without a medical background--is the overlap in the DSM criteria for *panic attack*; and those for what traditionally has been called the "fight or flight response" or "general adaptation syndrome" (GAS), first characterized by Hans Selye [8].

Most physiologists would indeed regard the GAS as an evolution-based adaptation to acute stress. But despite some overlapping features with panic attacks (e.g., adrenergic activation, tachycardia, increased respiratory rate, sweating), the GAS is a *fundamentally different process*. For example, the GAS usually lacks such panic-specific features as *a feeling of choking, chest pain, nausea, dizziness, fear of "going crazy," derealization, or paresthesias*—none of which is known to be "adaptive."

And although research is still incomplete, there is also reason to believe that the physiology of a panic attack differs from that of the prototypical "fight or flight" response. One of the foremost researchers in the area of panic disorder, Dr. Richard Maddock, notes that,

> "...panic attacks are *dysfunctional*, while ordinary fight or flight responses are generally adaptive. From the perspective of physiological data supporting this distinction, one difference immediately comes to mind. In the GAS response, elevated [serum] cortisol is the norm. However, elevated cortisol is distinctly the exception during panic attacks" (italics added; personal communication, November 16, 2012).

Indeed, panic attacks appear to share more features with *acute coronary syndrome* (ACS)—basically, myocardial ischemia—than with the general adaptation syndrome [9].

Moreover—unlike the GAS--panic attacks predict onset and severity of psychopathology beyond anxiety disorders [10]. In short, whereas the GAS is, by definition, *adaptive*—at least, in its earliest stages—it is far from clear that *any* panic attack, under any circumstances, is ever "normal" or "adaptive." In so far as it is experienced as terrifying, crippling, death-dealing, or debilitating, a panic attack is nearly *always* "pathological" (from *pathos*, meaning, "suffering") and disordered. That said, a single panic attack does not qualify as a *discrete* disorder or merit diagnosis of a specific disease entity. Thus, to diagnose *Panic Disorder*, DSM-5 requires additional features, such as recurrent attacks and maladaptive changes in behavior.

Notes

** As Dr. Maddock has pointed out, it is theoretically possible for a patient to meet DSM-IV panic attack criteria with only *four* of thirteen possible symptoms; e.g., tachycardia, sweating, sensations associated with increased respirations, and a fear of dying. In theory, under some threatening circumstances, these particular anxiety-related symptoms *might* be adaptive—but patients with such limited panic symptoms are almost never seen in clinical practice. As Dr. Maddock notes: "Although the simple DSM-IV definition of a panic attack can capture some adaptive fear or stress responses, I believe this has no bearing on clinical practice" (personal communication, November 25, 2012).

Part II: Context Does Not Determine "Disorderness" or Normality

In part I of this essay, I argued that panic attacks are nearly always pathological and disordered states, whether or not they occur in an "understandable context." I also distinguished the maladaptive aspects of panic attacks from the adaptive nature of the classic "fight or flight" response, sometimes known as the General Adaptation Syndrome. Indeed, because panic attacks per se appear predictive of subsequent psychopathology, one proposal for DSM-5 was to rate panic attacks as a separate dimension of pathology, across *all* mental disorders [11]; in fact, the manual actually indicates that "panic attack" may be used as a specifier in connection with any psychiatric disorder, such as PTSD, bipolar disorder, etc.

But the issue of "context" and its relationship to "disorderness" extends well beyond panic attacks: it arises in nearly all psychiatric diagnoses not explicitly *defined* contextually. Some DSM disorders, of course, are "context-bound," by definition; e.g., post-traumatic stress disorder requires a trauma, and adjustment disorders require some precipitating psychosocial stressor. For most other DSM diagnoses, however, the basic question arises: if we can "understand" the patient's presenting signs and symptoms, owing to *an explanatory psychosocial or environmental context*, are we entitled to regard the patient's condition as "normal," "non-pathological," or "non-disordered"?

I believe that such an explanatory context does not remove a psychiatric condition's *pathology*—or the need for treatment—*once the condition crosses a certain threshold of suffering and incapacity*. "Context" does not dissolve disorder, even if it seems to explain it. And often, we are quite wrong about such seeming "explanations" [12]. Indeed, if someone who climbed mountains for a living repeatedly and frequently experienced panic attacks whenever standing on the edge of a cliff—resulting in prolonged or pronounced suffering and incapacity—this state of affairs would be the (dys)functional equivalent of *disease*.

On this view, pathological states are constituted by pronounced or prolonged *suffering and incapacity*—or, if we prefer, by substantial or enduring *distress and disability*. While the term "disease" resists an *essential definition* [6]—i.e., one specified by necessary and sufficient criteria—most serious, clinical conditions called "disease" have pronounced or prolonged suffering (and some degree of incapacity) in common. These features constitute what the philosopher Ludwig Wittgenstein termed, "family resemblances" and may be compared to the overlapping fibers that make up a rope [13].

To be sure, not *all* pathological or disordered states constitute clinical *disease*. In our ordinary language, we usually don't apply the term "disease" to states of suffering and incapacity that are related to a *visible wound* or injury, such as a knife wound; i.e., we don't normally speak of "knife-wound disease." Nor do we usually apply the term "disease" to suffering and incapacity that is inflicted upon someone by *external malefactors*, such as terrorists or kidnappers. So, in this very limited sense, context *does* play some role in how we employ the term "disease," in our ordinary language.

There is another sense in which context plays a limited role in how we assess the "disorderness" of a condition. When a person experiences intense or prolonged suffering and incapacity "out of the blue"—i.e., in the *absence* of any known psychosocial precipitant or other explanatory context—*our clinical suspicions are usually raised*. We suspect some kind of internal disease process at work, such as a covert malignancy; or, in the case of major depressive symptoms, we suspect what used to be called an "endogenous" depression. In this very limited sense, then, the contextualists make a valid claim.

Where contextualists err is in supposing that the *presence* of an understandable, explanatory context—such as recent bereavement, job loss, or even hanging off a cliff—somehow renders a condition "normal," "non-pathological" or "non-disordered" [2], all other things being equal. Curiously, this fallacious reasoning seems more common in psychiatry than in general medicine. Consider the patient who, after abdominal surgery, develops clinically significant pain at the incision site. The pain—while entirely "understandable" and perhaps even statistically common—is nevertheless considered *pathological* and is quickly treated by diligent clinicians. The patient in such pain is *suffering* and is probably also incapacitated. Nobody argues that, "It's perfectly understandable that the patient is in pain—that's normal, coming out of surgery like that!" (Still fewer would argue that there is an "adaptive advantage" to be gained by being in pain after surgery—except in so far as crying out in pain may impel someone to relieve the patient's suffering!)

What about the "biological context" of a person's psychiatric symptoms? To be sure, the biological context affects our *diagnostic formulation*, but not the "disorderness" of a person's clinical signs and symptoms. The person running down the street naked, while screaming and breaking car windows, is in a *pathologically disordered state*, whether the "context" is recent cocaine intoxication, florid mania, or a terrible and understandable psychic trauma. To be sure: we need to pursue that differential diagnosis. *But our ability or inability to "understand" the genesis of the person's behavior is irrelevant to our determining that the condition is pathological and disordered.* Regardless of context, once a certain threshold of suffering and incapacity is crossed, physicians justifiably apply the term "disease" (or "disorder," "malady," etc.) to the person's condition. (For purposes of this discussion, I am using the terms "disease" and "disorder" more or less synonymously, though the medical literature is remarkably inconsistent in how these terms are applied [14].)

This is also true of maladaptive symptoms attributed to the patient's "developmental" context [15]. It is of course true that "temper tantrums" in a two-year old—or moodiness and impulsivity in an adolescent—is very often developmentally "normal." But once a certain threshold of suffering and incapacity is crossed, we rightly impute "disorderness" to the child's condition; make a diagnosis; and offer appropriate treatment. That the child's symptoms occur in an "understandable context" does *not* render our diagnosis a "false positive." Context helps *explain* pathology—it does not annul it.

Suffering and Incapacity

Finally, since I have highlighted the criteria of "suffering and incapacity," the reader may rightly ask, "How do we assess and quantify these features? And isn't any determination of this sort inherently subjective?" Indeed, I believe we have only limited tools for assessing suffering and incapacity, and often, these instruments are fairly crude. We do have objective, validated scales that help quantify the severity of *specific symptoms or mood states*; e.g., the Beck Depression Inventory, the Hamilton Depression Rating Scale, etc. In the DSM-IV, the Global Assessment of Function (GAF) scale provided a rough index of the patient's level of impairment and dysfunction. The DSM-5 offers what may be an improved assessment tool, making use of the World Health Organization Disability Assessment Schedule (WHODAS). This is a self-completed form that includes questions on how much difficulty the subject has had within the past 30 days, in such areas as: *concentrating on doing something for ten minutes; remembering to do important things; analyzing and finding solutions to problems in day-to-day life; generally understanding what people say...* etc. For subjects who indicate "none" or "mild" for each of the many domains, we may reasonably infer that they are functioning in the "normal" range for the human species. Similarly, the PHQ-15—a brief, self-administered questionnaire—seems to be useful in assessing somatic symptom severity, which, in turn, is correlated with the patient's functional status [16].

That said, it is harder to find assessment tools that get at the "inner world" of the patient, in the sense phenomenologists emphasize—tools that would help us appreciate not only incapacity and somatic pain, but "existential suffering" in a broader sense. To do so, I believe we need to move well beyond the symptom check-lists of the DSMs [17]. In my view, the first duty of all physicians is to relieve pronounced or prolonged suffering and incapacity. We must do so, regardless of how "understandable" the context in which this experience arises. This does not mean "medicalizing normality"—it means doing what caring physicians have done for countless centuries.

Acknowledgments

My sincere appreciation to Dr. Richard Maddock and Dr. Sidney Zisook for their helpful comments and suggestions on early drafts or portions of this essay. A slightly modified version of Parts 1 and 2 of this this piece appeared in the January 11 and January 15, 2013, issues, respectively, of *Psychiatric Times*.

References

[1] Zisook S, Corruble E, Duan N, et al. The bereavement exclusion and DSM-5. *Depress Anxiety*. 2012;29(5):425-443.

[2] Horwitz AV, Wakefield JC. *The Loss of Sadness*. Oxford: Oxford University Press; 2007.

[3] Kendler KS. Review of The Loss of Sadness: How Psychiatry Transformed Normal Sorrow into Depressive Disorder, by AV Horwitz, and JC Wakefield [book review]. *Psychological Medicine*. 2008;38:148-150. Available from: http://journals.cambridge.org/action/displayAbstract?fromPage=online&aid=1595220. Accessed March 8, 2014.

[4] Kendler KS. Grief exclusion. American Psychiatric Association; 2010. Available from: http://www.dsm5.org/about/Documents/grief%20exclusion_Kendler.pdf. Accessed March 8, 2014.

[5] Wakefield JC. Misdiagnosing normality: psychiatry's failure to address the problem of false positive diagnoses of mental disorder in a changing professional environment. *J Ment Health*. 2010;19:337-351.

[6] Lilienfeld SO, Marino L. Essentialism revisited: evolutionary theory and the concept of mental disorder. *J Abnorm Psychol*. 1999;108:400-411.

[7] Lilienfeld SO. Book Review of *The Loss of Sadness*, by AV Horwitz and JC Wakefield. *Soc Serv Rev*. 2009; 83:473-477.

[8] Selye H. Forty years of stress research: principal remaining problems and misconceptions. *Can Med Assoc J*. 1976;115:53-56

[9] Soh KC, Lee C. Panic attack and its correlation with acute coronary syndrome - more than just a diagnosis of exclusion. *Ann Acad Med Singapore*. 2010;39:197-202.

[10] Craske MG, et al. Panic disorder: A review of DSM-IV panic disorder and proposals for DSM-V. *Depress Anxiety*. 2010;27:93-112.

[11] Batelaan NM, Rhebergen D, de Graaf R, et al. Panic attacks as a dimension of psychopathology: evidence for associations with onset and course of mental disorders and level of functioning. *J Clin Psychiatry*. 2012;73:1195-1202.

[12] Pies RW. Depression and the pitfalls of causality: implications for DSM-V. *J Affect Disord*. 2009;116:1-3.

[13] Wittgenstein L. The Blue and Brown Books: Preliminary Studies for the Philosophical Investigations. New York: Harper Torchbooks; 1965.
[14] Pies R. Moving beyond the "myth" of mental illness. In: Schaler JA, ed. *Szasz Under Fire*. Chicago: Open Court, 2004: 327-353.
[15] Wakefield JC, First MB. Placing symptoms in context: the role of contextual criteria in reducing false positives in Diagnostic and Statistical Manual of Mental Disorders diagnoses. *Compr Psychiatry*. 2012;53:130-139.
[16] Kroenke K, Spitzer RL, Williams JB. The PHQ-15 is a brief, self-administered questionnaire that may be useful in screening for somatization and in monitoring somatic symptom severity in clinical practice. *Psychosom Med*. 2002;64:258-266.
[17] Pies R. After bereavement, is it "normal grief" or major depression? *Psychiatr Times*. 2012 February 21. Available from: http://www.psychiatrictimes.com/mdd/content/article/10168/2035804. Accessed March 8, 2014.

~~~~~~~~~~~~~~~~~

DSM-5: Petitions, Predictions, and Prescriptions

Some months ago, I received a stern admonition from my family doctor. My fasting blood sugar of 99 mg/dL was "right on the border", he said—and I had better work on bringing it down. "But," I protested, "when I was in medical school (in the 1970s), the normal FBS range went up to 110 mg/dl!"

"Well," he replied a bit impatiently, "they changed the criteria!"

Indeed, "they" did. The most recent criteria identify "pre-diabetes" (also called "impaired glucose tolerance") as an FBS between 100 and 125 mg/dl.

But isn't this what *psychiatrists* get accused of doing all the time—moving the diagnostic goal posts so as to broaden the inclusion criteria for various disorders? And doesn't this inevitably lead to over-diagnosis and over-prescription of potentially hazardous drugs? Such, at any rate, is the thinking by many of psychiatry's critics, including some prominent psychiatrists.

But the diabetes experts who promoted the new, lower threshold for an abnormal FBS did so based upon sound epidemiological and clinical data. As the American Diabetes Association website notes,

"[Prediabetes] puts you at a higher risk for developing type 2 diabetes and cardiovascular disease…For some people with prediabetes, early treatment can actually return blood glucose levels to the normal range. Research shows that you can lower your risk for type 2 diabetes by 58% by: Losing 7% of your body weight (or 15 pounds if you weigh 200 pounds) [and] exercising moderately (such as brisk walking) 30 minutes a day, five days a week" [1].

To the best of my knowledge, the prediabetes criterion change was not based on *predictions* of how much or how little anti-diabetes medication doctors were likely to prescribe, or how much "Big Pharma" would stand to gain or lose from the lower FBS threshold. Yet some in the mental health field would like the DSM-5 criteria sets to reflect and preempt such entirely hypothetical changes in prescribing patterns. Thus, the "Open Letter to the DSM-5" warns,

> "The proposal to lower diagnostic thresholds is scientifically premature and holds numerous risks. Diagnostic sensitivity is particularly important given the established limitations and side-effects of popular antipsychotic medications. Increasing the number of people who qualify for a diagnosis may lead to excessive medicalization and stigmatization of transitive [sic], even normative distress" [2].

Now, I would agree that several of the proposed changes in the DSM-5 are indeed "scientifically premature," in so far as they lack a sound foundation in long-term, epidemiological and clinical studies. (Others, such as dropping the "bereavement exclusion" in the diagnosis of major depressive disorder, are founded on quite good evidence, in my view). And, yes—psychiatrists must consider the overall health risks of their diagnostic system, as Dr. Allen Frances and others have repeatedly pointed out. But such deliberations must carefully weigh both the risks *and the benefits* of changes in the diagnostic system, based on *well-validated studies*—not on the basis of crystal ball gazing!

Objecting to a reduced threshold for a particular disorder based on the cynical prediction that "doctors will use it as an excuse to write more prescriptions" is neither good science nor good public policy. Furthermore, until we have universally accepted criteria for a given disorder, backed up by a veridical biomarker, it simply begs the question to assert that a lower threshold for a diagnosis will lead to "false positives" or "false epidemics." Without an unimpeachable criterion for "true", we cannot declare a finding to be "false"!

Absent empirical studies showing a *direct connection between the newly-proposed diagnostic threshold and actual harm to patients or the general public*, the "over-prescribing" argument amounts to social engineering—not scientifically-based disease classification. It is asking our diagnostic criteria to do the work of our continuing medical education—which, let us be frank, could certainly use improvement. If, for example, we want to discourage physicians from prescribing antidepressants for the very mildest cases of major depressive disorder (MDD), the best means of doing so is through enhanced training and education—not through manipulation of our diagnostic criteria for MDD. Of course, there may be perfectly sound reasons for "tightening" the MDD criteria, based on considerations of reliability, validity, and response to treatment—but these are scientifically-justified reasons for modifying *any* medical diagnostic criteria and have nothing to do with anticipated "misuse" of the criteria by over-zealous prescription writers.

Furthermore, there may be compelling public health reasons for identifying certain "pre-clinical" or "prodromal" psychiatric conditions, based on morbidity and mortality data, and on the longitudinal outcome of these conditions. Yes, the potential for inappropriate or premature pharmacotherapy exists with respect to these more subtle derangements--but that risk alone should not dictate our nosology. Moreover, it is fallacious to equate "treatment" in psychiatry with *medication,* even though rates of psychotropic prescriptions have been rising substantially in recent years—often owing to prescriptions written by primary care physicians rather than psychiatrists.

Indeed, some sub-clinical or prodromal states may respond well to various *non-pharmacological* interventions. For example, a study in the British Journal of Psychiatry [3] examined the construct of "early initial prodromal state (EIPS) of psychosis in which most of the disability and neurobiological deficits of schizophrenia have not yet occurred." The authors investigated the effects of an integrated psychological intervention (IPI), combining individual cognitive–behavioral therapy, group skills training, and other modalities, compared with "supportive counseling." The primary outcome was progression to psychosis at 12- and 24-month follow-up. IPI was found to be superior to supportive counseling in preventing progression to psychosis at 12-month follow-up.

Let's be clear: if confirmed, this would be a very important public health finding. It simply won't do for critics of DSM-5 to argue that such pre-clinical or prodromal syndromes will inevitably lead to over-use of antipsychotic or other medications—though, of course, this outcome is possible. These critics must also weigh the *potential benefits of early intervention*, as well as longitudinal studies examining *the risks of failing to intervene* early in pre-psychotic states.

There may also be a critical role for the FDA, in promulgating stricter prescribing indications for antidepressants and antipsychotics. Rather than jiggering our diagnostic criteria to discourage excessive medication prescribing, I believe we would make more progress with an FDA-mandated statement in the drug labeling information—a sort of "brown box" warning stating, for example,

> IMPORTANT: There are no convincing and consistent controlled data showing that antidepressants are superior to placebo or non-specific interventions for very mild instances of major depressive disorder (e.g., Hamilton Depression Rating <14). Antidepressants may carry a substantial side effect burden, and in mild cases of MDD, it is usually preferable to begin a form of psychosocial treatment. Antidepressants appear most effective in cases of moderate-to-severe MDD, and in cases involving melancholic or psychotic features [4].

Our diagnostic criteria should be guided by the best science we can muster, not by well-intentioned but misguided attempts to anticipate "bad behavior" on the part of clinicians. In short, if we are to change our diagnostic criteria in psychiatry, we should model our behavior on that of the diabetes experts, not the crystal ball gazers.

Acknowledgments

Thanks to James Knoll, MD, Nassir Ghaemi, MD, and Susan Kweskin for helpful comments on this piece. A slightly modified version of this piece appeared in the November 21, 2011, issue of *Psychiatric Times*.

References

[1] American Diabetes Association. Diagnosing diabetes and learning about prediabetes [online]. http://www.diabetes.org/are-you-at-risk. Accessed February 24, 2014.

[2] Society for Humanistic Psychology et al. Open letter to the DSM-5 [online]. Available from: http://www.ipetitions.com/petition/dsm5/. Accessed February 24, 2014.

[3] Bechdolf A, Wagner M, Ruhrmann S, et al. Preventing progression to first-episode psychosis in early initial prodromal states. *Br J Psychiatry*. 2012;200:22-29.

[4] Vöhringer PA, Ghaemi SN. Solving the antidepressant efficacy question? Effect sizes in major depressive disorder. *Clin Ther*. 2011;33:B49-61.

~~~~~~~~~~~~~~~~~

WHY PSYCHIATRY MAY SOMETIMES NEED FUZZY DIAGNOSES

Well, while I'm here, I'll do the work—and what's the work? To ease the pain of living...—Allen Ginsberg

Many words...don't have a strict meaning. But this is not a defect. To think it is would be like saying that the light of my reading lamp is no real light at all, because it has no sharp boundary.—Ludwig Wittgenstein, The Blue and Brown Books

As a general proposition, most scientists and physicians prefer sharpness to fuzziness, at least when it comes to defining terms. I generally share this view, as regards psychiatric diagnosis, but only up to a point. That point is defined by the well-being of my patient—and sometimes, this may call for a "fuzzy" diagnosis. To understand why this is so, consider the following thought experiment. Imagine that we have a set of psychiatric signs and symptoms, designated as A through F. Suppose that if we select "A,B,C,D,E" as constituting our identified "Syndrome X," we can correlate it with a specific pathophysiology, and even with a specific genetic anomaly. Sounds terrific, right? And all so very "scientific"! But suppose that the syndrome, so defined, corresponds poorly to our patients' subjective experience of distress; and furthermore, that the "ABCDE" syndrome does not lend itself well to any effective treatment.

Now imagine we start with the same A through F signs and symptoms, but we decide to group them as *either* "A,B,C,D,E" *or* as "B,C,D,E, F." We are, in other words, making our definition of Syndrome X "fuzzier." We now find that Syndrome X no longer corresponds as well to a particular pathophysiology or genetic defect—but that it better captures our patients' *subjective experience*, and also lends itself to an *effective treatment*. In short, the fuzzier syndrome allows us to reduce our patients' degree of suffering and incapacity to a greater extent than did the "sharp" ABCDE category. Which syndrome is more "real"—the "sharp" or the "fuzzy" one? Which is more pragmatically useful? And which syndrome leads us to *more humane medical care*, consistent with our ethical responsibilities as physicians?

Psychiatry often takes a beating for having "fuzzy" diagnoses that don't correspond to a specific pathophysiology, laboratory test, biomarker, or genetic defect. In this regard, we are held up to considerable scorn, in contrast to the "precise" and pathophysiology-based diagnoses in the hallowed world of "real" medicine—for example, the world supposedly inhabited by pathologists, internists, and neurologists. This is certainly the conventional wisdom of the lay press, and—more frequently than I care to admit—even of many psychiatrists. But this narrative is mostly bunk.

In the first place, there is an extraordinary degree of subjectivity and "fuzziness" in general medicine, neurology, and—yes—even in general pathology. I learned this recently when a family member underwent a prostate biopsy, only to be told by two pathologists that he had a "suspicious" nest of cells in one quadrant of his prostate. Suspicious? *Was it cancer or not?* my relative wanted to know. Nobody, including his urologist, could tell him. The specimen was sent off to an "expert" at Johns Hopkins, who, presumably, was either smarter than the first two pathologists, or nearer the Mind of God. The two puzzled pathologists were not trying to be evasive—there was simply an irreducible amount of uncertainty in their observation. Prostate cells sometimes show microscopic features that are neither clearly benign nor clearly malignant. This is because Nature itself is inherently "fuzzy," notwithstanding our sincere desire, as diagnosticians, to "carve Nature at its joints," as Plato put it (*Phaedrus* 265d-266a). Ideally, we will eventually learn what degree of cellular fuzziness we need to preserve—or cast aside—in order to provide patients like my relative with the right kind of care.

Nature may be equally uncooperative when it comes to psychiatric disorders. Our patients' suffering may not correspond to some Platonic "essence" that has a well-defined set of necessary and sufficient criteria. Nor are such precise criteria sets necessarily more "real" than other constructions we might use as disease categories—any more than a sharply-focused beam of light is more "real" than the fuzzy beam coming from Wittgenstein's reading lamp. Of course, it is worth trying to be precise—but not necessarily "as precise as possible". A better and more ethically defensible goal for physicians is to be as precise *as is clinically useful*. We are not physicists, we are physicians: our primary goal ought to be to reduce suffering and incapacity, and to enhance life in all its healthy and creative dimensions. For that matter, even the physicists speak only of "probability" and "uncertainty" at the quantum level—they still can't say precisely where that elusive electron is hiding.

To be sure: it is generally laudable, in psychiatry, to develop diagnostic criteria with high inter-rater reliability; good sensitivity and specificity; and a strong association with specific biogenetic markers. But if our diagnostic categories can't capture our patients' felt experience—the *phenomenology* of their illness—what good is "carving Nature at its joints"? If biomarkers and genotypes do not allow us to alleviate our patients' suffering and incapacity, what service have we rendered them? I'm with the beatnik poet on this one: we are in this profession to ease the pain of living.

Acknowledgment

A slightly modified version of this piece appeared in the December 1, 2009, issue of *Psychiatric Times*.

~~~~~~~~~~~~~~~~~

WESTERN PSYCHIATRIC IMPERIALISM, OR SOMETHING ELSE?

In a very long essay in the Sunday New York Times Magazine of November 10, 2010, entitled, "The Americanization of Mental Illness," Ethan Watters suggests that a kind of psychiatric-cultural imperialism has been foisted on other countries and cultures by "the West." Specifically, Watters claims that,

> "For more than a generation now, we in the West have aggressively spread our modern knowledge of mental illness around the world.... There is now good evidence to suggest that in the process of teaching the rest of the world to think like us, we've been exporting our Western "symptom repertoire" as well. That is, we've been changing not only the treatments but also the expression of mental illness in other cultures."

Watters claims, for example, that as the general public and mental health professionals in Hong Kong "…came to understand the American diagnosis of anorexia," the presentation of the illness in Hong Kong actually became more "virulent."

Though the Watters thesis has its merits, it is also glib and simplistic in many of its assumptions and conclusions. To be fair: Watters rightly calls attention to the ways that culture and ethnicity can shape both the diagnosis and expression of psychiatric conditions and symptoms. But this is hardly news to psychiatrists: the late Dr. Ari Kiev advanced much the same thesis in his 1972 book, *Transcultural Psychiatry*.

Watters' more controversial claim is that the exportation of American psychiatric nosology and "biomedical ideas" has changed the way symptoms are diagnosed and expressed in some other cultures. But this claim is very hard to validate. The "American" diagnostic system is, in the first place, not terribly different from the World Health Organization's *International Classification of Disease* (ICD), whose descriptions of "mental and behavioral disorders" evolved almost contemporaneously with those of the last two DSMs. It would be very hard to tease out the cross-cultural influence of the DSM classification from that of the ICD, over the past 30 years. More important, Watters fails to consider alternative explanations for his "findings"; for example, rising rates of DSM-type anorexia nervosa in Hong Kong could be due largely to *increased recognition of a long-standing, indigenous disorder* that heretofore had not been fully appreciated by Chinese clinicians.

An example from American history helps make the point. Many of the basic symptoms of post-traumatic stress disorder (PTSD) have been recognized for centuries—at least since the U.S. Civil War, and probably much earlier—and have gone by various names, such as "soldier's heart," "combat fatigue," "shell-shock," etc. But it took the efforts of troops returning from the Vietnam War to "push" psychiatry toward recognition of PTSD as a bona fide disorder. Understandably, *apparent* PTSD prevalence rates have soared since the diagnosis entered American nosology in 1980, with the advent of DSM-III. But it is entirely possible that the *actual* prevalence of PTSD symptoms in the U.S. has not changed markedly over many generations.

To return to Mr. Watters' thesis: it would not be surprising to find that, as clinicians in other cultures began to familiarize themselves with DSM or ICD psychiatric disease criteria, the *apparent* prevalence rates of certain psychiatric conditions increased in those countries. It is quite another thing to imply that the *actual* prevalence of these conditions has increased—

and that their morphology has changed—as a result of Western influences. Yet Watters seems to imply just this, when he asserts that

> "...a handful of mental-health disorders—depression, post-traumatic stress disorder and anorexia among them—now appear to be spreading across cultures with the speed of contagious diseases. These [Western-based] symptom clusters are becoming the lingua franca of human suffering, replacing indigenous forms of mental illness."

We would need several generations of very sophisticated epidemiological studies, carried out using identical diagnostic criteria, to substantiate this "contagion-replacement" hypothesis. Anecdotal claims, such as those presented in the Watters article, are utterly inadequate. But even if Watters is correct, his claims do not answer the fundamental medical-ethical question: *will adopting "Western" diagnostic criteria ultimately lead to a net reduction in suffering, and a net increase in well-being, in other cultures?* If, after careful systematic study, the answer to this question turns out to be no, our Western paradigms will have failed. If the answer turns out to be yes, we might conclude that we have been exporting a very valuable commodity.

Acknowledgment

A slightly modified version of this piece appeared in the January 12, 2010, issue of *Psychiatric Times*.

~~~~~~~~~~~~~~~~

Is Bigotry a Mental Illness?

> *The Second Temple was destroyed because of causeless hatred. Perhaps the Third will be rebuilt because of causeless love.*—Rav Abraham Isaac Kook.

There were only three Jewish students in my high school, and I was one of them. In the small, western New York town where I grew up, most people were fairly tolerant. But a tiny clique of anti-Semites made life tough for us Jewish kids. Most of the time, we just shrugged off the jokes and insults, or came right back at these louts with a snappy retort. (Prejudice may have its unexpected benefits, in the sharpening-of-wits department.) Sometimes, the bigotry grew more menacing. I still remember Robin Hicks (not his real name) walking up to me in the hallway, looking me squarely in the eyes, and very calmly saying, "Jews don't live long, you know."

This brief autobiographical vignette is simply a way of saying that the issue of bigotry is more than of merely academic interest to me. I am therefore quite invested in the outcome of a controversy that has arisen recently in our profession; namely, whether or not "pathological bigotry" should be considered a psychiatric disorder. I use the term "pathological bigotry" to encompass a variety of related terms, including "pathological hatred," "racial paranoia," "extreme racial bias," and "pathological bias."

A piece in the *Washington Post* [1] provided an excellent snap-shot of how opinion on this issue has divided members of the psychiatric and academic communities—including several esteemed colleagues whom I greatly respect. As the *Post* reporter notes, the stakes are high:

> "Advocates have circulated draft guidelines [for making pathological bias an official DSM diagnosis] and have begun to conduct systematic studies...if [the proposal] succeeds, it could have huge ramifications on clinical practice, employment disputes, and the criminal justice system. Perpetrators of hate crimes could become candidates for treatment, and physicians would become arbiters of how to distinguish 'ordinary prejudice' from pathological bias."

Those who advocate making pathological bigotry a formal psychiatric diagnosis argue along these lines: "Psychiatrists and other mental health professionals regularly confront extreme forms of racism, homophobia, and other forms of irrational hatred. Many patients holding these views are very troubled and sometimes even disabled by them. Some individuals with pathological bigotry are frankly delusional, perceive themselves as 'under attack,' and become overtly dangerous to themselves or others. We should diagnose and treat these individuals because we may be able to help them, just as we can with other troubled patients. For example, some extremely hateful patients may be helped with psychotherapy or antipsychotic medication. Psychiatric diagnosis cannot avoid the social context of mental illness, and the mere fact that our diagnoses may be misused in the criminal justice system should not deter us from applying them."

Those who oppose "medicalizing" these forms of bigotry argue roughly as follows:

> "It is a mistake to pathologize a widespread form of human stupidity. Psychiatrists have enough trouble now, justifying the reality of ADHD and 'conduct disorder'—do we really need the added woes attendant to our declaring bigotry a mental disorder? How would we differentiate mere *dislike* of some minority groups from pathological bigotry? Would we want this diagnosis to be a mitigating factor in, say, a violent crime against a member of a minority group? Most people who hold these bigoted attitudes are not psychotic; most probably learned their attitudes from their parents. Moreover, these individuals are rarely troubled by their beliefs. What motivation would they have for seeking or accepting 'treatment'? When faced with such hateful individuals, psychiatrists should focus on diagnosing and treating well-validated, co-morbid conditions, such as paranoid schizophrenia."

Both sides make good points. In order to resolve these seemingly irreconcilable views, I believe we first need to build a conceptual framework for determining what counts as "disease" in psychiatry. We can then can compare "pathological bigotry" to our paradigm, and try to determine to what degree it coincides. We must then consider how the general construct of "disease" relates to the further determination of whether a particular set of signs and symptoms constitutes *a specific disease*. Finally, we need to examine the preliminary empirical data that have emerged from some recent studies of "pathological bias."

I have argued for more than 30 years [2] that our concept of "disease" grew out of an ancient tradition based on the recognition of *suffering and incapacity*. Disease is not diagnosed, in the first place, by medical specialists using high-tech imaging devices or laboratory tests—though these may help determine the *specific disease entity*. In psychiatry, as in general medicine, it is often a family member or the soon-to-be patient who first recognizes that something is terribly wrong. This is based on our ordinary perception of *suffering and incapacity in the absence of an obvious external cause* (such as a knife wound). A mother who observes that her son has been tormented for months by "voices telling him to kill himself"; has stopped eating and bathing; and has barricaded himself in his room for two weeks does not need a specialist to tell her that her son is "sick" or "diseased." Indeed, the term "disease" arose from our everyday awareness that certain pathological states leave us *without ease* or comfort—hence, the now obsolete word "diseasy," to describe such individuals. While there is no written-in-stone, "essential" definition of the term *disease*—that is, no list of necessary and sufficient conditions that invariably applies—I believe that the presence of marked suffering and incapacity is a good starting point for defining what philosopher Ludwig Wittgenstein might have called the "family traits" of disease entities [3].

On this account, a person presenting to a psychiatrist with pronounced suffering and incapacity due *directly* to intense, irrational hatred of a race, religion, or ethnic group would, indeed, be "diseased." I hasten to add that the kind of "suffering" I am positing must not be due solely to the *punitive consequences* of acting on bigoted beliefs, such as being thrown in jail for a racially-motivated assault. The suffering must be, at least in part, intrinsic or "primary"; that is, a direct consequence of *experiencing one's own pathological bias*. Suppose, for example, a patient presented with the complaint, "Doc, I have these incredibly intense feelings of anger and hatred toward people from [Country X]. I know it's crazy, and I'd like to change, but I can't. The feelings and thoughts are shameful to me, and they torment me night and day. I can hardly eat or sleep, feeling this way." I would argue that to just the extent such a hypothetical patient meets our broad criteria for disease—suffering and incapacity—he or she is worthy of our compassion and care.

But what about those individuals—like my old nemesis, Robin Hicks—who are apparently *neither suffering nor incapacitated* as a direct result of their bigoted beliefs? Are they, nevertheless, "sick" or "diseased"? My personal response is, "Not in any sense that is relevant to the practice of clinical psychiatry." (As *concerned citizens*, of course, we may rightly and vigorously oppose such people on purely moral grounds.) It is true that we are sometimes asked—usually by the legal system—to deal with individuals who have committed antisocial acts, but who do not seem in any way bothered or incapacitated by their behaviors per se; e.g., sexual predators whose pedophilia is completely "ego-syntonic." These sociopathic individuals represent a medico-legal dilemma, and I have no easy answers as to how our profession should deal with them. However, I would argue that they do not represent individuals with *disease*.

But now: even if we agree that pathological bigotry accompanied by suffering and incapacity represents "disease" in a generic sense, we must still ask if it represents *a specific disease* that might warrant inclusion in the DSM-5?

Here, I believe, psychiatry must draw on the history of general medicine. Historically, physicians usually begin the conceptual-empirical march toward "disease" by first identifying a *syndrome*; that is, a specific set of signs and symptoms that we observe with great consistency and regularity. Such a syndrome—for example, central obesity, muscle weakness, hypertension, and amenorrhea-- may ultimately be understood as a *specific disease* when one or more of the following criteria are met:

1) A pattern of genetic transmission is discovered, sometimes leading to the identification of a specific genetic locus.
2) The syndrome's pathophysiology and/or pathologic anatomy becomes reasonably well-understood.
3) The syndrome's course, prognosis, and response to treatment are seen to be relatively predictable and uniform across many populations.

Indeed, when the features of Cushing's *Syndrome* (noted above) were traced to *pituitary dysfunction*, that particular condition became known as Cushing's *Disease*.

Of course, there have been innumerable debates as to whether "classical" psychiatric disorders or diseases, such as schizophrenia, fully meet any of the three criteria just described [4-6]. But whatever one's view of such controversies, it seems to me that the construct of "pathologic bigotry" has not yet reached even the *syndromal* level, much less the status of a specific "disease." Nonetheless, our present diagnostic schema would allow us to treat such individuals under a number of existing diagnostic categories, depending on the nature and severity of their "pathology." For example, one might consider a diagnosis of *obsessive-compulsive disorder*, if the patient's ruminations about "race" or ethnicity were ego-alien and intrusive, and he or she maintained a modicum of "reality testing." On the other hand, the person might qualify as having "delusional disorder, persecutory type" if his bigoted beliefs reached the proportions of a paranoid psychosis.

All that said, there are some preliminary but intriguing data emerging from the work of Prof. Edward Dunbar, at U.C.L.A. that may someday form the foundation for a "pathological bias syndrome." Dunbar has developed a scale (the Outgroup Hostility Scale, OHS) for measuring the dimensions of pathological bias—for example, experiencing panic and anxiety in response to benign contact with members of a racial or ethnic group. In a study of psychotherapy outpatients who sought treatment for problems unrelated to such bias [7], Dunbar found that OHS scores were correlated with measures of hypomania, hostility, panic symptoms, and lower scores on the GAF (Global Assessment of Functioning). A history of psychological trauma was also a factor in some pathologically biased patients. Earlier work by Dunbar found that high ratings of "outgroup bias" were significantly associated with Axis II criteria for Paranoid, Borderline, and Antisocial Personality Disorders [8].

Nonetheless, Dunbar stops short of concluding that pathological bias should be considered a "stand alone disorder." As he notes, "...the identification of specific symptoms of such a diagnostic category would need to demonstrate, via clinical research, *an independence from other recognized diagnostic categories, and to... [confer] serious impairment to the individual such as to warrant mental health treatment*" (italics added). [7] Moreover, Dunbar acknowledges that, as yet, "...there are no established practice guidelines for the treatment of pathologically biased patients."

Carl Bell, MD, a psychiatrist who has written extensively in this area, rightly argues that "... racism most likely has biological, psychological., and sociological origins..." He adds, however, that racism is "...mainly a product of learned behavior and that "....a majority of explicitly racist persons do not have any psychopathology" [9]. In my view, it is at best premature to create a new diagnostic category for racism or bigotry. Still, to the extent that subgroups of those with pathological bias may have co-morbid psychopathology—and to the extent that these individuals are willing to undergo diagnosis and treatment—psychiatrists should remain actively interested and involved.

Acknowledgments

I wish to thank Sally Satel, MD, and Edward Dunbar, PhD, for their helpful comments on this piece. A slightly modified version of this piece appeared in the May 1, 2007, issue of *Psychiatric Times*.

References

[1] Vedantam S. Psychiatry ponders whether extreme bias can be an illness. *The Washington Post*. 2005 December 10, p. A01. Available from: www.washingtonpost.com/wp-dyn/content/article/2005/12/09/AR2005120901938.html. Accessed March 8, 2014.

[2] Pies R. On myths and countermyths: more on Szaszian fallacies. *Arch Gen Psychiatry*. 1979;36:139-144.

[3] Wittgenstein L. The Blue and Brown Books: Preliminary Studies for the Philosophical Investigations. New York: Harper and Row; 1958.

[4] Pies R. Moving beyond the "myth" of mental illness. In: Schaler JA, ed. *Szasz Under Fire*. Chicago: Open Court Publishing; 2004: 327-353.

[5] Szasz TS. *Schizophrenia: The Sacred Symbol of Psychiatry*. New York: Basic Books, Inc; 1976.

[6] Schramme T. The legacy of antipsychiatry. In: Schramme T, Thorne J, editors. *Philosophy and Psychiatry*. New York: Walter de Gruyter; 2004: 94-119.

[7] Dunbar E. Examining the problems of pathological bias: syndrome, disorder, or social norm? Available from: http://edunbar.bol.ucla.edu/papers/Clinical_Bias_Study%20OneJAP%20%20ms%20Dec%202005PDF.pdf

[8] Dunbar E. The relationship of DSM diagnostic criteria and Gough's Prejudice Scale: exploring the clinical manifestations of the prejudiced personality. *Cult Divers Ment Health*. 1997;3:247-257.

[9] Bell C. Racism: a mental illness? *Psychiatr Serv*. 2004;55:1343.

~~~~~~~~~~~~~~~~

Chapter 3

GRIEF, DEPRESSION, AND THE BEREAVEMENT CONTROVERSY

DEPRESSION IS A THIEF, EVEN WHEN YOU LEARN FROM IT

Writer Jonah Lehrer caused quite a stir with his recent article in the N.Y. Times Magazine, with the unfortunate title, "Depression's Upside" [1]. I have a detailed rejoinder to Lehrer's article, posted on the Psych Central website [2]. While I found the piece misleading and credulous, the fault is not entirely Mr. Lehrer's, and I believe he undertook the article in good faith and with good intentions. Alas, Mr. Lehrer, to my knowledge, does not have any medical training; and he relied heavily on a strained and dubious argument known as the "analytical-rumination hypothesis" (ARH). This holds, in effect, that major depression has certain "adaptive" advantages, including the enhancement of some problem-solving skills [3].

Lehrer apparently spent little time talking to mood disorder specialists or evolutionary biologists, regarding the gaping evidentiary holes in this hypothesis. In fairness, Mr. Lehrer has stated that he did speak with "…numerous working psychiatrists…and, not surprisingly, got a wide range of reactions to the analytic-rumination hypothesis" [4]. Indeed, this is not surprising, given the wide range of psychiatric practices and patient populations. I believe that most mood disorder specialists, upon hearing the essence of the ARH, would respond with either a dropped jaw or a barnyard epithet.

But is there any sense in which depression might have an "upside"? So much of the debate turns on what is meant by the term "depression." A major problem with Mr. Lehrer's original piece is that he did not fully clarify what he meant by "depression." In contrast, it is quite clear that the paper [3] on which Lehrer bases his evolutionary claims used the term "depression" to describe DSM-IV major depressive disorder—not a brief period of pensive, poetic reverie. Unfortunately, even the DSM-IV construct of major depression is so elastic, one can wrap it around almost anyone presenting with a couple of weeks of depressed mood and a few changes in sleep, appetite, and functioning.

To answer the "upside" question, we first need to distinguish three related yet distinct concepts and claims: (1) major depression is "instructive"; (2) major depression is "adaptive"; and (3) major depression is "conducive to significant mental health (or physical health) benefits."

I would not deny that major depression, like other serious challenges in life, may be "instructive" for some unknown proportion of individuals. Just as one may learn from the experience of having chronic heart disease, or cancer, one may also learn from depression. A bout of depression may demonstrate, for example, one's own "inner strength" in the face of adversity, or reveal who one's true friends are. Yet I'll gladly wager that few who have experienced severe depression would recommend it to friends and family as a "great learning experience."

I also have very serious doubts that major depression is "adaptive" in any significant way, though it is notoriously difficult to prove claims about what traits are or are not useful evolutionary adaptations. Perhaps grief—or very mild, brief bouts of depression—could confer some modest advantages in an evolutionary sense; e.g., by increasing one's empathy toward others, which could be highly adaptive in many cultures. In my view, this is not likely the case when we consider severe and debilitating major depressive illness. Perhaps the distinction between grief and major depression is what Rabbi Bunam of Pzysha (1767–1827) had in mind when he observed, "*A broken heart prepares man* for the *service* of God, but dejection corrodes *service*" [5].

For more severe depression, I believe that whatever adaptive advantages it might provide are overwhelmed by the maladaptive aspects of the illness. For example, the rate of completed suicide in major depression—roughly 4 in 100, averaging outpatient and inpatient rates—is many magnitudes greater than the rate in the general U.S. population, of about 11 per 100,000 [6].

I have suggested elsewhere that major depression may be "conserved" in the human species not because it is adaptive, but because it is a *spandrel*—essentially, *a non-adaptive trait that exists only by virtue of underlying, adaptive traits*. A spandrel is a kind of evolutionary "hitch-hiker" that doesn't really contribute anything to the cost of the ride. One example, drawn from paleontologist Steven J. Gould, is the fact that our bones are white. "Whiteness" per se has no adaptive value—it simply happens to be a property of the adaptive constituents of our bones (calcite and apatite) [7]. My colleague, Peter Kramer, MD, also put forth the "spandrel" hypothesis, in his book, *Against Depression*. For a searching critique of the ARH, I recommend the essay by University of Chicago evolutionary biology professor Jerry Coyne, PhD [8].

As regards mental health benefits, such as increased clarity of thought or problem-solving ability issuing from depression, this strikes me as, well--unlikely in the extreme. We have numerous studies [9] pointing to the significant cognitive deficits present in those with major depressive episodes—so much so that in my residency days, we used to speak of "depressive pseudodementia." We now know that there is nothing "pseudo" about these mood-related deficits; rather, they represent bona fide abnormal brain function [10]. As for any putative physical benefits to major depression–on the contrary, major depression is associated with substantially increased health risks, such as cardiovascular disease and diabetes [11].

I also think it's helpful to ask, in philosopher William James's terms: what is the "cash value" of the idea that major depression confers an adaptive advantage by improving our problem-solving skills? Let's stipulate such an advantage. So what? Where does that information get us, in our attempt to help people live better, more productive lives? How does it help our severely depressed patients? Should we encourage patients to prolong their depressive bouts in order to increase their analytic abilities?

We have known for decades that the sickle-cell *trait* provides a survival advantage over people with normal hemoglobin in regions where *malaria* is endemic—but this trait also increases rates of painful and debilitating sickle-cell *disease*. If, in a malaria-rich environment, we had the means both to reverse the sickle cell trait and to prevent malaria, would we not do so? By analogy: if we could prevent major depression with all its disadvantages, but still find ways to improve people's "problem-solving skills," would we not do so? Surely there are ways of teaching people how to "analyze" their problems without asking them to bear the immense burdens of major depression!

Some have suggested [4] that by informing patients of the supposed "upside" to their depression, we may somehow encourage them, or relieve some of the "stigma" associated with this illness. I remain unconvinced. I believe that for every patient who brightens up upon hearing of the supposed "upside" to her depression, there will be ten who wonder why they are *not* experiencing depression's wondrous benefits, such as an improved ability to analyze their problems. I think many severely depressed patients would find such "Rah-rah, depression!" talk eminently non-empathic, and might well ask, "Is there something wrong with me? Can't I even do *depression* right?" This, certainly, is my strong clinical intuition, based on the last nearly 30 years of working with seriously depressed patients. But it is a matter of empirical research to confirm these clinical impressions.

In truth, all the academic theorizing in the world regarding depression's "upside" won't alter the painful reality of major depression for people like Rose, who recently wrote as follows:

> *"I have resistan[t] major depression. I suffer constantly, daily with worthlessness, guilt, crying, and helplessness. I have been working with my doctors for years. I just received disability without benefits (no insurance due to pre-existing conditions)... I have tried suicide and I know it was me reaching out for help...I am desperate for any help. I am a burden for my family and I hate feeling sorry and pitying myself. I just want appropriate help to get this disease cured or at least to achieve relief for myself and my life. Please give any advise... this is a major cry for help"* [12].

None of this is to say that people who are depressed are in any way "broken" and must be "fixed." One should never confuse a person's mood state or illness with his or her value or goodness as a human being! Nor is it to say that, if a depressed patient has found meaning and benefit in his depression, we should quash his sense of hope or gratitude. But in all the years I sat with severely depressed patients, I can't recall one who praised the "upside" of their depression—at least, while in the midst of it.

The Talmud teaches us that we should learn from all persons, even a thief. For example, thieves work hard at night! I see severe major depression as a kind of thief. Now, to be sure: being robbed (of happiness, pleasure, ease of mind and body, etc.) may indeed be instructive–one learns courage, resilience, caution, and the need to take care of oneself. But a thief is still a thief—and few of us would recommend a "good burglary" to our friends or family, as a means of instruction in life's lessons.

Acknowledgment

A slightly modified version of this piece appeared in the March 5, 2010, issue of Psychiatric Times.

References

[1] Lehrer, J. Depression's upside. *New York Times Magazine*. 2010 February 28. Available from: http://www.nytimes.com/2010/02/28/magazine/28depression-t.html. Accessed March 9, 2014.

[2] Pies R. The myth of depression's upside [online]. Psych Central. World of Psychology blog. 2010 March 1. Available from: http://psychcentral.com/blog/archives/2010/03/01/the-myth-of-depressions-upside/. Accessed March 9, 2014.

[3] Andrews PW, Thomson JA. The bright side of being blue: depression as an adaptation for analyzing complex problems. *Psychological Review*. 2009;116:620-654. Available from: http://sites.google. Accessed March 9, 2014.

[4] Lehrer J. More on depression [online]. The Frontal Cortex blog. 2010 March 5. Available from: http://scienceblogs.com/cortex. Accessed March 9, 2014.

[5] Besserman P. *The Way of the Jewish Mystics*. Boston: Shambhala; 1994: 115-117.

[6] National Research Council. *Reducing Suicide: A National Imperative*. Washington, DC: The National Academies Press, 2002. http://books.nap.edu/openbook.php?record_id=10398 & page=71

[7] Gould, SJ. *The Structure of Evolutionary Theory*. Cambridge, MA: Belknap Press; 2002.

[8] Coyne J. Is depression an evolutionary adaptation? Available from: http://whyevolutionistrue.wordpress.com/2009/08/30/is-depression-an-evolutionary-adaptation-part-2/. Accessed March 9, 2014.

[9] DeBattista, C. Executive dysfunction in major depressive disorder. *Expert Rev Neurother*. 2005;5(1):79-83.

[10] Hosokawa T, Momose T, Kasai K. Brain glucose metabolism difference between bipolar and unipolar mood disorders in depressed and euthymic states. *Prog Neuropsychopharmacol Biol Psychiatry*. 2009;33:243-250.

[11] Lett H, Blumenthal J, Babyak M, et al. Depression as a risk factor for coronary artery disease: evidence, mechanisms and treatment. *Psychosom Med*. 2004;66:305-315.

[12] Comment on: The myth of depression's upside] [online]. Psych Central. World of Psychology blog. Available from: http://psychcentral.com/blog/discuss/8113/#comment-642718 Accessed March 9, 2014.

~~~~~~~~~~~~~~~

IS MAJOR DEPRESSION "ADAPTIVE"? CLINICAL DATA SAY NO

The poet Denise Levertov was no stranger to sorrow and loss. In her poem, "Stepping Westward" [1], she writes of the aging process, as both a burden and a gift. The poem begins,

"What is green in me/darkens, muscadine..."

Muscadine is a woody vine that produces a musk-scented purple grape, used to make wine. Levertov's image is one of growing darkness, but also of emotional growth and maturation. With old age comes "the fruit of the vine"—wisdom and awareness. Levertov's poem goes on to observe, *"If I bear burdens/ they begin to be remembered/ as gifts..."*
We all know that sorrow can bring insight, if it is properly and deeply understood. This "gift" may also emerge from the pensive reflection of ordinary grief and bereavement. I begin with Levertov's poetic images because I want to distinguish what Thomas a Kempis called "the proper sorrows of the soul" from what psychiatrists know as *major depression*. I would never argue against the claim that, on some level, *ordinary grief* may be adaptive—in fact, in a series of articles, Dr. Sidney Zisook and I have stated as much [2, 3].

But when the same claim is made with regard to *major depressive disorder* (MDD), as in the so-called *Analytical (or Adaptive) Rumination Hypothesis* (ARH) [4, 5, 6], I am left shaking my head. In its simplest formulation, the ARH asserts that "...depression is nature's way of telling you that you've got complex social problems that the mind is intent on solving"; and that "depression is in fact an adaptation, a state of mind which brings real costs, but also brings real benefits" [4]. In effect, the ARH asserts that the "analytical" and ruminative cognitive processes of the depressed person facilitate complex, social problem-solving. A number of experimental manipulations are cited to support the ARH (e.g., see Hertel et al. [7]), but few psychometric studies of *clinically-depressed* patients (e.g., meeting DSM-IV MDD criteria) are adduced as evidence. (Let's leave aside the simplistic notion that depression arises from unresolved "social problems"—of course, this is sometimes so, but in many cases, interpersonal problems are the *consequence* of pre-existing depression [8].)

The basic claims of the ARH do not square with anything in my experience as a specialist in mood disorders for over 25 years, nor with the overwhelming majority of *clinical* studies of cognitive function in MDD, to be reviewed presently. But first, it is critical that we distinguish studies of *clinical populations* from *experimental manipulations* involving non-clinical test subjects--usually described as being "sad" or in a "depressed mood state"—who are asked to solve various artificial "problems" (e.g., see Hertel et al. [7]). These test subjects—e.g., college student volunteers [4]—are usually "induced" to have very brief periods of depressed mood, using some experimental intervention. These subjects have virtually nothing in common with the seriously depressed patients psychiatrists treat, who have often been ill for weeks, months, or even years.

To be clear: I have many problems with the DSM-IV construct of MDD, such as its almost risible elasticity—MDD is a diagnosis that can be stretched around almost anyone with two weeks, or two years, of depressive symptoms [9]. But when carefully applied to someone with *a month or more of severe depression; one or more melancholic features; pronounced suffering; and substantial social-vocational incapacity*, "MDD" describes a very real disease entity, with a lifetime suicide rate of about 4 in 100 [10]. The notion that such a condition is in *any* sense "adaptive" flies in the face of clinical experience; the reports of most severely depressed patients; and, as I hope to show, most studies of cognitive and social function in depressed individuals.

As to "evolutionary" arguments for and against the ARH, I will leave those to authorities in the field of evolutionary biology [11], though I am deeply skeptical of some recent claims regarding the supposed benefits or adaptive advantages of "analytical rumination" [6]. My intention here, however, is to examine the published studies of cognitive function in patients with major depression, and to pose the following questions: (1) Is there credible evidence showing that MDD (or clinically significant depression) enhances any specific types of cognitive skills or mental processes? (2) Is there credible evidence that *rumination* in MDD enhances any type of "problem-solving" skills? and (3) Is there credible evidence showing that depressed individuals possess enhanced social or interpersonal skills, such that they might be at some kind of "adaptive advantage"? These questions, of course, cannot address whether those who have endured an episode of severe MDD are or are not "wiser" for the experience; or whether they were able to find life-enhancing "meaning" or valuable perspectives in the course of their suffering. These are fundamentally philosophical and spiritual—not scientific--determinations. Finally, I will not address the controversial matter of antidepressant treatment, other than to note this: the claim that MDD is not "adaptive"—indeed, that it is pervasively *mal*adaptive—is surely *not* to claim that all persons with MDD require, or benefit from, antidepressant treatment. Simply put, some do, and some probably do not [12]. In any case, the issue of pharmacotherapy would take us far afield.

Clinical Studies of Cognition in Depression

Dr. Charles DeBattista, in a recent review, concluded that, "The types of executive deficits seen in depression include problems with planning, [as well as] initiating and completing goal-directed activities" and that such "executive dysfunction" tends to worsen in direct proportion to the severity of depression [13]. Similarly, a review by French investigators concluded that "...executive deficits associated with frontal lobe dysfunction may be prominent in depression" and that "...unipolar depressed patients mainly exhibit cognitive inhibition deficits, problem-solving impairments and planning deficits" [14]. Furthermore, unipolar depressed patients tend to show "...difficulties in hypothesis testing with a loss of spontaneous and reactive cognitive flexibility," attributable to dysfunction in the dorsolateral prefrontal cortex (DLPFC). (Ironically, proponents of the ARH suggest that prefrontal brain regions show *enhanced activity* in major depression, thus facilitating "analytic rumination"; in fact, the brain imaging evidence in MDD is complex and often conflicting, perhaps reflecting slightly differing sub-regions of the prefrontal cortex [15]). Cognitive problems may be especially pronounced in older depressed individuals, as Alexopoulos and colleagues have shown. They note that "depressed patients often have disturbances in attention, speed of processing, and executive function even in the absence of dementing disorders." Moreover, "...executive dysfunction and related cognitive abnormalities *confer significant disability and add to adversity* experienced by the depressed elderly person" (italics added) [16]. Collectively, these findings do not suggest any salient adaptive advantages in the cognitive state of most clinically depressed patients. Quite the contrary: as Alexopoulos et al., note, citing the work of Nezu and Ronan, *problem-solving therapy* (PST) for geriatric depression actually "...originated from the observation that depressed patients *use inadequate or inappropriate approaches in addressing their problems...*" (italics added) [16].

Rumination: Friend or Foe?

There is little disagreement with the observation that clinically depressed patients tend to ruminate; i.e., to focus repetitively on the same issue, problem, or thought (the term comes from the Latin *ruminari*, "to chew cud"). In general, the research literature points to the deleterious effects of depressive rumination. As Rimes and Watkins [17] observe, citing the work of Nolen-Hoeksema [18] and others,

> "Increasing evidence suggests that rumination plays a role in the maintenance of depression...Experimental studies have found that in dysphoric participants, compared to [use of] distraction, rumination increases depressed mood, cognitive distortions and...impairs problem-solving skills..." [17].

These findings are consistent with those of Donaldson and Lam [19], who found that patients with major depression who were made to ruminate experienced a *deterioration* in their mood and *gave poorer problem solutions*. Similarly, Park et al. [20] found that experimentally induced rumination, as compared with distraction, increases depressed mood and negative memories in adolescents with a first episode of MDD.

Taken in toto, these findings flatly contradict the central claim of the ARH; i.e., that rumination is helpful and adaptive in addressing one's problems, social or otherwise. But there is a complication we need to consider: rumination appears to be subdivided into *analytical self-focus* (ASF) and *experiential self-focus* (ESF). In essence, ASF involves thinking analytically "about" oneself and one's symptoms; for example, "How did I get so depressed? Why do I feel so guilty?" In contrast, ESF involves a "here and now" focus, on the *direct experience* of one's thoughts, feelings and sensations in the present moment; e.g., "Right now, I'm feeling hurt and angry that John left me for someone else." Rimes and Watkins [17] studied these two types of rumination in 30 depressed participants (MDD by DSM-IV critiera) and 30 never-depressed volunteers. Participants were randomly allocated to "analytic" (high analysis) or "experiential" (low analysis) self-focused manipulations. The study found that in depressed participants, *analytical self-focus increased ratings of feeling "worthless" and "incompetent.*" The experiential self-focus condition resulted in no significant change in such judgments. (Neither mode of rumination had a significant effect in the non-depressed controls.) The authors concluded that "...an analytical mode of self-focused rumination may be particularly maladaptive in depression" [17]. Once again, no support for the ARH is provided. Indeed, in direct contradiction of the ARH, Watkins et al. have shown that *treating* depressive rumination with cognitive-behavioral therapy "...appears to yield generalized improvement in depression and co-morbidity" [21]. If rumination were indeed adaptive and productive, we would expect the opposite result.

Social and Interpersonal Skills in Depression

Does being clinically depressed somehow make one more empathic, or improve one's ability to "read" the social cues of others? Might depression enhance social bonding in a way that could be "adaptive"—if not on an "evolutionary" time scale (e.g., by increasing the depressed person's reproductive potential), at least in the here-and-now? Some preliminary answers have emerged from studies of the ability to recognize *facial expression*. What does facial expression have to do with social and interpersonal skills? A good deal, according to Yoon and colleagues (2009). They note that, "Biases in the processing of subtle facial expressions of positive affect may...contribute to the interpersonal difficulties that maintain [depression]" [22]. Put in more colloquial terms: if you can't tell that someone is smiling at you, the two of you are not likely to hit it off. Indeed, in their study of subjects with Major Depressive Disorder (MDD), Yoon et al. found that major depression interferes with "reading" subtle expressions of positive affect, such as the famous "Mona Lisa smile." It is hard to see any adaptive advantage in this perceptual bias.

A core argument of the ARH is that unresolved "social problems" *precede* clinical depression, which is said to be an adaptive *response* to these problems. But as Segrin observes in his review,

> "Three different theoretical relationships between disrupted social skills and depression [have been] described...[namely] poor social skills as a cause of depression, depression as a cause of poor social skills, and poor social skills as a vulnerability factor in the development of depression. Currently, there is some evidence to support each of these conceptualizations" [8].

Despite this ambiguity, there is little doubt that clinically depressed individuals show a variety of social and interpersonal deficits, including, according to Segrin,

> "...inhibition in initiating new relationships and interactions with others; problems in expressing themselves clearly to others; inappropriately and excessively self-disclosing information, especially if it is negatively toned, to others; and sometimes being overly negative and perhaps even hostile around other people" [8].

Once again, it is hard to imagine any short-term, adaptive advantage emerging from these widespread interpersonal difficulties in depression, much less an enhanced "evolutionary" advantage that would favor attracting a mate, engaging in sexual activity, reproducing, etc. But these are matters of debate for the evolutionary biologists.

Conclusion

I would wager that the great Renaissance artist, Albrecht Durer, understood clinical depression far better than some modern-day proponents of the Analytic Rumination Hypothesis. In his 1514 depiction of "Melencolia 1," Durer shows the pensive goddess sitting amidst an array of unused analytic tools and instruments, staring somberly into space. As one commentator observed, "...her fixed state is one of intent though fruitless searching. She is inactive not because she is too lazy to work but because work has become meaningless to her; her energy is paralyzed not by sleep but by thought" [23].

A psychiatrist could hardly have described severe depression more accurately, or refuted the ARH more succinctly.

I do not doubt that for some MDD patients, there are indeed "remembered gifts" that are appreciated upon *recovery* from their depression. Many formerly depressed patients are able to reflect productively on their periods of depression, and express the view that they learned important "life lessons" from these depressive bouts. But this is not to say that MDD *itself* is "adaptive" during the course of the patient's illness. Virtually all the evidence I have reviewed leads to precisely the opposite conclusion. Nonetheless, the final word has not been written on this controversy. It would be instructive to do a carefully-designed, empirical study that examined the question of depression's "upside" from the patient's point of view—controlling for possible confounds, such as the type of depression; whether or not the patient is hospitalized; how much support the patient is receiving from significant others; when in the course of illness the patient is evaluated, etc. I'm not aware of such studies, whereas I have countless experiences hearing about the hellish suffering brought on by major depression. I remain open to the possibility that brief periods of mild depression may sometimes permit useful reflection on one's problems, and perhaps even lead to some helpful solutions. But in my experience, it is usually *despite*—not because of—serious depression that solutions to life's problems are found. We owe our patients more than specious theories regarding the "upside" of their depression; we owe them careful diagnosis and safe, effective, and readily-available treatment [12].

Acknowledgments

I would like to express my appreciation to Dr. Katharine Rimes and Dr. Rebecca Park for their helpful comments and references; and to Dr. George Alexopoulos and Dr. Emily Becker-Weidman for providing their papers. I also want to acknowledge the seminal research of Dr. Helen Mayberg in studying regional brain imaging in MDD. However, this commentary represents solely my own analysis and conclusions. A slightly modified version of this piece appeared in the November 4, 2010, issue of *Psychiatric Times*.

References

[1] Levertov D. Stepping Westward [online]. Available from: http://www.chriscorrigan.com/parkinglot/levertov.htm#_Toc23572766. Accessed March 9, 2014.

[2] Zisook S, Simon NM, Reynolds CF 3rd, et al. Bereavement, complicated grief, and DSM, part 2: complicated grief. *J Clin Psychiatry*. 2010;71:1097-1098.

[3] Pies R, Zisook S. Grief and depression redux: response to Dr. Frances's "compromise." *Psychiatr Times*. 2010 September 28. Available from: http://www.psychiatrictimes.com/dsm-5/content/article/10168/1679026. Accessed March 9, 2014.

[4] Andrews PW, Thomson JA. Depression's evolutionary roots. *Scientific American*. 2009 August 25. Available from: http://www.scientificamerican.com/article/depressions-evolutionary/. Accessed March 9, 2014.

[5] Andrews PW, Thomson JA. The bright side of being blue: Depression as an adaptation for analyzing complex problems. *Psychological Review*. 2009;116:620-654.

[6] Andrews PW, Thomson JA. Coyne battles Darwin, many other evolutionary biologists—and himself. *Psychiatr Times*. 2010 September 23. Available from: http://www.psychiatrictimes.com/articles/coyne-battles-darwin-many-other-evolutionary-biologists%E2%80%94and-himself. Accessed March 9, 2014.

[7] Hertel G, Neuhof J, Theuer T et al. Mood effects on cooperation in small groups: does positive mood simply lead to more cooperation? *Cogn Emot*. 2000;14:441-472.

[8] Segrin C. Social skills deficits associated with depression. *Clin Psychol Rev*. 2000;20:379-403.

[9] Ghaemi SN. Why antidepressants are not antidepressants: STEP-BD, STAR*D, and the return of neurotic depression. *Bipolar Disord*. 2008;10:957-968.

[10] Ruter TJ, Davis M. Suicide prevention efforts for individuals with serious mental illness: roles for the state mental health authority. In: Litts DA, Radke AQ, Silverman MM, editors. Series of Technical Reports. National Association of State Mental Health Program Directors Medical Directors Council. Available from: www.sprc.org/library/SeriousMI.pdf

[11] Coyne JA. The evolutionary calculus of depression. Psychiatr Times. 2010 August 5. Available from: http://www.psychiatrictimes.com/depression/content/article/10168/1633704. Accessed March 9, 2014.

[12] Pies R. Antidepressants work, sort of—our system of care does not. *J Clin Psychopharmacol*. 2010;30:101-104.

[13] DeBattista C. Executive dysfunction in major depressive disorder. *Expert Rev Neurother*. 2005; 5:79-83.

[14] Fossati P, Ergis AM, Allilaire JF. Executive functioning in unipolar depression: a review. *Encephale*. 2002;28:97-107.

[15] Hosokawa T, Momose T, Kasai K. Brain glucose metabolism difference between bipolar and unipolar mood disorders in depressed and euthymic states. *Prog Neuropsychopharmacol Biol Psychiatry*. 2009;17;33:243-250.

[16] Alexopoulos GS, Raue PJ, Kanellopoulos D et al.: Problem solving therapy for the depression-executive dysfunction syndrome of late life. *Int J Geriatr Psychiatry*. 2008;23:782-788.

[17] Rimes KA, Watkins E. The effects of self-focused rumination on global negative self-judgments in depression. *Behav Res Ther*. 2005;43:1673-1681.

[18] Nolen-Hoeksema S. The role of rumination in depressive disorders and mixed anxiety/depressive symptoms. *Abnorm Psychol*. 2000;109:504-511.

[19] Donaldson C, Lam D. Rumination, mood and social problem-solving in major depression. *Psychol Med*. 2004;34:1309-1318.

[20] Park RJ, Goodyer IM, Teasdale JD. Effects of induced rumination and distraction on mood and overgeneral autobiographical memory in adolescent Major Depressive Disorder and controls. *Child Psychol Psychiatry*. 2004;45:996-1006.

[21] Watkins E, Scott J, Wingrove J, et al. Rumination-focused cognitive behaviour therapy for residual depression: A case series. *Behav Res Ther*. 2007;45:2144-2154.

[22] Yoon KL, Joorman J, Gotlib IH. Judging the intensity of facial expressions of emotion: depression-related biases in the processing of positive affect. *J Abnorm Psychol*. 2009; 118:223-228.

[23] Panofsky E, *The Life and Art of Albrecht Dürer*, 4th ed. (Princeton University Press, 1955), 160.

~~~~~~~~~~~~~~~~~

MAJOR DEPRESSION AFTER RECENT LOSS IS MAJOR DEPRESSION — UNTIL PROVED OTHERWISE

Suppose your new patient, Mr. Jones, tells you he is feeling "really down." He meets all DSM-IV symptomatic and duration criteria for a major depressive episode (MDE) after having lost his wife to cancer, two weeks ago. Should you diagnose, "Major Depressive Disorder"? I'm guessing most psychiatrists would be reluctant to do so. Indeed, DSM-IV permitted a "bereavement exclusion" in such circumstances, provided the patient lacks "…certain symptoms that are not characteristic of a 'normal' grief reaction." But say another week has gone by. Mr. Jones tells you tearfully, "Doc, I caused my wife's cancer. I'm thinking of driving my car into a tree. I'm just not worth keeping around." He shows marked psychomotor retardation and has missed work this last week. Is this just "normal grief"? Maybe not, now that Mr. Jones has those "certain symptoms" that would override the bereavement exclusion. These vexing issues are nicely discussed in a recent editorial by Maj [1].

Psychiatric Times recently published a "Commentary" [2] by Professors Alan V. Horwitz, PhD, and Jerome C. Wakefield, PhD, authors of *The Loss of Sadness: How psychiatry transformed normal sorrow into depressive disorder* [3]. Essentially, the Horwitz-Wakefield (H-W) thesis holds that the "decontextualized" criteria for MDE set forth in DSM-III (1980) and DSM-IV have created a "seeming epidemic of depression" and spuriously high depression prevalence rates. By "decontextualized," Horwitz and Wakefield mean, *without considering the context of loss or bereavement that makes the person's depressive symptoms "normal" or understandable*. The second linchpin in the H-W thesis is the claim that psychiatrists can, and should, determine how "proportionate" the depressed person's response is to the recent loss—based on so-called "evolutionarily derived criteria" [3, p. 221].

The Loss of Sadness is a thoughtful book with honorable intentions. But I believe the H-W thesis puts the conceptual "cart" many years before the evidentiary "horse"; and that its practical effect could be to undermine our care of some bereaved patients *who also meet MDE criteria*.

What Is At Issue Here?

Let me be clear: after a major loss, many people will experience intense sadness and isolated depressive symptoms (e.g., tearfulness, insomnia, poor appetite) that often do not constitute "disease" or "mental disorder." Many will feel better with simple support and "tincture of time," after 1-2 months. As Maj notes, "A depressive state is an expectable and culturally sanctioned response to the death of a loved one and…does not represent a mental disorder" [1]. This much is not in dispute.

Rather, the controversies arising from the H-W thesis are these: (1) are there *controlled, prospective data* showing that recent loss or bereavement per se *predicts a benign, self-limited course,* when the patient meets all symptomatic and duration criteria for a MDE? (2) Are there controlled data showing that major depressive symptoms after recent loss or bereavement differ in fundamental ways, including treatment response, from typical depressive symptoms *without loss or bereavement?* And finally, (3) do we have any *clinically-validated instruments*, based on "evolutionarily-derived" criteria, by which to judge how "proportionate" a patient's depressive reaction is to a putative stressor? In our present state of very limited evidence, I believe the answer to these questions is *no* [1, 4].

Common Sense or Theoretical Bias?

Horwitz and Wakefield make much of "common sense" in their book. Thus, they believe, "…a wealth of evidence supports the commonsense judgment that many people who develop symptoms of depression after a loss, *even when they meet DSM criteria for a disorder*, are not disordered, but are experiencing a *biologically designed* response" (italics added) [3, p. 51]. First, we would do well to recall Einstein's well-known dictum: "Common sense is the collection of prejudices acquired by age eighteen." As for the supposed "wealth of evidence," a careful search for controlled, prospective studies reveals only a poverty of data.

Now consider the following "common sense" view of depressive symptoms in the context of bereavement. Common sense tells us that bereavement-related depression (BRD) will abate on its own within a few weeks or months, as the patient copes with the loss. Common sense tells us that BRD symptoms will more closely resemble those of "normal sadness" than those of non-bereaved ("standard") major depression. And, because BRD is precipitated by a unique loss, common sense tells us the depression is not likely to recur, all other things being equal. Finally, common sense might tell us that BRD is a normal, "adaptive" response to loss, whose "biology" and response to antidepressants would differ considerably from that of standard major depression.

This is all quite commonsensical—and all quite without convincing controlled evidence. For example, Brent et al. [5] studied depressive reactions in youths exposed to a friend's suicide. The study found that the exposed subjects developed symptoms most consistent with *major depressive episodes*—not uncomplicated bereavement—on the basis of both *course* and *risk of recurrence*. The median duration of depression in the 37 subjects who became depressed was *8 months!* Compared with controls, the exposed subjects also had a higher rate of *depressive recurrence* during the follow-up period, even after adjusting for previous history of depression and other risk factors.

Similarly, Karam et al. [6] compared features of bereavement-related and non-bereavement related major depression in a prospective community study (N=685). The global "symptom profile" of depressed individuals and their risk for depressive recurrence was similar in bereaved and non-bereaved subjects. Moreover, the *duration of illness was actually longer in the bereaved group.* The authors concluded that "…the descriptive and etiologically neutral approach the DSM presumes in reaching a diagnosis should be applied in the case of [major depression] until more convincing data point to the contrary."

We have very limited data on the neurobiology of BRD versus "standard" major depression. However, Zisook and Kendler [7] found that, in general, BRD has biological features that resemble those of "standard" major depression, including impaired immune function and excessive adrenocortical function. And, it is far from clear that these abnormalities represent merely an "adaptive" response to loss.

Some features may distinguish BRD from depression triggered by *other* losses or stressors; for example, lower rates of seeking professional treatment [8] and less interference with life activities in BRD [9]. However, there are deep clinical and epistemological problems in the notion of a unique "trigger" for a depressive episode; e.g., chronological distortions in a patient's recollection of depression onset [1, 4] and the presence of underlying medical factors [4]. Indeed, I believe the construct of a depressive "trigger" is nebulous and empirically unverifiable, except perhaps in highly unusual scenarios; e.g., a euthymic subject is injected with a powerful, short-acting biogenic amine-depleting agent; develops severe depressive symptoms within 2 hours; then spontaneously remits over the next 12 hours.

The Appeal to "Tradition"

Horwitz and Wakefield repeatedly invoke what they call the "2500 year history of psychiatric medicine" [2, 3] in defending their depression "with cause" versus "without cause" distinction. Citing Aristotle, Felix Platter, and Emil Kraepelin, Horwitz and Wakefield argue that only depressive syndromes "without cause" were considered "mental disorders" throughout most of medical history [3, p. 58]. Our modern diagnostic schema, they maintain, "radically diverges from what has traditionally been considered appropriate" [3, p. 53].

Let us put aside the suspicion that this argument is essentially an appeal to "eminence-based medicine." We must still ask whether the "with cause/without cause" distinction is truly representative of how most physicians have reasoned *and acted* during the entire 2500 year history of medicine. H. C. Erik Midelfort, Professor of History at the University of Virginia, and author of the book, *A History of Madness in Sixteenth Century Germany* (Stanford University Press) comments on this as follows:

> "... for ancient and early modern physicians, there was *no clear, bright line between disease and health*. They did not, generally, decide that someone was suffering an understandable and proportionate sadness and was not therefore 'ill.' They generally decided that if one were suffering, *for whatever reason and whether proportionate or disproportionate*, they would do what they could to help...[and their remedies] did not depend upon a strict decision that so-and-so was fundamentally 'ill' while someone else was merely sad for good, sufficient, and proportionate reasons" (italics added; personal communication, October 12, 2008).

Indeed, the physician's primary role has always been to *relieve suffering and incapacity*—not to act as an amateur evolutionary biologist and sit in lofty judgment, as regards how "proportionate" a patient's response is to some putative stressor. And when ethnic, cultural, and religious factors are considered, the notion of computing a "proportionate" response becomes even less tenable.

Is There Really an "Epidemic" of Depression?

Epidemiological data from the 1980s [10] indeed suggested that the incidence of depressive disorders in cohorts born since WW II has been increasing in some countries, such as the U.S., Sweden, and Germany. However, recent, multi-decade epidemiological data from both the Baltimore ECA Study [11] and the Lundby Study [12] from Sweden strongly suggest that the incidence of depression over the past 30-50 years has remained more or less the same, with the possible exception of rising rates in women. Both these studies used criteria similar to the "precipitant-neutral" criteria of DSM-III and DSM-IV.

To be sure, Horwitz and Wakefield do not claim that that there has been an "actual increase" in rates of depressive illness [3 p. 4]. Rather, they point to "...the recent pandemic of seeming depressive disorder," which they unambiguously attribute to "...changes in the psychiatric diagnostic system presented in DSM-III..." [2]. Furthermore, they believe that virtually all community-based epidemiologic studies of depression since the late 1970s are contaminated by "false positive" diagnoses of depression, owing to use of "decontextualized" DSM criteria [3].

But this notion of "false positives" is troubling on several levels. First, we do not have a veridical "test" for depression—akin to, say, detecting *treponema pallidum* in syphilis—that would demonstrate that subjects have been "falsely" diagnosed as depressed, by DSM criteria. Nor, as healers, should we insist on such a test. Furthermore, the claim that epidemiological studies of depression produce many "false positives" is entirely circular. It *assumes as true precisely what Horwitz and Wakefield have failed to prove*: namely, that we should not "count" cases of bereavement-related depression as depression. This would be analogous to a cancer researcher arguing that we should exclude mesothelioma cases that appear to be "provoked" by environmental carcinogens, without *first* demonstrating that such "precipitated" cases differ in their *pathophysiology, course, outcome, response to treatment*, etc., compared with spontaneous cases.

As for reports of rising rates of "depression" as a psychiatric diagnosis, and increased antidepressant prescribing rates in recent years [3, p. 187], these trends are probably driven by numerous factors, including increased public awareness of depression; increased help-seeking; exposure of both patients and physicians to "Big Pharma" advertising; and pressure exerted by third-party payers to provide "reimbursable" diagnoses. These trends are certainly worrisome, *but they cannot confidently be attributed to changes in our diagnostic criteria for depression*. Indeed, I believe that over-diagnosis of depression—to the extent it occurs—often results from a *failure to apply DSM criteria stringently*, rather than to their use. This, however, is a conundrum that requires much more study.

objections to the H-W thesis should not be misconstrued as a blanket endorsement of DSM-IV (or DSM-5) criteria for major depressive disorder (MDD). Among several problems with these criteria [13], the *two-week duration criterion may be too brief*. (Dr. Sidney Zisook, personal communication, November 7, 2008). Extending it to 3-4 weeks might slightly decrease sensitivity, but could increase *specificity* for MDD. Only carefully conducted, longitudinal studies of MDD outcome will decide the matter. But extending the duration criterion for MDD has nothing to do with attributing "special properties" to depression in the context of loss. It simply reflects the clinical observation that some patients with depression of only 1-2 weeks duration *may spontaneously remit*, given another 2-3 weeks.

Neither do I mean to suggest that the DSM's categorical system of diagnosis represents the pinnacle of psychiatric wisdom. I and many others have long believed that a "dimensional," psychodynamic, spiritual, and phenomenological understanding of grief and depression should complement and enrich the DSM categories [14-18].

A Heart Attack Is a Heart Attack

Dr. Zisook has observed that when someone has a myocardial infarction (MI), physicians regard it as a probable manifestation of cardiac *disease*, regardless of its "context." The MI may have occurred in the context of the patient's poor diet, smoking, and high levels of psychic stress—but it is still an expression of *disease*. We do not try to "normalize" the MI by saying, "Well, *you'd* have a heart attack, too, if *you* had been exposed to that much stress!" (This is a version of what I call the "Fallacy of Misplaced Empathy" [19].) To be sure, knowing the medical and psychosocial context helps us *counsel and treat* the post-MI patient, just as knowing the experiential and socio-cultural context of a patient's depression facilitates holistic treatment, as Dr. Zisook observes *(*personal communication, November 7, 2008). And, in so far as Horwitz and Wakefield have shown us the importance of "context" *in these respects*, they have performed a useful service. One hopes their book may also spark much-needed research, since there is a paucity of rigorous, controlled studies of bereavement- vs. non-bereavement related depression.

Nevertheless, as Maj concludes, "At the present state of knowledge, it may be…unwise to disallow the diagnosis of major depression in a person meeting the severity, duration, and impairment criteria for that diagnosis just because the depressive state occurs in the context of a significant life event" [1]. Depression is a potentially *lethal* condition. It would be tragic if we inadvertently discouraged recently bereaved persons from seeking professional help, on the dubious presupposition that their depressive symptoms are merely "normal adaptations" to loss.

Ackowledgments

I wish to thank the following for their helpful comments on various aspects, or early drafts, of this commentary: Prof. H. C. Erik Midelfort, Mario Maj, MD, Sidney Zisook, MD, Michael B. First, MD, David Brent, MD, Dr. Cecilia Mattisson, Prof. Nancy Siraisi, William W. Eaton, PhD, and Richard A. Friedman MD. A slightly modified version of this piece appeared in the December 1, 2008, issue of *Psychiatric Times*.

References

[1] Maj M. Depression, bereavement, and "understandable" intense sadness: should the DSM-IV approach be revised? *Am J Psychiatry*. 2008;165:1373-1375.

[2] Horwitz AV, Wakefield JC. An Epidemic of depression. Major depressive disorder or normal sadness? *Psychiatr Times*. 2008 25 November.

[3] Horwitz AV, Wakefield JC. *The Loss of Sadness.* New York: Oxford University Press; 2007.

[4] Pies R. Depression and the pitfalls of causality: implications for DSM-V. *J Affect Disord.* 2009;116(1-2):1-3.

[5] Brent DA, Perper JA, Moritz G et al. Major depression or uncomplicated bereavement? A follow-up of youth exposed to suicide. *J Am Acad Child Adolesc Psychiatry.* 1994;33:231-239.

[6] Karam E, Tabet CC, Alam D et al. Bereavement related and non-bereavement related depressions: A comparative field study. *J Affect Disord.* 2009;112(1-3):102-110.

[7] Zisook S, Kendler KS. Is bereavement-related depression different than non-bereavement-related depression? *Psychol Med.* 2007;37:779-794.

[8] Kendler KS, Myers J, Zisook S. Does bereavement-related major depression differ from major depression associated with other stressful life events? *Am J Psychiatry.* 2008;165:1449-1455.

[9] Wakefield JC, Schmitz MF, First MB, Horwitz AV. Extending the bereavement exclusion for major depression to other losses: evidence from the National Comorbidity Survey. *Arch Gen Psychiatry.* 2007;64:433-440.

[10] Klerman GL, Weissman MM. Increasing rates of depression. *JAMA.* 1989;261:2229-2235.

[11] Eaton WW, Kalaydjian A, Scharfstein DO, et al. Prevalence and incidence of depressive disorder: the Baltimore ECA follow-up, 1981-2004. *Acta Psychiatr Scand.* 2007;116(3):182-188.

[12] Mattisson C, Bogren M, Nettelbladt P, et al. First incidence depression in the Lundby Study: A comparison of the two time periods 1947-72 and 1972-1997. *J Affect Disord.* 2005;87:151-160.

[13] Zisook S. Four questions and an alternative. Commentary on Chapter 1, "Diagnosis of Depressive Disorders," by Professor Gordon Parker. In: Herrman H, Maj M, Sartorius N, editors. *Depressive Disorders.* 3rd ed. Volume 9 of WPA series *Evidence and Experience in Psychiatry.* Hoboken, NJ: Wiley-Blackwell; 2009:27-31.

[14] Geppert C. *The value of nothing. Psychiatr Times.* 2009 Jun 2. Available from: http://www.psychiatrictimes.com/articles/value-nothing. Accessed March 9, 2014.

[15] Genova P. Dump the DSM! *Psychiatr Times.* 2003 April 1. Available from: http://www.psychiatrictimes.com/display/article/10168/47316. Accessed March 9, 2014.

[16] Pies R. The anatomy of sorrow: a spiritual, phenomenological, and neurological perspective. *Philos Ethics Humanit Med.* 2008;3:17.

[17] Schwartz MA, Wiggins O. Science, Humanism, and the Nature of Medical Practice: A Phenomenological View. *Perspect Biol Med.* 1985, 28:231-261.

[18] Ghaemi SN. Feeling and time: the phenomenology of mood disorders, depressive realism, and existential psychotherapy. *Schizophr Bull.* 2007;33:122-130.

[19] Pies R. Is grief a mental disorder? No, but it may become one [online]. Psych Central. World of Psychology blog. Available from: http://psychcentral.com/blog/archives/2008/10/04/is-grief-a-mental-disorder-no-but-it-may-become-one/. Accessed February 26, 2014.

For Further Reading

Clayton PJ, Herjanic M, Murphy GE, Woodruff R Jr. Mourning and depression: their similarities and differences. *Can Psychiatr Assoc J*. 1974;19:309-312.

Karam EG. The nosological status of bereavement-related depressions. *Br J Psychiatry*. 1994;165:48-52.

Kramer PD. Bereavement-related-depression is depression [online]. Psychology Today. In Practice blog. 2008 September 16. Available from: http://www.psychologytoday.com/blog/in-practice/200809/bereavement-related-depression-is-depression.

Accessed February 26, 2014.

GW Brown. Life events and affective disorder: replications and limitations. *Psychosomatic Med*. 1993;55:248-259.

Almeida DM, Wethington E, Kessler RC. The daily inventory of stressful events: an interview-based approach for measuring daily stressors. *Assessment*. 2002; 9:41-55.

Akiskal HS, Bitar AH, Puzantian VR, et al. The nosological status of neurotic depression: a prospective three- to four-year follow-up examination in light of the primary-secondary and unipolar-bipolar dichotomies. *Arch Gen Psychiatry*. 1978;35:756-766.

~~~~~~~~~~~~~~~~~

AFTER BEREAVEMENT, IS IT "NORMAL GRIEF" OR MAJOR DEPRESSION?

The capacity to be consoled is a consequential distinction between grief and depression.
—Kay Jamison, PhD, Nothing Was the Same

The relationship between grief and depression following recent bereavement has turned into one of the most contentious debates in psychiatry—and has made front-page news in the New York *Times* [1]. Much of the controversy has focused on whether the so-called "bereavement exclusion" in DSM-IV should be eliminated, as some have proposed, in the DSM-5. My colleagues and I have discussed this in several different venues, and have argued that there is no convincing scientific or clinical basis for retaining the bereavement exclusion (BE). In contrast, several prominent clinicians and scholars have argued forcefully for retaining the BE (see references and suggested reading list below). The debates have sometimes shed more heat than light, with one group arguing that the BE confuses clinicians and interferes with the diagnosis and treatment of potentially serious depression (my position); and the other group insisting that eliminating the BE will "medicalize normal grief" and lead to over-prescription of antidepressants. (For those who want to delve into the debate, please see the collegial exchange Dr. Sidney Zisook and I had with Dr. Michael B. First [2].)

In the mean time, the average clinician may be wondering, "What am I supposed to do with my bereaved patients, while the so-called experts are battling it out? How do I distinguish a normal grief reaction, after a loss, from a major depressive episode?" As a small step toward addressing this conundrum, I have developed an assessment tool that I call the *Post-Bereavement Phenomenology Inventory* (PBPI). The tool can be found as an addendum at the end of this chapter. It is based on the premise that the DSM symptom checklists simply do not permit an in-depth understanding of the different "world views" represented by ordinary ("productive") grief and major depression [3-5]. Thus, the term "phenomenology" is used in the philosophical sense, in reference to the subjective experience of the patient—in effect, the structure and contents of the patient's mental life [6].

The PBPI represents neither a *categorical* nor a *dimensional* model of psychiatric evaluation; rather, it is an example of "prototype matching," an approach that has shown promise in the diagnosis of bipolar disorder [7, 8]. Although the PBPI is aimed primarily at assessing response to *bereavement* (the death of a loved one), it is my hope that it will also be of use after any major loss, such as divorce, job loss, the break-up of an intimate relationship, etc. First, though, some caveats about the PBPI:

1) I offer this preliminary screening instrument without any claim that it has been validated in clinical studies; that it replaces a conventional "DSM" approach to diagnosis; or that it may be used in forensic assessments.
2) The PBPI is not intended as a substitute for a full psychiatric evaluation, including the use of validated screening instruments, such as the Beck Depression Inventory or other depression rating scales.
3) The PBPI is expected to be most useful when the results are *combined with more empirical clinical findings in major depression*, such as the absence or presence of early morning awakening, pronounced weight loss, visible psychomotor agitation or retardation, diurnal mood variation, etc.
4) The interpretation of patients' response to the PBPI has not yet been quantified, and there is as yet no "scoring system" for the results. Eventually, the items on the PBPI may be converted to a 4- or 5-point Likert-type scale.
5) The PBPI is not directly "translatable" into a DSM or ICD diagnosis; rather, it is intended to raise (or lower) the clinician's *index of suspicion* that a bereaved patient may be experiencing a major depressive episode.

I am hoping that the PBPI will serve a heuristic purpose, in stimulating research on post-bereavement grief and depression. Indeed, the PBPI lends itself to many testable hypotheses and empirically falsifiable predictions. For example, I would hypothesize that patients who show a prominently "left-sided" profile of responses are more likely to represent cases of major depressive disorder (MDD), as determined by a complete diagnostic evaluation. Further, I would hypothesize that patients with a strong left-sided profile would prove to be at a relatively higher risk of suicide, psychiatric hospitalization, and social-vocational impairment, compared with patients showing a prominent right-sided profile. In contrast, I would predict that those with a prominent right-sided profile would usually prove to be experiencing ordinary or "productive" grief, in response to a recent major loss.

Based on the premise that grief and major depression are distinct constructs (albeit with some overlapping symptoms [5]), I would expect that most bereaved patients will produce something close to an "en bloc" response profile; i.e., either most of the left-sided *or* most of the right-sided responses will be checked off. However, human emotional responses are notoriously prone to defying our constructs! It is certainly possible that some patients will produce a "mixed" or "left/right" response pattern. It is not clear what condition this would represent, though, in theory, patients who are experiencing "complicated grief" [5] (sometimes called "pathological grief") might produce such variegated responses. This is a question that will need to be settled with careful, empirical research.

It also seems plausible that a variety of biological, psychological, and social variables might cause a "shift to the left" or to the right, if the same patient were to complete the PBPI several times, over a period of weeks or months. For example, a person early in the course of bereavement who receives supportive counseling could—in principle—show a shift to the right (toward ordinary or productive grief) in the course of treatment. Conversely, a bereaved patient whose grieving process is somehow thwarted or overwhelmed by a supervening major depressive episode might show a "shift to the left," given serial PBPIs. Thus, sequential PBPIs might prove useful in the ongoing assessment of bereaved patients.

From the standpoint of clinical management, however, clinicians should assume that *left-sided responses "trump" right-sided ones*. For example, any patient checking off item 8 ("persistent thoughts or impulses about ending my life") will require immediate and thorough clinical evaluation, regardless of the patient's having checked off several items on the right. Similarly, a pattern of "5,9,10" checked off on the left—suggesting feelings of worthlessness, anhedonia, and psychomotor retardation—ought to serve as a "red flag" for the clinician. A patient with a "left 5,9,10" pattern merits careful evaluation, in order to rule out a major depressive disorder—even if he or she checks several responses on the right.

Clearly, the particular patterns of responses and their interpretation will require careful longitudinal studies of post-bereavement grief and depression. Ultimately, I would like to see these two profiles of responses correlated with such indices as *number of psychiatric hospitalizations; frequency of suicide attempts; impairment in vocational function; and biomarkers of major depression*, such as neuroendocrine and inflammatory responses. Hence, I welcome feedback from clinicians who might wish to use the PBPI as part of a research study of post-bereavement grief or depression, and I place no restrictions on its professional use. (However, it is not intended as a "self-screening" instrument, and those experiencing pronounced depressive symptoms should, as always, be guided by a thorough professional evaluation.)

It is my hope that the PBPI may point the clinician toward the need for further clinical assessment—and will perhaps provide a deeper understanding of the bereaved patient's "inner world" than that obtained from symptom check lists.

Acknowledgments

I would like to thank Sidney Zisook, MD, and M. Katherine Shear, MD, for their helpful comments on an earlier draft of this scale, and for their seminal contributions to this area of research. A slightly modified version of this piece appeared in the February 21, 2012, issue of *Psychiatric Times*.

References

[1] Carey B. Grief could join list of disorders. *The New York Times*. 2012 January 24. Available from: http://www.nytimes.com/2012/01/25/health. Accessed March 8, 2014.

[2] First MB, Pies RW, Zisook S. Depression or bereavement? Defining the distinction [online]. Medscape Psychiatry. 2011 April 8. Available from: http://www.medscape.com/viewarticle/740333. Accessed February 24, 2014.

[3] Pies R. The anatomy of sorrow: a spiritual, phenomenological, and neurological perspective. *Philos Ethics Humanit Med*. 2008; 3:17. Available from: http://www.ncbi.nlm.nih.gov/pmc/articles/PMC2442112/. Accessed February 24, 2014.

[4] Pies R. The two worlds of grief and depression [online]. Psych Central. World of Psychology blog. Available from: http://psychcentral.com/blog/archives /2011/02/23/the-two-worlds-of-grief-and-depression/. Accessed February 24, 2014.

[5] Zisook S, Shear K. Grief and bereavement: what psychiatrists need to know. *World Psychiatry*. 2009; 8(2):67-74.

[6] Schwartz MA, Wiggins O. Science, humanism, and the nature of medical practice: a phenomenological view. *Perspect Biol Med*. 1985;28:331-366.

[7] Zimmerman M, Galione JN, Ruggero CJ et al. A different approach toward screening for bipolar disorder: the prototype matching method. *Compr Psychiatry*. 2010;51:340-346.

[8] Ghaemi SN, Miller CJ, Berv DA, Klugman J, Rosenquist KJ, Pies R. Sensitivity and specificity of a new bipolar spectrum diagnostic scale. *J Affect Disord*. 2005; 84:273-277.

For Further Reading

Grohol J. Will depression include normal grieving too? [online] Psych Central World of Psychology blog. Available from: http://psychcentral.com/blog/archives/2012/01/25/will-depression-include-normal-grieving-too/. Accessed March 9, 2014.

Zisook S, Reynolds CF 3rd, Pies R, et al. Bereavement, complicated grief, and DSM, part 1: depression. *J Clin Psychiatry*. 2010;71:955-956.

Zisook S, Simon N, Reynolds C, et al. Bereavement, complicated grief, and DSM, part 2: complicated grief. *J Clin Psychiatry*. 2010;71:1097-1098.

Bonanno GA, Wortman CB, Lehman DR, et al. Resilience to loss and chronic grief: A prospective study from pre-loss to 18 months post-loss. *J Pers Soc Psychol*. 2002;83: 1150-1164.

Frances A. Good grief. *The New York Times*. 2010 August 14. Available from: http://www.nytimes.com/2010/08/15/opinion/15frances.html. Accessed March 1, 2014.

Ghaemi SN. Feeling and time: the phenomenology of mood disorders, depressive realism, and existential psychotherapy. *Schizophr Bull*. 2007;33:122-130.

Jamison KR. *Nothing Was the Same*. New York: Vintage Books; 2011.

Pies R, Zisook S. Grief and depression redux: Response to Dr. Frances's "Compromise" *Psychiatr Times*. 2010 September 28. Available from: http://www.psychiatrictimes.com/dsm-5/content/article/10168/1679026.

Accessed February 24, 2014.

Clayton PJ. Bereavement and Depression. *J Clin Psychiatry*. 1990;51:34-38.

Pies R. Once again: Grief is not a disorder, but it may be accompanied by major depression: *A Response to Dr John Grohol. Psychiatr Times*. 2012 January 27. Available from:

http://www.psychiatrictimes.com/blog/pies/content/article/10168 /2023007. Accessed March 9, 2014.

Wakefield J. DSM-5: proposed changes to depressive disorders. *Curr Med Res Opin.* 2012;28:335-343.

Lamb K, Pies R, Zisook S. The Bereavement Exclusion for the diagnosis of major depression: to be or not to be? *Psychiatry (Edgemont).* 2010;7(7):19-25.

Addendum

The Post-Bereavement Phenomenology Inventory (PBPI)

Instructions to patient: People who have experienced a recent, major loss react in a variety of ways. There are no "right" or "wrong" responses to this questionnaire. After each numbered item, please check the sentence (either in the left *or* right column) that *better describes* how you have been feeling, thinking, or behaving for the past 1-2 *months*. Please check only *one* box for each numbered item:

Which fits you better:

The sentence on the left:	Or... The sentence on the right?
1. I am filled with despair nearly all the time, and I almost always feel hopeless about the future ☐	I feel sadness a lot of the time, but I believe that eventually, things will get better ☐
2. My sadness or depressed mood is nearly constant, and it isn't improved by any positive events, activities or people. ☐	My sadness or depressed mood usually comes in "waves" or "pangs", and there are events, activities or people who help me feel better. ☐
3. When I am reminded of my loss (of a loved one, friend, job, etc.) I feel nothing but pain, bitterness, or bad memories ☐	When I am reminded of my loss (of a loved one, friend, job, etc.) I often feel intense grief or have painful memories; but sometimes, I have good thoughts and pleasant memories. ☐
4. I will probably never get back to feeling like my "old self" again. ☐	Things are really tough now, but I'm hopeful that, with time, I will feel more like my "old self." ☐
5. I feel like a worthless person who has done mostly bad things in life, and let my friends, family and loved ones down. ☐	I feel like I'm basically a good person and that in general, I have done my best for my friends, family and loved ones. ☐

(Continued)

The sentence on the left:	Or... The sentence on the right?
6. All I can think about lately is myself, and how miserable I feel; I hardly think about friends, family or loved ones, except to blame myself for some failing. ☐	Even though I'm less social and outgoing since my loss, I still think a lot about friends, family and loved ones, often with good feelings about them. ☐
7. When friends or family call or visit, and try to cheer me up, I don't feel anything, or I may feel even worse. ☐	When friends or family call or visit and try to cheer me up, I usually "perk up" for a while and enjoy the social contact. ☐
8. I often have persistent thoughts or impulses about ending my life, and I often think I'd be better off dead. ☐	I sometimes feel like a part of me has been lost, and I wish I could be re-united with the person or part of my life I am missing; but I still think life is worth living. ☐
9. Almost nothing that I used to like doing (reading, listening to music, sports, hobbies, etc.) is of any comfort or consolation to me anymore. ☐	The things that I have always liked doing (reading, listening to music, sports, hobbies, etc.) give me some comfort and consolation, at least temporarily. ☐
10. I feel "slowed down" inside, like my body and mind are stuck or frozen, and like time itself is standing still. ☐	My concentration isn't as good as usual, but my body and mind aren't slowed down, and time passes in the usual way. ☐

Source: Ronald Pies, MD, 2012.

~~~~~~~~~~~~~~~~~

GRIEF AND DEPRESSION: THE SAGES KNEW THE DIFFERENCE

There is nothing as whole as a broken heart.—the Kotzker Rebbe

In the intense debate over elimination of the "bereavement exclusion" from the DSM-5, a persistent claim among those who opposed the elimination was that intense grief and mild major depression are virtually indistinguishable—at least, shortly following the death of a loved one [1]. But while it is true that the intense grief of bereavement and major depressive disorder (MDD) often share some features—for example, tearfulness, insomnia, low mood, and decreased appetite--there are many substantive differences [2, 3]. This is true not merely in terms of the DSM's "check lists" of symptoms, but also in *phenomenological* terms; i.e., *how the affected person experiences herself and the world* [4]. For example, unlike the person with MDD, most recently bereaved individuals are usually not preoccupied with feelings of worthlessness, hopelessness, or unremitting gloom; rather, self-esteem is usually preserved; the bereaved person can envision a "better day"; and positive thoughts and feelings are often interspersed with negative ones [2, 3, 4].

It is striking that many sages and scholars of ancient and early modern times seem to have appreciated these differences far better than some modern-day writers. Indeed, the distinction between severe ("clinical") depression and ordinary sorrow seems to be as old as recorded history. Thus, in the Old Testament, the figure of King David presents us with portraits of *both* severe depression *and* normal bereavement. In Psalm 38, conventionally ascribed to David, the psalmist laments his sins. He tells us that "There is no soundness in my flesh...no health in my bones because of my sin...my wounds grow foul and fester because of my foolishness, I am utterly bowed down and prostrate; all the day I go about mourning...I groan because of the tumult of my heart" [5]. Modern diagnosticians would see in this description a picture quite consistent with an episode of severe (perhaps melancholic) major depression. In contrast, after the death of his beloved friend, Jonathan, the very same King David is moved to write a passionately stirring dirge, known as "The Lament of the Bow" (2 Samuel 1:17-27), addressed to his lost friend: "How have the mighty fallen...I grieve for you, my brother Jonathan, you were most dear to me..." [5]. There is no trace, in David's lament, of the self-loathing and bodily decay found in Psalm 38. David's period of mourning after Jonathan's death represents roughly what modern-day mental health professionals would call "uncomplicated bereavement"—not clinical depression.

Fast-forward nearly three millennia to 19th century Europe, in the area of present-day Belarus, where the Jewish mystical movement known as *Hasidism* was developing. There we find the remarkable figure of Rabbi Schneur Zalman of Liady (1745-1812), known as "The Alter Rebbe"—the founder of what became known as *Chabad* [6]. (The term "Chabad" is an acronym of three Hebrew words that mean "wisdom, understanding, and knowledge"). Chabad—also known as the *Lubavitch* movement—represented a synthesis of the rational and mystical elements of Judaism. While a detailed discussion of Chabad would take us far afield, it is quite extraordinary to find that Rabbi Schneur Zalman (RSZ) described a typology of grief and depression that bears an uncanny resemblance to our modern-day understanding of these conditions. In his classic work known as the *Tanya*, RSZ distinguished between two conditions, called *merirut* and *atzvut* [6]. While these terms are variously translated, their rough, English equivalents are, respectively, *sorrow* and *melancholy*. They are also sometimes distinguished as *constructive grief* vs. *destructive grief*; or as *bitterness* vs. *dejection*. In distinguishing *merirut* from *atzvut*, Rabbi Aryeh Kahn puts it this way:

> "The first is active, the second—passive. The first one weeps, the second's eyes are dry and blank. The first one's mind and heart are in turmoil; the second's are still with apathy and heavy as lead. And what happens when it passes, when they emerge from their respective bouts of grief? The first one springs to action: resolving, planning, taking his first faltering steps to undo the causes of his sorrow. The second one goes to sleep" (based on *Tanya*, ch.31) [7].

Table 1. Comparison of Mood States

	Merirut	Atzvut	Melancholia
Definition, alternate terms	Constructive grief, sorrow, bitterness	Destructive grief, "black depression," melancholy, dejection, "bottomless pit"	"Black bile"
Mood, feeling tone	Sadness, weeping, mind and heart in turmoil	Misery, apathy, numbing, feelings blocked, eyes dry and blank, mind and heart "heavy as lead"	Blunted emotional response, unremitting apprehension, no mood reactivity
Energy/psychomotor Change	Vibrant, awakened, active, "springs to action" to undo cause of sorrow	Passive, no initiative	Psychomotor retardation (anergia, torpor) or agitation
Vegetative functions	? No clear change	Excessive sleep	Disturbance in sleep (usually early a.m. awakening) decreased appetite/weight diurnal mood variation (mood, energy, usually worse in a.m.)
Somatic experience or expression	? No clear somatic abnormalities	Heart is "constricted" and "dull as a stone"	Reduced facial and vocal reactivity
Self-image	"Springboard" for self-improvement; soul-searching arising from one's spiritual stocktaking	Despair toward oneself; person nurses awareness of misfortunes, feels worthless, disgraced	Nihilistic convictions of hopelessness, guilt, sin, ruin; psychosis sometimes present
Social function	No severe impairment described	Focused on self, no desire to emerge, neither initiating nor welcoming communication; "No mood to face the world and its obstacles."	Social withdrawal
World view	Basic optimism toward life is retained	Despair toward mankind, drained of hope	Morbid thoughts, nihilistic convictions of hopelessness, guilt, sin, ruin;
Course/outcome	Followed by joy	Deteriorating course w/ further depression	Poor outcome unless treated effectively

Source: Ronald Pies, MD, April, 2013.

Merirut, in other words, is constructive; *atzvut*, destructive. The epigram at the beginning of this essay—"There is nothing as whole as a broken heart"—expresses a crucial paradox: when we grieve in a "healthy" and adaptive way, we ultimately integrate the loss into the larger fabric of our life. We learn and grow, even as we ache with sorrow. In contrast, with severe depression, we are beaten down and sometimes broken. Indeed, *atzvut*—destructive grief—bears some striking resemblances to our modern-day conception of melancholia, as described by Fink and Taylor [8, 9]. Table 1 summarizes some of the main features of *merirut, atzvut*, and melancholia.

Perhaps if Rabbi Schneur Zalman had been around during the recent, vitriolic debate over the bereavement exclusion, we would have seen more light and felt less heat!

Acknowledgment

I wish to thank Rabbi Bezalel Naor for pointing out RSZ's distinction between *merirut* and *atzvut*. A slightly modified version of this piece appeared in the April 29, 2013, issue of *Psychiatric Times*.

References

[1] e.g., see Russell Friedman : "Not even the best trained clinicians can distinguish grief from mild depression." (If this were true, of course, then no clinician could ever be accused of having been *mistaken* in diagnosing *either* grief *or* mild major depression, shortly after bereavement.) Quoted in: Frances A. Last plea to DSM-5: save grief from the drug companies [online]. Huffington Post blog. 2013 January 7. Available from: http://www.huffingtonpost.com/allen-frances/saving-grief-from-dsm-5-a_b_2325108.html. Accessed March 9, 2014.

[2] Zisook S, Shear K. Grief and bereavement: what psychiatrists need to know. *World Psychiatry*. 2009;8(2):67-74.

[3] Lamb K, Pies R, Zisook S. The bereavement exclusion for the diagnosis of major depression: to be, or not to be. *Psychiatry (Edgmont)*. 2010;7(7):19-25.

[4] Pies R. After bereavement, is it "normal grief" or major depression?

[5] *Psychiatr Times*. 2012 February 21. Available from:

[6] www.psychiatrictimes.com/mdd/content/article/10168/2035804. Accessed March 9, 2014.

[7] Oxford Annotated Bible, Revised Standard Version. Oxford: Oxford University Press; 1962.

[8] Mindel N. *The Philosophy of Chabad*. Brooklyn, NY: Kehot Publication Society; 1985.

[9] Kahn A. Good grief. Available from: http://caje33.wikispaces.com/file/view/Dreskin_bettertishab%27avhandout.pdf. Accessed March 9, 2014.

[10] Kaplan A. Whither melancholia? *Psychiatr Times*. 2010 January 8. Available from: http://www.psychiatrictimes.com/print/article/10168/1508125. Accessed March 9, 2014.

[11] Taylor MA, Fink M. *Melancholia: The Diagnosis, Pathophysiology, and Treatment of Depressive Illness*. Cambridge: Cambridge University Press; 2006.

For Further Reading

Rabbi Adin Steinsaltz. *Understanding the Tanya: Volume Three in the Definitive Commentary on a Classic Work of Kabbalah by the World's Foremost Authority.* San Francisco: Jossey-Bass; 2007.

Rabbi Zushe Greenberg. Sadness [online]. Chabad Jewish Center of Solon. Monthly Messages 2001. Available from: http://www.solonchabad.com/templates/articlecco_cdo/aid/254698/jewish/Monthly-Messages-2001.htm. Accessed February 26, 2014.

Rabbi Yisroel Cotlar. I sinned and repented: now what? [online]. Chabad.org. Available from: http://m.chabad.org/m/article_cdo/aid/1600121. Accessed February 26, 2014.

~~~~~~~~~~~~~~~~~

BEREAVEMENT AND THE DSM-5, ONE LAST TIME

It's now official: to the satisfaction of some and the consternation of others, the DSM-5 has eliminated the so-called bereavement exclusion in the diagnosis of major depressive disorder (MDD). As a specialist in the treatment of mood disorders for over 30 years, I was pleased to see National Public Radio covering this important development [1], but disappointed that only one side of the debate was given prominent coverage. I believe it's important for the public to understand why the DSM-5 will drop the bereavement exclusion—and equally, for clinicians to appreciate the complexities of diagnosing post-bereavement depression, under the new guidelines.

The bereavement exclusion was eliminated from the DSM-5 for two main reasons: (1) there have never been any adequately-controlled, clinical studies showing that major depressive symptoms following bereavement differ in nature, course, or outcome from depression of equal severity in any other context—or from MDD appearing "out of the blue" [2]; and (2) major depression is a potentially lethal disorder, with an overall suicide rate of about 4% [3]. Disqualifying a patient from a diagnosis of major depression simply because the clinical picture emerges after the death of a loved one risks closing the door on potentially life-saving treatment.

True, the "old" DSM-IV criteria provided a mechanism to "override" the bereavement exclusion; for example, if the depressed, bereaved patient were psychotic, suicidal, preoccupied with feelings of worthlessness, or functioning very poorly in daily life. Unfortunately, there are many bereaved patients whose depressive symptoms are *severe*, but who would not "qualify" for the DSM-IV override criteria; for example, those with profoundly impaired concentration, significant weight loss, or severe insomnia. Under the DSM-IV "rules," these bereaved patients probably would not have received a diagnosis of MDD and been provided appropriate treatment. The new DSM-5 criteria will no longer pose the risk of shunting these patients out of the mental health treatment setting.

To be sure, ordinary grief is not a disorder, and does not require professional treatment--nor should any arbitrary time limit be placed on grief, whether after the death of a loved one or any other tragic loss. Contrary to many misleading claims in the lay press, the DSM-5 does *not* impose a time limit on "grief"—a universal and generally adaptive response to loss.

DSM-5 will merely ensure that a particular *subset* of persons with MDD—those who meet full symptom-duration criteria within the first few weeks after the death of a loved one—will no longer be *excluded* from the set of MDD patients as a whole.

The 2-week minimum duration for diagnosing MDD has been carried over from DSM-IV to DSM-5. To be sure, this is sometimes too little time to permit confident diagnosis of MDD. But this is true regardless of the "context" in which the depressive symptoms occur—whether after the death of a loved one; the loss of house and home; or in the absence of any clear precipitant. In ambiguous cases, a patient's prior history of MDD, or a strong family history of depression, can help clinch the diagnosis. And, of course, the prudent clinician always has the option of deferring the diagnosis of MDD for a week or two, in order to see what "trajectory" the bereaved patient's depression takes. Some patients will improve spontaneously, while others will need only a brief, supportive intervention. And nothing in DSM-5's criteria for MDD will deny grieving patients the love and support of family, friends, or clergy.

Furthermore, contrary to insistent cries of alarm by some, "treatment" of post-bereavement depression need not involve antidepressant medication, except in the most severe cases. Psychotherapy alone is appropriate in mild-to-moderate cases, though it is true that this option is not readily available in our dysfunctional health care system—if "system" is not too charitable a term [4]. But this is a societal problem that requires deep, structural changes in how we deliver health care; it is *not* a problem to be solved by jiggering with our diagnostic criteria for major depression.

The text of DSM-5 (e.g., see footnote on p. 161) helps explain some of the important and recognizable differences between uncomplicated ("normal") grief and major depression. For example, bereaved persons with normal grief often experience a mixture of sadness and more pleasant emotions, as they recall memories of the deceased. Anguish and pain are usually experienced in "waves" or "pangs," rather than continuously, as is usually true in major depression [5]. The grieving person typically remains hopeful that things will get better, and is "consolable" with love and support. In contrast, the clinically depressed patient's mood is almost uniformly one of gloom, despair, and hopelessness—nearly all day, nearly every day—and rarely responds to consolation [6].

The person with moderate, uncomplicated grief is unlikely to seek professional or psychiatric help, within the first few weeks after the death of a loved one. Thus, the much-ballyhooed claim that clinicians using the DSM-5 will declare a normally grieving person "mentally ill" after just two weeks is exaggerated and misleading. (The normally grieving patient may be given the "V" code diagnosis of "Uncomplicated Bereavement," V62.82.) In contrast, the grieving person *who develops MDD* often senses that something has gone terribly wrong, and may *then* seek professional help. Providing effective treatment for the grieving person's major depression may actually help in "working through" the grief itself. Indeed, when symptoms of major depression intervene and go untreated, working through grief-- and integrating it into one's life-- is made all the more difficult [5].

The line between health and disease is not always clear, either in psychiatry or in general medicine. In truth, we do not find Nature "carved at its joints", neatly delineating disease from health. Ultimately, physicians must decide how broadly or narrowly to define disease and disorder, with the ultimate aim of *relieving human suffering and incapacity* [7]. There will always be an element of clinical judgment in rendering our diagnoses, and we need to view our diagnostic systems with humility. Moreover, the elimination of the bereavement exclusion will require improved communication between psychiatrists and primary care physicians, who now provide most of the treatment (such as it is) for depressed patients [4]. We need to ensure that PCPs are aware that there are fundamental differences between grief and major depression—and that normal grief must not be "medicated away." Indeed, we must all remain mindful of Erich Fromm's teaching: "To spare oneself from grief at all costs can be achieved only at the price of total detachment, which excludes the ability to experience happiness."

Acknowledgment

A slightly modified version of this piece appeared in the December 11, 2012, issue of Psychiatric Times.

References

[1] Psychiatrists to take new approach in bereavement [online transcript]. All Things Considered. National Public Radio. 2012 December 6. Available from: http://www.npr.org/2012/12/06/166682774/psychiatrists-to-take-new-approach-in-bereavement#commentBlock. Accessed March 9, 2014.
[2] Zisook S, Corruble E, Duan N, et al. The bereavement exclusion and DSM-5. *Depress Anxiety*. 2012;29:425-443.
[3] Coryell W, Young EA. Clinical predictors of suicide in primary major depressive disorder. *J Clin Psychiatry*. 2005;66:412-417.
[4] Pies R. Antidepressants work, sort of—our system of care does not. *J Clin Psychopharmacol*. 2010;30:101-104.
[5] Zisook S, Shear K. Grief and bereavement: what psychiatrists need to know. *World Psychiatry*. 2009;2:67-74. Available from: http://www.ncbi.nlm.nih.gov/pmc/articles/PMC2691160/. Accessed March 9, 2014.
[6] Jamison KR. *Nothing Was the Same*. New York: Knopf; 2009. Also: an excellent video with Dr. Kay R. Jamison explains some of the key differences between grief and depression: http://bigthink.com/ideas/16707
[7] Pies R. Toward a concept of instrumental validity: implications for psychiatric diagnosis. *Dial Phil Ment Neuro Sci*. 2011;4(1):18-19. Available from: http://www.crossingdialogues.com/Ms-D11-01.pdf. Accessed February 26, 2014.

For Further Reading

Pies R. Bereavement does not immunize the grieving person against major depression [online]. GeriPal blog. Available from: http://www.geripal.org/2012/12/bereavement-does-not-immunize-grieving_4.html. Accessed March 9, 2014.

Zisook S, Pies R, Corruble E. When is grief a disease? *The Lancet*. 2012;379:1590.

Bonanno GA, Wortman CB, Lehman DR, et al. Resilience to loss and chronic grief: a prospective study from preloss to 18-months postloss. *J Pers Soc Psychol*. 2002;83:1150-1164.

Chapter 4

PSYCHIATRY IN CRISIS

IS PSYCHIATRY NOW A "HOUSE

Every kingdom divided against itself is brought to desolation; and every city or house divided against itself shall not stand.—Matthew 12:25

Judge the whole of the person charitably.—Talmud (Pirke Avot, 1:6)

"Hired guns." "Whores." "Greedy, insensitive bastards." These are some of the more printable epithets used to describe psychiatric physicians who (allegedly) have "sold out to Big Pharma"—for example, by failing to disclose conflicts of interest, or to report large sums of money earned through their work with pharmaceutical companies. It may surprise some—but perhaps not many—that these terms of abuse were hurled not by members of some anti-psychiatry group, but by *psychiatrists,* writing on a well-known "watchdog" blog site. To be clear: I have no wish to excuse or rationalize the actions of some in our field who indeed have abused the public trust by engaging in any of the actions described. Anger—even outrage—is appropriate and healthy, with respect to their *behavior*. But must we also *demonize* these individuals, some of whom (notwithstanding their transgressions) have made important contributions to clinical care and scientific research?

The late Dr. Albert Ellis—the psychologist who originated Rational Emotive Behavioral Therapy—always insisted that we distinguish between a person's *behavior*, and the individual's *value as a human being*. Writing in their classic 1961 book, *A Guide to Rational Living*, Ellis and his colleague, Robert Harper argued that, "…A person's (good or bad) acts are the *results* of his being, but they are never that being itself" (italics added) [1, p. 104).

We often tell our patients they should not condemn the totality of their being on the basis of a selfish or hurtful act they have committed—yet some of us seem all too ready to condemn a colleague in the most sweeping and dehumanizing terms, because he or she is guilty (or is believed guilty) of one or more ethical lapses. By all means, let us condemn the transgressions! But let's also retain a scintilla of human sympathy and understanding for the flawed human beings who committed them.

The problem of "demonizing rhetoric" is obviously not confined to the field of psychiatry, where it seems to be the effluvium of a few particularly bilious individuals. The language of demonization is all too prevalent in the narratives of many political and religious groups, who attack their opponents as infidels, heretics, traitors, or even worse. Carried to an extreme, we find terms like "vermin" applied to ethnic or religious groups who are the objects of hatred or persecution—the Nazis were infamous in their use of this term. Yes, I know—there is a difference between calling someone a "drug company whore" and reducing the person to the status of vermin. But the distance between the terms is not as wide as some would persuade themselves. And when one moves from the psychiatry blog sites to the rabid anti-psychiatry websites (e.g., http://outlawpsychiatry.blogspot.com), one sees in no uncertain terms how easily an unflattering epithet can morph into a dehumanizing slur.

The divisions within psychiatry extend far beyond concerns over "conflicts of interest" and "Big Pharma"—where there are, at least, valid ethical issues to be raised. Unfortunately, the profession continues to be mired in the same fruitless arguments over "biology" versus "psychology" that anthropologist Tanya Luhrmann documented in her classic investigation, *Of Two Minds: The Growing Disorder in American Psychiatry* (2000). And, all too often, one hears proponents of the "biomedical" model disparaging advocates of the "psychodynamic" model—or vice verse. This sterile debate persists, despite the heroic efforts of "pluralistic unifiers," such as my *Psychiatric Times* colleagues Nassir Ghaemi, James Knoll, Glen Gabbard and Cynthia Geppert—to mention just a few. These clinician-scholars have refused to buy into the Manichean world of the "splitters"; rather, they espouse a scientific-humanistic perspective that comfortably embraces both molecules and motives. This broad-based, pluralistic model was the one I imbibed during my residency at Upstate Medical University, where a fledgling resident could —as my revered teachers, Robert Daly and Eugene Kaplan might put it—"do theology in the morning and biology in the afternoon."

Psychiatry as a profession faces many challenges, and no small number of genuine threats. From excessive involvement with "Big Pharma" to the diminished role of psychotherapy; from managed care's fifteen minute "med checks" to controversies over DSM-5, psychiatry understandably feels besieged, these days. No doubt, we have contributed to many of these problems through our own missteps or inaction. Yet, for all its flaws, psychiatry remains the most comprehensive and humanistic of the medical specialties—and has a great deal to offer the suffering individuals who seek our help. In 1858, Abraham Lincoln—addressing the issue of slavery—warned the nation that, "A house divided against itself cannot stand." It would be a genuine tragedy if psychiatry becomes "a house divided" by the rancor of its own rhetoric.

Acknowledgment

A slightly modified version of this piece appeared in the December 15, 2009, issue of *Psychiatric Times*.

Reference

Ellis A, Harper RA. *A Guide to Rational Living.* Chatsworth, CA: Wilshire Book Company; 1961.

WE ARE ALL DSM5 DIAGNOSTICIANS—WE ARE NOT ALL PHYSICIANS

Another life-time ago—just after leaving residency—I took a job as a psychiatric consultant at a large, university mental health center. Had I known the poisoned politics of the place, I would have headed for someplace safe—like, say, Afghanistan. The mental health center was directed by a very jovial psychologist, who, nominally, was my boss. But the mental health center was a subdivision of the "Student Health Service," which was run by a crusty old internist who may have trained with William Harvey. He steadfastly refused to let the psychologists hospitalize a student in crisis, without first obtaining "medical approval." He wasn't much more respectful of my role, as "Consulting Psychiatrist," and once muttered, within earshot, "A psychiatrist is nothing but a damn psychologist with "M.D." after his name!" I left the job after two frustrating years. My time wasn't wasted, though—I learned a lot about psychopathology in the college-age population, and gained considerable respect for clinical psychologists. (My respect for psychiatric social workers evolved much earlier—the legacy of my late mother, Frances Pies Oliver, ACSW.)

My time at the university clinic also prepared me for the kinds of disagreements we are now facing, as psychiatrists, psychologists, and other mental health professionals weigh in on the DSM-5—and on who is "qualified" to be a DSM-5 "diagnostician." As comments by respected colleagues like Dr. H. Steven Moffic and Dr. Daniel Carlat demonstrate—and as comments by Drs. Charles Huffine, John Riolo, and other fine clinicians reinforce [1]—this is truly a hot-button issue. Though distinct from the substantive controversies surrounding the new DSM-5 criteria, the argument over who "owns" DSM-5 diagnosis is clearly related to the nature of the manual itself.

So let's step back for a moment and ask a fundamental question: what is "diagnosis"? The word may be understood through its Greek origins: *dia-* means "across" or "between"; *gnosis* means "knowledge." So diagnosis may be understood as "knowing the difference between" condition "A" and condition "B." Diagnosis is therefore an inherently *relational* term: you cannot "know" that a patient has schizophrenia without knowing that he or she does *not* have another condition that could also account for the symptom picture—like, say, chronic amphetamine abuse. ("Knowing", of course, is a tad grandiose—I really mean something like, "having a very high degree of factually-based confidence.")

This is one reason that the recent DSMs have incorporated *exclusionary criteria* for the principal (and usually, most serious) psychiatric disorders. Thus, in the DSM-5 criteria for schizophrenia, the "E" criterion states, *"The disturbance is not attributable to the physiological effects of a substance (e.g., a drug of abuse, a medication) or another medical condition."* The clear implication is that one must rule out a variety of "medical conditions" in order to diagnose schizophrenia. Similar exclusion criteria are built into the constructs of major depressive and manic episodes. To *diagnose* schizophrenia or mania, therefore, is to *know the difference between* these states and, for example: Wilson's Disease; complex partial seizures; phencyclidine or cocaine intoxication; corticosteroid toxicity; CNS lupus; and a tumor of the left temporal lobe.

Is it "elitist," parochial, or merely defending one's "turf" to claim that only physicians, among mental health professionals, have the requisite training and expertise to make such determinations? I believe the answer is *no*. But is it elitist to claim that only physicians—

especially psychiatrists—can contribute in valuable ways to a patient's DSM-5 diagnosis? I'd shout "Yes!" to that one.

As a psychiatry resident, I learned valuable diagnostic wisdom from a number of my psychologist supervisors. The psychologists will often pick up personality traits and psychodynamic issues that I sometimes miss; and the neuropsychologists, in particular, are better than I am at picking up subtle deficits related to regional brain dysfunction. Psychiatric social workers are also better than I am at delving into the patient's family systems issues, social supports, economic pressures, housing problems, and marital stressors that used to be coded on that woefully neglected, multi-axial stepchild, Axis IV. (The DSM-5, of course, has done away with the entire multi-axial system). And let's not forget about the clinical nurse specialists, physician's assistants, psychiatric nurses, and mental health aides—all of whom have valuable knowledge and experience to contribute to the patient's care.

But before we all break out into the proverbial chorus of "Kumbaya," let me be clear: respect for the knowledge and wisdom of other professionals does not mean creating a false "democracy" of interchangeable diagnosticians. Ultimate responsibility for the patient's diagnosis will inevitably reside with the identified attending physician. And by "inevitably," I mean something like: *you*, as the attending physician and "Captain of the Ship," will be the one hauled up in front of the judge and jury to explain why Mr. Jones's temporal lobe tumor was called "paranoid schizophrenia" for four years—until Mr. Jones keeled over dead, from elevated intracranial pressure.

Does this mean that psychiatrists are infallible diagnosticians, or that we routinely perform up to our own standards of medical training? Alas, no. Too many psychiatrists, in my view, have forgotten how to inflate that blood pressure cuff to check for postural hypotension; and too many of us prematurely reach a "psychiatric" diagnosis before obtaining routine laboratory tests, such as thyroid functions. To this day, I am still haunted by a case of neurosyphilis I missed many years ago, in a hospitalized patient diagnosed with chronic schizophrenia.

We can all do better. We are all "diagnosticians." And we can all contribute in important ways to the DSM-5 diagnostic process. But we are not all physicians.

Acknowledgment

A slightly modified version of this piece appeared in the February 17, 2010, issue of *Psychiatric Times*.

Reference

[1] Moffic HS. CAUTION! Who should be the DSM-5 diagnostician? *Psychiatr Times*. 2010 February 3. (See comments by Drs. Huffine and others.) Available from: http://www.psychiatrictimes.com/caution-who-should-be-dsm-5-diagnostician. Accessed March 9, 2014.

For Further Reading

Simon RI, Shuman DW. *Clinical Manual of Psychiatry and Law.* Washington DC: American Psychiatric Publishing; 2007. (See in particular the concept of *respondeat superior*, pp. 25-26.)

Pies R, Summergrad P. Dementia, delirium and other cognitive disorders. In: WikiBooks Textbook of Psychiatry [online]. Most recent review 2013 March 21. Available from: http://en.wikibooks.org/wiki/Textbook_of_Psychiatry. Accessed March 9, 2014.

Oyebode F. The neurology of psychosis. *Med Princ Pract.* 2008;17:263-269.

~~~~~~~~~~~~~~~~~

DOCTOR: ARE YOU "DRUGGING" OR "MEDICATING" YOUR PATIENTS? ANTIPSYCHIATRY AND THE WAR OF WORDS

Philosophical problems begin when language goes on holiday.—Ludwig Wittgenstein [1]

You have read the blogs and seen the placards a dozen times: *doctors prescribe too many "drugs" for too many patients.* Psychiatrists, in particular, are popular targets of politically-motivated language that seeks to conflate the words "medication" and "drug"—thereby tapping into the public's understandable fears concerning "drug abuse" and our need to carry out a "War on Drugs." Misleading radio ads promise "drug-free" treatment of panic disorder (certainly possible, but not always achievable) and the internet bristles with the phrase, "psychiatric drugging" (my February 7, 2014, Google search pulled up 27,000 results). And, all too predictably, any physician who argues that psychotropic medication is often an effective and life-saving intervention is hustled off to the perp-line of "drug company shills."

All this will not surprise students of language, history, and philosophy. Those who control language are well positioned to control thought and behavior. If government officials can persuade the public that killing innocent civilians is merely "collateral damage," they have gone a long way toward justifying the carpet-bombing of a village. If anti-psychiatry groups and bloggers can persuade the public that psychiatry is "drugging" people, they have gone a long way toward marginalizing and discrediting the profession. To understand how powerful the words "drug" and "drugging" are, imagine the feckless campaign that would be waged if the perennial protesters in front of the APA's Annual Meeting carried signs that read, "Psychiatrists: Stop Medicating Your Patients!"

Is this all merely a matter of "semantics" or—in the parlance of postmodernism—"competing narratives"? Is there any scientific reason to distinguish "drugs" from "medications"? And finally, what are our ethical obligations as healers when medication is administered, either voluntarily or—far less frequently—involuntarily?

There is, of course, a qualified scientific case to be made against overuse of some psychotropic medications. In the first place, we have far too many medications using the same old mechanism of action, with only modest efficacy, and too many unacceptable side effects. The so-called atypical antipsychotics (AAPs) are good examples. With the clear exception of clozapine—and possibly risperidone and olanzapine, according to one meta-analysis [2]—the AAPs are not substantially more effective than the first-generation neuroleptics. Meta-analyses, of course, must be viewed cautiously, since the studies that compose them may be flawed or biased, and unpublished "negative" studies may be excluded, as my colleague Nassir Ghaemi, MD, has pointed out [3]. Thankfully, decreased rates of tardive dyskinesia with the AAPs are a bright spot in this otherwise downbeat assessment, and this is no trivial gain.

Nonetheless, the metabolic side effects of the AAPs (weight gain, lipid and glucose dysregulation, etc.) are substantial problems, and call into question the goal of expanding the labeled "non-psychotic" indications for these medications [4]. We sorely need to escape from the "D2-5HT2-me too" paradigm—antipsychotics that block mainly dopamine-2 and various serotonin receptors—and uncover more fundamental mechanisms of antipsychotic action. Critics of psychiatry are indeed justifiably skeptical regarding "Big Pharma's" concerted efforts to expand the use of AAPs to the treatment of non-psychotic conditions, for which effective and better-tolerated medications are already available. And yes—many of these same critics are quite properly alarmed at the decreasing use of psychotherapy in psychiatric practice [5].

In short, our antipsychotic pharmacopeia is nothing to brag about. And yet, psychiatrists must resist those who would hijack language in the service of their narrow political agenda—that of discrediting psychiatry and psychiatric treatment. We must begin by pushing back against the campaign to eliminate psychiatric "drugs," by pointing out that there are substantial biochemical and clinical differences between many life-enhancing *psychotropic medications* and *drugs of abuse,* such as heroin and cocaine. For example, contrary to the notion that antidepressants produce only "cosmetic" changes that "cover up symptoms," we now have compelling evidence from animal models that antidepressants are working at the deep, structural level of the gene. Thus, antidepressants are known to increase production of various nerve growth factors, and to enhance the "connections" between neurons. Indeed, a recent review by Schmidt & Duman concluded that "...hippocampal atrophy is observed in patients with depression, and this effect is blocked or reversed by antidepressant treatments" [6]. A similar case for benign neurotrophic effects can also be made for lithium and possibly some of the atypical antipsychotics.

Let me be clear: as physicians and healers, psychiatrists have an ethical responsibility to see that medications are prescribed and administered in a compassionate and non-coercive way, consistent with the principles of informed consent and respect for personal autonomy. When informed consent from the patient is not possible—in certain emergency situations, or when the patient lacks the cognitive capacity to make informed medication decisions—we must ensure that medication decisions proceed through "due process of law." This may require obtaining a legal guardianship, or seeking a judicial determination that involuntary medication is justified. And, beyond informed consent, our medication decisions should consider the patient's personal, cultural, and spiritual needs, as articulated by my colleague, Cynthia Geppert, MD [7].

Yes, one can argue that, in today's setting of "mis-managed care," psychotropic medication is sometimes prescribed too readily, when psychotherapy would be the preferred treatment. And, yes: we need more effective medications in psychiatry, used in more judicious ways—particularly in children, adolescents, and those with dementia, for whom our evidence-base is often shaky. We should be wary of attempts to expand both our disease categories and the labeled indications for psychotropic medications. But to lump all psychotropic medications in with drugs of abuse is to embrace junk science and junk rhetoric. Psychiatrists need to find a gentle but persuasive language of resistance, in the face of this linguistic ploy.

Acknowledgment

A slightly modified version of this piece appeared in the October 29, 2009, issue of *Psychiatric Times*.

References

[1] Wittgenstein L. The Blue and Brown Books: Preliminary Studies for the Philosophical Investigations. New York: Harper and Row; 1958: 1, 38.
[2] Leucht S, Corves C, Arbter D, Engel RR, Li C, Davis JM. Second-generation versus first- generation antipsychotic drugs for schizophrenia: a meta-analysis. The Lancet. 2009;373:31-41.
[3] Ghaemi SN, Shirzadi AA, Filkowski M. Publication bias and the pharmaceutical industry: the case of lamotrigine in bipolar disorder. *Medscape J Med*. 2008;10(9):211.
[4] Pies R. Should psychiatrists use atypical antipsychotics to treat nonpsychotic anxiety? *Psychiatry (Edgmont)*. 2009;6(6):29-37.
[5] Mojtabai R, Olfson M. National trends in psychotherapy by office-based psychiatrists. Arch Gen Psychiatry. 2008;65:962-970.
[6] Schmidt HD, Duman RS. The role of neurotrophic factors in adult hippocampal neurogenesis, antidepressant treatments and animal models of depressive-like behavior. *Behav Pharmacol*. 2007;18(5-6):391-418.
[7] Geppert CMA, LW Roberts. *The Book of Ethics*. Center City, MN: Hazelden; 2008.

~~~~~~~~~~~~~~~~~

MOVING BEYOND HATRED OF PSYCHIATRY: A BRAVE VOICE SPEAKS OUT

Sometimes I wonder if hatred of psychiatrists is one of the few remaining forms of acceptable bigotry. If the vitriol on many anti-psychiatry websites is any indication, the answer may be yes.

No, I'm not comparing psychiatrists to ethnic or racial minorities, or claiming that we deserve anybody's sympathy. And I'm not talking about vigorous but constructive criticism of psychiatry, much of which is justified [1]. I'm talking about the kind of visceral, rage-ridden hatred that makes the hairs on your neck stand up, or sends your heart plummeting to your stomach.

"I hate shrinks. Shrinks should die. Shrinks are evil." These are the kinds of comments recently cited by a brave, young woman who blogs under the *nom de plume*, Natasha Tracy. I generally oppose the use of pseudonyms among bloggers, particularly health care professionals who hide behind fake names to launch cowardly attacks on their colleagues. But "Ms. Tracy," who is not in the health care field, convincingly explains the safety concerns that have led her to adopt this pen name.

It turns out that Ms. Tracy has been diagnosed with bipolar disorder, and has been writing about her illness with courage and candor for several years [2]. As a specialist in bipolar disorders, I can say that Natasha's understanding of this illness is more accurate and sophisticated than that of many physicians I have encountered over the past thirty years. But more than that: she shows uncommon wisdom and deep compassion, when it comes to discussing psychiatrists and psychiatry. Here are a few excerpted remarks from Natasha's essay, "Hatred of Psychiatry Doesn't Create Change" [2].

"'I hate shrinks. Shrinks should die. Shrinks are evil.' ...OK I get it, you don't like psychiatrists. Personally, I would find a more intelligent way to express an argument, but your point is clear nonetheless. You're ranting. I get that. I rant. We all do. It's a healthy expression of the frustration seen when dealing with so many things outside of our own control. But at some point you have to stop hating, wishing for murder, and committing moral condemnation and actually do something useful... When we say we 'hate' something what we really mean is our emotions have overwhelmed us to the point where we no longer think rationally. Something you 'hate' can't be redeemed, can't be made better and contains no shades of grey... Hatred is a mucky darkness that lets you scream and yell all day but doesn't let you move on to affect the thing you 'hate.'

"...I have to engage with psychiatry I understand [that] for all its faults, and yes, there are many, psychiatry saves lives every day. I understand [that] psychiatry gave me, and so many others, a life. And I understand blind hatred doesn't help me get any better...people need to engage the psychiatric system to treat their mental illness I believe in: educating people, empowering people...encouraging patients to take their doctors to task...making people more active in their own health care [and] reducing prejudice."

Those last two words are particularly important. Prejudice is a net that ensnares not only those who suffer from severe psychiatric illness, but also many of us who care for these individuals [3]. Natasha is a member of the *Society of Participatory Medicine,* a non-profit organization dedicated to "...a cooperative model of health care that encourages and expects active involvement by all connected parties (patients, caregivers, healthcare professionals, etc.) as integral to the full continuum of care..." [4]. This is certainly a worthy model of healthcare, and one that ought to inform—and *re*form—psychiatry. But it is a model supported by *mutual respect*—it cannot stand on a foundation of hatred and prejudice.

The Roman statesman and Stoic philosopher, Seneca (4 BCE – 65 CE) lived in turbulent times and knew firsthand of hatred's toxic effects. He wrote that,

> "Hatred is not only a vice, but a vice which goes point-blank against Nature....Hatred makes us destroy one another. Love unites, hatred separates. Love is beneficial, hatred is destructive. Love succors even strangers; hatred destroys the most intimate friendship. Love fills all hearts with joy; hatred ruins all those who possess it. Nature is bountiful; hatred is pernicious. It is not hatred, but mutual love, that holds all mankind together" [5].

I do not know if Natasha Tracy has ever gone through the philosophy of Seneca; but Seneca's philosophy has clearly gone through her.

Acknowledgments

My thanks to Dr. Glen Gabbard for his counsel on the premise of this piece; and to the website Healthyplace.com for permission to quote from Natasha Tracy's blog. A slightly modified version of this piece appeared in the May 24, 2012, issue of Psychiatric Times.

References

[1] Pies R. How *American psychiatry* can save itself: Part 2. *Psychiatr Times*. 2012 March 1. Available from: www.psychiatrictimes.com/display/article/10168/2040753. Accessed March 9, 2014.

[2] Tracy N. Hatred of psychiatry doesn't create change [online]. HealthyPlace blog. 2001 May 2. Available from: http://www.healthyplace.com/blogs/breakingbipolar/2011/05/hatred-of-psychiatry-doesn%E2%80%99t-create-change/. Accessed February 25, 2014.

[3] Sartorius N. Guidance on how to combat stigmatization of psychiatry and psychiatrists. *World Psychiatry*. 2012;11:61-62.

[4] Society for Participatory Medicine. Available from: http://participatorymedicine.org/. Accessed February 25, 2014.

[5] Davis C. *Greek and Roman Stoicism*. Boston: Herbert B. Turner & Co., 1903.

~~~~~~~~~~~~~~~~~

DECONSTRUCTING "CONFLICTS OF INTEREST": A USER'S GUIDE

He who proclaims will proclaim flat.—Lionel Ziprin

The debate within the medical profession over "conflicts of interest" (COI) has often been shrill, and sometimes seems to be based on misunderstandings or myths about what COI entails. In this psychiatrist's view, it is helpful to step back from flat proclamations; acknowledge that the issues involved are complex; and aspire to some semblance of humility. Nobody has cornered the market on "the right way" to deal with COI in the realms of medical research, publication, and education [1]. At the same time, as Prof. Alan Stone has noted (personal communication, August 27, 2009), *ethical* considerations lie at the heart of any debate on COI; in particular, the ancient dictum, "Do no harm." Indeed, ethicist James M. DuBois has pointed out a direct connection between some types of COI and harm to the general public: "Mental health consumers are at risk when studies that involve questionable scientific and publication practices are translated into therapeutic practice" [1, p. 205].

What follows are simply the views of this educator, editor, and erstwhile psychiatric researcher—views strongly held, but not intended as "proclamations." With that prologue, here is my "User's Guide" to conflicts of interest, written in the form of questions and answers.

> In the health care field, what is the professionally-accepted definition of "conflict of interest?"

There is no single, universally-accepted definition of COI, though there is substantial convergence around a few general definitions of the term. Therefore, when someone is alleged to have a "conflict of interest," the first order of business is asking the person making the allegation to define "conflict of interest."

> But aren't professional journals and organizations providing reasonably clear definitions of COI?

Yes, but the definitions differ in important ways, and are sometimes difficult to interpret. Most definitions of COI—both outside and within the medical profession—follow one of three underlying paradigms, which we might call the "3 Ps": *perception, potential,* and *probability*. These are founded, respectively, on judgments regarding how observers *perceive* the situation in question; on whether the situation has any *potential* for conflict of interest; and on whether the situation is *more likely than not* to lead to such conflict. For example, one definition of COI from the business world emphasizes *perception*: "We can define a conflict of interest as a situation in which a person has a private or personal interest *sufficient to appear* to influence the objective exercise of his or her official duties as, say, a public official, an employee, or a professional" (italics added) [2].

Note that this definition does not require any *actual* influence upon the person's objective exercise of duties. Neither does it require either the *potential* or the *probability* of an actual conflict of interest arising—rather, it falls under the rubric of "having the *appearance* of impropriety." Of course, one might suspect that if there *is* such an appearance, there must *also* be a reasonable likelihood of COI ("Where there's smoke, there's fire!"), but this line of reasoning fallaciously assumes that all perceptions of COI are necessarily *accurate* or *objective*, and are not themselves influenced by all manner of motives and biases.

Another widely-cited definition of COI from Columbia University emphasizes the *potential* of some situation to compromise one's objectivity: "The simplest working definition [of COI] states: A conflict of interest is a situation in which financial or other personal considerations *have the potential* to compromise or bias professional judgment and objectivity" [3].

The Columbia definition of COI, like that of MacDonald et al., does not require that any decision *actually* be biased, or even that such bias be *likely*; on the contrary, the Columbia doctrine is clear that "...a conflict of interest exists *whether or not decisions are affected* by a personal interest; a conflict of interest implies only the *potential* for bias, not a likelihood" (italics added) [3].

Incorporating the word "potential" into the core definition of COI appears to create logical and syntactic problems for the Columbia position, when it later comes to defining "potential conflict of interest" [3]. The Columbia position also seems internally contradictory, as when it states, "There are many varieties of conflicts of interest, and they appear in different settings and across all disciplines. While conflicts of interest apply to a 'wide range of behaviors and circumstances,' they all involve the *use* of a person's authority for personal and/or financial gain" [3].

The word "use" implies that the situation has gone beyond merely a *potential* action, and has veered over into an *actual abuse of power or authority*. Finally, it is important to note that in the Columbia definition, "...a conflict of interest is *not considered misconduct* in research, since the definition for misconduct is currently limited to fabrication, falsification, and plagiarism" (italics added) [3].

Probability- or *tendency-* based definitions of COI imply that in a certain set of conditions, an individual's judgment, *more likely than not*, will be influenced by some secondary interest. ("Potential" COI might entail a 2%, 30%, or 60% probability; "tendency" or "likelihood," as I use the terms, implies a >50% probability). This is exemplified in the definition offered by Harvard ethicist Dennis Thompson, for whom a COI is "...a set of conditions in which professional judgment concerning a primary interest (such as a patient's welfare or the validity of research) *tends to be unduly influenced* by a secondary interest (such as financial gain)" (italics added) [4].

Note that this definition avoids the term "potential" altogether. Rather, it emphasizes the *likelihood* or *probability* of a bias developing ("...tends to be unduly influenced"). Importantly, Thompson also includes a semi-quantitative "specifier" for COI; that is, there must be an *undue degree* of influence. This is conceptually very important, because it implies that a COI may not be present if the degree of influence remains modest or moderate; i.e., within some unspecified parameters of acceptability. On this view, not every situation in which bias *might* occur—or be *perceived* by others as existing—would be a full-blown conflict of interest. Indeed, in theory, Thompson's definition even allows for the possibility that in a situation in which someone stood to gain financially by compromising objectivity, but was literally not "interested" in financial gain, a full-fledged conflict of interest might not exist.

One important caveat, however, applies to Thompson's definition. As philosopher Arthur Schafer has observed, all "interests" are not created equal, in terms of the physician's moral and fiduciary obligations. Thus, as ethicist Dr. Howard Brody (citing Schafer) tartly observes: "The physician has a professional duty to care for the patient at a level of reasonable competence and fiduciary commitment. By contrast, the physician has no duty to make more money" [5 p. 34].

> Is a COI an "either-or" thing? That is, is it a binary or categorical term, like "on" or "off," such that either one does or does not have a COI? Or are there "degrees" of COI?

Thompson's definition implies the latter; i.e., that there may be "minor" or "low-level" conflicts that do not rise to the level of full-blown COI. Indeed, this is also implied in the definition of COI provided by the International Committee of Medical Journal Editors (ICMJE), in their Uniform Requirements for Manuscripts Submitted to Biomedical Journals:

> "Conflict of interest exists when an author (or the author's institution), reviewer, or editor has financial or personal relationships that inappropriately influence (bias) his or her actions (such relationships are also known as dual commitments, competing interests, or competing loyalties). *These relationships vary from negligible to great potential for influencing judgment. Not all* [financial or personal] *relationships represent true conflict of interest"* (italics added) [6].

That said, ICMJE appropriately cautions that the reviewer or editor is not necessarily the best judge of whether a COI is present, and, indeed, may not even be conscious of an actual or incipient COI:

> "...the potential for conflict of interest can exist *regardless of whether an individual believes* that the relationship affects his or her scientific judgment...[therefore] All participants in the peer-review and publication process must disclose all relationships that *could be viewed* as *potential conflicts of interest.* Disclosure of such relationships is also important in connection with editorials and review articles, because it can be more difficult to detect bias in these types of publications than in reports of original research" (italics added) [6].

Thus, the ICMJE guidelines would require disclosure of putative conflicts that might not rise to the level of COI, but which might be *perceived* even as *potential* conflicts of interest. This highlights the difference between a *definition* of COI that invokes "inappropriate influence"; and *guidelines for disclosure*, which may use a lower threshold.

What Are the Main Types of COI?

It is important to distinguish two types of COI: *financial* and *non-financial*. In theory—and assuming honest financial self-disclosure by authors and researchers—financial COI is "detectable"; e.g., by evaluating an individual's declared stock holdings. *Non*-financial COI, however, may be nearly impossible to detect, if it involves, say, an editor's intense dislike of a particular author—or a peer reviewer's wish to thwart a competitor's academic goals by summarily rejecting the researcher's submission. The only real protection against this type of "stealth" COI is to submit papers to a *double-blind review* (neither author nor reviewer knows the identity of the other) ideally by several reviewers. Alternatively, some journals have an "open review" policy, in which reviewers actually *sign* their reviews. This approach, used in some Biomed Central journals, has pros and cons. On the one hand, it may reduce the likelihood of anonymous "slash and burn" reviews; on the other hand, it may constrain the reviewer's candid assessment of a manuscript.

Some authorities [1] also distinguish "inherent" from "induced" conflicts of interest. For example, some might argue that the medical research enterprise inherently involves a tension between a "selfless" dedication to benefitting mankind, and a not-so-selfless interest in advancing one's career (see below, re: "vested interest"). Other conflicts of interest are "induced"; for example, when a researcher knowingly creates situations of financial dependency that may compromise judgment.

Is a "Vested Interest" the Same Thing As a "Conflict of Interest"?

No. A particular individual's motivation virtually always contains an element of *self-interest,* or a *vested interest* in promoting the well-being of one's family, friends, employer, religious or civic group, etc. (I am not using "vested interest" in the legal sense; but rather, to denote *a special interest in protecting or promoting that which is to one's personal advantage*.) For example, an editor may be highly motivated to present his or her journal in a positive light (it would be a peculiar editor who would seek to do otherwise!). In so doing, the editor's "bias" may indeed work to the journal's advantage; e.g., by attracting readers, advertisers, etc. But by itself, this does not necessarily entail a *conflict* of interest. That is, there is not necessarily a conflict between one's *primary professional and fiduciary obligations*, and one's *secondary interests*, such as securing an income, promoting one's career, etc. The crucial question is whether one fulfills one's professional and fiduciary obligations ethically and responsibly. Indeed, it may be in the interest of *all* parties concerned (editors, writers, readers, the scientific community, etc.) to see a journal, professional organization, or company flourish. In short, a *vested interest* is not necessarily a *conflict* of interest, though in some cases it may become one.

Does Having a COI Inherently Mean One Is Behaving Unethically?

No. If we accept the concept that a COI represents a *set of conditions*, it is not possible to ascribe moral qualities to a set of conditions. A COI is not an *action* or *behavior*; therefore, it cannot be "ethical," "unethical," or of any moral character at all. Indeed, in their widely-cited study of industry-sponsored research in psychiatry, Perlis et al. state, "Conflict of interest need not imply unethical behavior or wrongdoing" [7]. Similarly, DuBois notes that COI "…does not in itself imply wrongdoing" [1, p. 204].

On the other hand, one might *deliberately engage in behaviors that create a conflict of interest* (cf. "induced" COI). For example, one might set oneself up as the direct financial beneficiary of some company (condition "A"), then subsequently agree, in some other setting, to render ostensibly impartial verdicts on the quality of that company's goods or services (condition "B"). *Knowingly* creating such a conflict of interest would be unethical in itself; failure to disclose condition A to those involved in Condition B would greatly compound the ethical lapse. Indeed, as Dr. Daniel Carlat has argued, "…choosing to participate in a potentially damaging incentive structure is, by itself, morally wrong in a way that is even 'worse' than simply calling it a conflict of interest" (personal communication, August 30, 2009).

In short, what is ethical or unethical is whether or not one *knowingly creates* a COI; whether or not one *discloses* the conflict to the appropriate parties; and how one *manages* the conflict.

Example: A psychiatrist, Dr. Smith, agrees to join a "speaker's bureau" for a large pharmaceutical company (Company A). In return, she receives periodic stipends from the company, for her talks. She then accepts a position at a community mental health center, where Dr. Smith is named to be Chair of the Pharmacy Committee. It is the committee's job to decide which medications to include on the center's formulary; "candidate" medications include several drugs produced by Company A. Dr. Smith does not inform her clinical supervisor at the health center of her affiliation with Company A.

Q. Does a conflict of interest exist for Dr. Smith?
A. Yes, clearly.
Q. Did Dr. Smith act unethically in accepting the Pharmacy Committee position?

A. That depends on whether she knew, or should have known, that drugs produced by Company A were likely to be "candidate" drugs for the formulary. If she had such knowledge but accepted the position anyway, she acted unethically to the extent that she *knowingly created a COI for herself*. If Dr. Smith did *not* know and could not reasonably have foreseen that the committee would be considering drugs made by Company A, she may have acted *imprudently* or naively, but not necessarily unethically, in accepting the position.

Q. Having accepted the committee chair, did Dr. Smith act unethically by failing to inform her clinical supervisor, and the committee, of her affiliation with Company A?

A. At the very least, Dr. Smith did not fulfill her professional and ethical obligations; i.e., her affiliation certainly should have been disclosed. Even if Dr. Smith was unsure of what drugs might come before the Pharmacy Committee, her affiliation with Company A should have been disclosed to her supervisor and the committee. Had Dr. Smith disclosed the COI to her supervisor, they might have worked out an agreement whereby Dr. Smith would *recuse herself* from any committee decisions regarding drugs produced by Company A.

Does having a COI mean that a doctor or researcher has made a faulty decision, produced inaccurate results, or rendered a judgment that is biased or unfair?

No, not necessarily. Again: a COI is a *set of conditions*, not a behavioral outcome or "verdict" on the quality of one's work. To be sure, those conditions that create a COI do, by definition, *predispose* one toward bias, inaccuracy, or unfair judgments, but none of these outcomes necessarily follows from the COI per se.

Example: Dr. Jones is a medical researcher who has written a review paper on the efficacy of the drug "nullotropin," and the writing has been funded by an "unrestricted writing grant" from the pharmaceutical company that produces nullotropin. Dr. Jones carries out a careful review of all the placebo-controlled, randomized studies of nullotropin, including several unpublished studies that found no significant effect or benefit from the drug. During the writing of the paper, Dr. Jones has no contact with the underwriting company, and is subject to no "monitoring" or "feedback" from the company. His paper ultimately concludes that "Nullotropin appears to be moderately effective for its indicated use, notwithstanding two unpublished, negative studies." The drug company does not require "pre-authorization" or "right of refusal" with respect to Dr. Jones's work, and the paper is submitted to and accepted by a peer-reviewed journal that uses "blinded" reviews. The financial support for Dr. Jones is disclosed in the appropriate section of the paper.

Q. Did a conflict of interest exist with respect to Dr. Jones writing and submitting the paper? If so, was it a major conflict of interest?

A. Arguably, a COI did exist, using Thompson's definition, if Dr. Jones believed (correctly or not) that his writing grant might be withheld by the company—or that the company would never again support his writing—if the outcome of his paper was unfavorable to nullotropin. If that was the case, then there existed "a set of conditions in which [Dr. Jones's] professional judgment concerning a primary interest (such as a patient's welfare or the validity of research) tends to be unduly influenced by a secondary interest (such as financial gain)." In theory—however implausibly—if Dr. Jones *held no such belief* about the company; or, for whatever reason, had no need at all to concern himself with financial support in the future (let's posit that Dr. Jones is fabulously wealthy!), some might argue that no COI was actually present. Nevertheless, erring on the side of caution, *one should assume a COI in a case such as this, and disclose the financial relationship.*

Given the many safeguards built into this vignette—e.g., no contact between Dr. Jones and the company during the writing; no "pre-approval" of the paper by the company, etc.—one could argue that the COI in this case was not a serious or major one. But that is often not the case. One can easily imagine (and sometimes, document) instances in which the pharmaceutical sponsor puts considerable pressure on the writer/researcher to "play ball" and produce a paper consistent with the corporate interests of the company. Recently, there have been disturbing reports in which some companies are alleged to have concealed "negative studies" of their product from the very physicians who were speaking or writing about them [8].

Are studies underwritten by pharmaceutical companies inherently biased, owing to financial conflict of interest?

No, though it is easy to become cynical about such studies. For example, there has been much written about the disproportionate number of "positive" (favorable) drug studies associated with pharmaceutical-company underwriting. However, there remains some question as to the underlying basis for this finding. For example, one widely-cited study found that industry sponsorship is disproportionately linked with positive results, in published studies of psychiatric drugs [7]. This is certainly of great concern and importance. However, Perlis et al. also acknowledged the possibility that

> "...industry sponsorship may allow larger and better-designed studies, with greater statistical power to identify significant differences if such differences exist. Indeed, the median number of subjects was larger among studies in which conflict of interest was present. Industry-funded trials would naturally examine drugs already suggested to have efficacy in earlier-stage trials" [7].

Similarly, a comprehensive review of pharmaco-economic studies, carried out at the Centre for Health Economics, University of York (UK), concluded that while there are some causes for concern, given the fact that most pharmacoeconomic studies report positive findings for the sponsor's drug,

> "... a more detailed analysis suggests that, while the methodological quality of some published studies may be poor, the main reason for positive results is that companies only sponsor economic studies where a positive outcome is likely" [9].

It has been argued that the best defense against inaccurate and misleading scientific presentations lies in the accurate, scientific scrutiny of the article's methods, design, statistical analysis, and conclusions [10]. As Klein and Glick aptly observe, "...the important issue is whether the presentation truthfully reflects the known scientific facts and draws justifiable conclusions..." [10]. If a study or article meets this test, the issue of financial underwriting is not of great public health importance. If the study fails this test, the research is certainly not redeemed by its independent funding source.

A number of authorities have argued in favor of transparent access to all ongoing clinical studies; pharmaceutical company disclosure of any "negative" studies; availability of the researchers' "raw data" to journal editors [10]; and, as this writer once suggested, a national online "clearing house" of data, disclosing all financial ties between researchers and the pharmaceutical industry. Daniel J. Carlat MD has also called upon journals to "…require authors to disclose all financial ties to any health care–related company, whether seemingly relevant or irrelevant to the topic of the article. It would then be up to the readers to decide whether these ties represented true conflicts" [11].

These ideas all have points in their favor. Yet it remains true that a researcher utterly without any conflict of interest may still produce an atrocious and misleading piece of research. Conversely, a researcher or writer who has an acknowledged (or even unacknowledged) conflict of interest may produce an article or study that is accurate, meticulously-designed and scrupulously analyzed. Journals can do only so much to assess COI in submitted articles, given limited time, staff and financial resources. As Klein and Glick observe, "…the complex COI issue cannot be dealt with by an editorial fix" [10].

Conclusion

In summary, there is no single, universally accepted definition of conflict of interest. In this writer's view, Thompson's definition [4]—which emphasizes *likelihood* of COI and *undue* influence—is perhaps the least problematic, notwithstanding its failure to distinguish moral obligations from mere "interests." A COI per se does not indicate wrongdoing, but whether one *discloses* a COI, and how one *manages* COI, does have important moral implications. The presence of pharmaceutical company sponsorship of a research study warrants careful scrutiny for COI, but there is no valid reason to assume that sponsored studies are inherently biased or unreliable. Ultimately, physicians need to equip themselves with the analytic skills and understanding that will allow them to distinguish real science from "junk science" [10,12].

Acknowledgments

I wish to thank Marc D. Schwartz, MD, for stimulating my thinking on these issues; as well as Alan Stone, MD, Daniel J. Carlat, MD, and Prof. James M. DuBois for their helpful comments on early drafts. The opinions expressed herein, however, are the author's alone. A slightly modified version of this piece appeared in the November 24, 2009, issue of Psychiatric Times.

References

[1] DuBois J. *Ethics in Mental Health Research*. Oxford: Oxford University Press; 2008.
[2] MacDonald C, McDonald M, Norman W. Charitable conflicts of interest. *Journal of Business Ethics*. 2002;39:67-74.
[3] Ruth F, Plaza J. Conflicts of interest: responsible conduct of research [online]. Columbia University. Available from: http://ccnmtl.columbia.edu/projects/rcr/rcr_conflicts/foundation/index.html#1_1. Accessed February 25, 2014.

[4]   Thompson DF. Understanding financial conflicts of interest. *N Engl J Med.* 1993;329:573-576.
[5]   Brody H: Hooked. Ethics, the Medical Profession, and the Pharmaceutical Industry. Lanham, MD: Rowman & Littlefield; 2007.
[6]   ICMJE: Conflicts of Interest. Accessed at: http://www.icmje.org/ethical_4 conflicts.html
[7]   Perlis RH, Perlis CS, Wu Y et al. Industry sponsorship and financial conflict of interest in the reporting of clinical trials in psychiatry. *Am J Psychiatry.* 2005;162:1957-1960.
[8]   Kaplan A. Forest under fire. *Psychiatr Times.* 2009 April 8. Vol. 26 No. 4. Accessed at: http://www.psychiatrictimes.com/display/article /10168 /1399086
[9]   Drummond M, Barbieri M. Conflict of interest in industry-sponsored economic evaluations: real or imagined? *Curr Oncol Rep.* 2001;3:410-413. Available from: http://www.upf.edu/cres/_pdf/interest.pdf. Accessed March 9, 2014.
[10] Klein DF, Glick ID. Conflict of interest, journal review, and publication policy. *Neuropsychopharmacology.* 2008;33:3023-3026.
[11] Carlat DJ. Conflict of interest in psychiatry: how much disclosure is necessary? *Psychiatr Times.* 2006 November 1. Available from: http://www.psychiatrictimes.com /articles/conflict. Accessed March 9, 2014.
[12] Ghaemi SN. Good clinical care requires understanding statistics. *Psychiatr Times.* 2009 March 6, 2009. Available from: http://www.psychiatrictimes.com/display/article/10168 /1385693. Accessed March 9, 2014.

For Further Reading

Dubovsky AN, Dubovsky SL. Psychotropic Drug Prescriber's Survival Guide: Ethical Mental Health Treatment in the Age of Big Pharma. New York: WW Norton; 2007.

~~~~~~~~~~~~~~~~~~

WRITING ABOUT PATIENTS: THE PERENNIAL DILEMMA

Here is the conundrum: You have completed treatment with a fascinating and complex patient. Mr. A has bipolar depression, Marfan syndrome, and hypothyroidism. You managed not only to navigate around the rocks of his medical problems, but also to stabilize Mr. A's bipolar disorder using a combination of lithium (Eskalith, Lithobid), thyroxine, and interpersonal therapy. You would now like to share your experience with colleagues, so you write up the case history; then suddenly, you are seized with misgivings.

Do you need Mr. A's permission before submitting the case, even though you were careful to disguise his identity? Is it legal and ethical to proceed with publication without such explicit permission? After all, you want to respect the patient's autonomy and privacy. Then again, what if the patient refuses to give his or her consent? Do you really want to "kill" the case report? Don't you have a professional obligation to teach the art and science of psychiatry through such reports? Of course, the patient may have some important insights that could enhance the report, but what if he insists on making changes that contradict your medical opinion? Even worse, what if merely *presenting* your write-up to the patient opens old wounds and actually precipitates a relapse of his depression? Finally, is informed consent even possible, given that your patient will undoubtedly feel an obligation to assist and please you?

On the other hand, if you *do not* obtain permission, aren't you misappropriating the "patient's story" as your own? Shouldn't an empowering and collaborative approach be preferred in writing about the "shared experience" of treatment? Furthermore, suppose you do not obtain Mr. A's consent and he then recognizes himself in your case report. After all, some patients read our professional journals or find our articles on the Internet. What reaction will that bring? Will the patient be flattered that you thought enough of him to publish the case? Or will the patient be furious with you, and possibly even sue you? Come to think of it: Was that part about "Mr. A is 7 feet, 2 inches tall" so accurate and specific that he could easily be identified as the subject of your report? Maybe you should just drop the whole publication idea and go to a movie!

A Historical Perspective

This is a conundrum, indeed. From a historical perspective, of course, psychiatrists have been writing about their patients for more than a century. Indeed, Freud maintained that analysts have an affirmative duty to publish what they learn from treating patients [1]. In publishing his case history of Dora in 1905, Freud took care to conceal the patient's identity; for example, the patient he wrote about was not from Vienna; nobody knew that Freud was treating her; and Freud used no names that would be recognizable. He also believed (correctly or not) that the patient, whose treatment had been completed four years earlier, would "no longer be interested in the events he reported" [1].

Yet ultimately, despite Freud's precautions, Dora's identity was discovered.

Today

Clearly, there are compelling legal and ethical reasons for routinely obtaining a patient's permission to publish his or her case history. As Alan Stone, MD, a member of *Psychiatric Times'* editorial board, succinctly put it: "Why not get the patient's consent? For example, [say], 'Here is the disguised, brief account of your illness. Is there anything you would like me to change or further disguise?' Get a signed consent that solves the legal and ethical questions." (personal communication, September 6, 2007). Dr. Stone is in good company. Richard A. Friedman, MD, an academic psychiatrist who writes for the *New York Times*, routinely obtains patients' permission for his case write-ups. "The reason is that I don't want them to feel in any way surprised or exploited. I don't do it for legal reasons, but more because it's the way I'd like to be treated if someone were writing something about me" (personal communication, September 6, 2007). Some medical writers will seek more informal *assent* on the patient's part, without going through a formal *consent* procedure.

But psychiatrists Stephen B. Levine, MD, and Susan J. Stagno, MD, offer another perspective, arguing that, at times, obtaining the patient's permission to publish may actually be *un*ethical [2]. With respect to patients still in treatment, Levine and Stagno argued, "Asking for permission crosses a professional boundary by inserting the doctor's professional agenda into the treatment. The agenda consumes the patient's time and energy. It temporarily transforms the therapy into a discussion of the therapist's issue." These authors observed that "publication has nothing to do with why the patient came for therapy," and that strong negative emotions may be unleashed when publication is raised.

Although Levine and Stagno discussed this in the context of patients under active treatment, I see no reason why the same ethical issue could not arise even with some former patients—particularly those with a fragile recovery who might easily be overwhelmed by having to grapple with the therapist's "professional agenda." On the other hand, as Dr. Stone reminds us, "informed consent was imposed by courts on a resistant medical profession who said it disrupted the doctor-patient relationship and burdened the patient with information he or she could not handle" (personal communication, September 6, 2007).

In truth, the whole notion of "confidentiality" is more complex than it may appear at first glance. Confidentiality is not a binary term. Rather, we can define several levels of confidentiality with respect to a given case report (Table 2).

Table 2. Conceptual Levels of Confidentiality

I.	**Average reader cannot recognize the identity of the patient after reading the article.**
II.	**Average reader cannot discover the patient's identity after casual investigation (e.g., Google search).**
III.	**Determined reader cannot discover patient's identity after extensive attempts (extensive on-line search, phone calls to potential informants, etc.).**
IV.	Professional private investigator cannot discover patient's identity after determined effort.
V.	I-IV criteria met, plus: family and close friends cannot recognize identity of patient, based on the case report.
VI.	I-V criteria met, plus: patient him/herself does not recognize that case is about him or her.

Boldface: The author believes *all* case reports written without the patient's consent should meet *at least* the first three levels of confidentiality.

At the most rudimentary level, the average reader of a case report should not be able to recognize the identity of the patient after a casual perusal of the text. At the most stringent level of confidentiality, *even the patient described* would not be able to recognize himself in the case report. But in the latter instance, would the case be of much merit? Surely, there is something a bit perverse in creating a case history so estranged from the patient's own experience that the patient himself cannot recognize the subject of the report!

In theory, the ideal case report might be recognizable by the patient but by *no one else*— not even close friends, family, or members of the patient's treatment team, for patients whose care is managed in clinics or inpatient units. I suspect that in practice, this ideal is rarely achieved. In my view, however, case reports should provide *at least* "level 3" protection; that is, even a determined reader should not be able to discover the patient's identity, even after extensive efforts (such as an online search, phone calls to possible informants, and so forth).

What Is Confidentiality?

But wait—what, exactly, are clinicians required to keep "confidential"? It is clear that the medical record per se is nearly sacrosanct. Indeed, whereas the physical ("paper" or electronic) record is the property of the psychiatrist, *the information contained in the medical record belongs to the patient* [3]. Such information cannot be released to third parties without the patient's explicit consent, absent a subpoena or other compelling legal requirement. The patient has what I call "intercessory prerogatives"; for example, if you plan to send a letter to the patient's insurer discussing her "substance abuse," the patient may justifiably intercede and say, "No way! I don't want that letter to go out."

Table 3. Twelve Dos and Don'ts When Publishing a Case Report or Treatment Narrative

• DO get patient's informed consent if the case material cannot be presented accurately without revealing patient's identity or making identification likely.
• DO focus on the "internal dynamics" of the case (i.e., non-discoverable features rather than physical or biographical information).
• DO disguise, alter, or omit critical information about the patient that would likely reveal his or her identity, consistent with publication requirements*
• DO consider obtaining consultation from a colleague, prior to submitting case for publication.
• DO evaluate your counter-transference, potential negative feelings about patient, etc.
• DO write respectfully and sensitively about the patient; carefully consider the patient's likely reaction in the event he/she reads the piece and recognizes himself/herself.
• DO be prepared to deal with emotional (and possibly legal) repercussions of publication, if patient reads the piece.
• DO NOT provide geographical, institutional and temporal clues that could aid in identifying patient (location of clinic, year/month of treatment, etc.).
• DO NOT provide unique physical features of patient unless medically relevant (in which case, informed consent may need to be obtained if features are very unusual or exceptional).
• DO NOT provide more ethnic or demographic information than is absolutely necessary to make the essential teaching points.
• DO NOT drop "bombshell" revelations about the patient that were not already discussed and worked through when the patient was in treatment.
• DO NOT make derogatory, defamatory, or potentially libelous statements about the patient.

*Some publications insist that *no* facts about the patient may in any way be altered, including name, ethnicity, age, etc. In such cases, omitting certain critical identifying information is the only option, if patient's consent is not obtained.

It is less clear, however, that physicians are ethically required to subject *written accounts of their own clinical experience* to a sort of "prior restraint" process that is governed by the patient's preferences. It seems to me that the *physician's narrative*—whether a case study, an essay, or a poem—is properly understood as the intellectual or artistic work-product of the physician. In effect, it is *the doctor's property*. Far from presuming to tell "the patient's story" (as some patients' rights advocates put it), the physician's narrative is quintessentially *the physician's story;* it is about how the doctor perceived and experienced the patient's condition, care, and treatment.

I do not assume that the legal system would agree with my analysis, but on ethical grounds, I believe this is a defensible position—*provided that the doctor's narrative adequately conceals the patient's identity from other parties.* (If the doctor fails in this regard, he or she must be held accountable, both ethically and legally.)

To be sure, obtaining the patient's permission to publish is certainly required in *some* circumstances, but it is not clear that this is true in *all* cases. If, for example, the physician writes a poem about a patient 5 to 10 years after treatment has ended (as this writer has), is the physician ethically required to obtain the patient's permission? (Let's leave aside the practical difficulties in tracking down former patients or contacting the family members of patients who are deceased!) Furthermore, if our ethical responsibility extends to "protecting" a patient from a possible adverse reaction to reading about himself, does it also extend to very similar patients in one's practice who may read the case and *mistakenly believe it is about them?* Must we obtain *their* permission in advance, too, or reassure them after the fact that "This case report was not about you"?

Alas, there may be no good options in the matter of writing about our patients—only less bad ones.

In Table 3, I have suggested some do's and don'ts when submitting a patient's case for publication.

Conclusion

It is my view that *if accurate presentation of the case requires details that would probably reveal the patient's identity to others, the patient's informed consent must be obtained.* In some instances, careful revision may avert the problem; in questionable cases, I recommend asking a trusted colleague to read the case and provide consultation. (Institutional review boards may also provide such oversight for psychiatrists associated with medical facilities.) I also recommend the self-administration of what I call the "sleep test": if you lie awake at night wondering whether you should publish a patient's case, you probably should not!

Some psychiatrists may choose to collaborate with patients in writing up the case report, as was suggested by Michael A. Schwartz, MD (personal communication, September 17, 2007). Others (e.g., psychiatrists who intend to publish clinical cases) might consider an informed-consent process at or near the beginning of treatment. (A *process* of informed consent, documented periodically, is almost always preferable to the patient's simply signing a "consent form" of some kind.) This might involve a statement such as, "Ms. Jones, I want you to know that I am committed to protecting the confidentiality of the information in your record. From time to time, I do publish case reports based on patients I treat. I take great care to make sure that the identity of the patient cannot be determined by others. But, I do not necessarily show the patient the report or seek the patient's permission to publish it. How do you feel about that arrangement? If you are in any way uncomfortable with it, you should feel free now, or at any time, to 'opt out' of that arrangement. No matter what you decide, you will continue to get the very best care I can provide."

Of course, this sort of preemptive discussion might also create complications of its own: perhaps the patient will think, "Here I come in with all these problems, and this joker is already talking about writing me up for some damn magazine!"

In the final analysis (pardon the pun), I believe Dr. Glen Gabbard [4, 5] had it about right: "No approach is without its problems. A clinically based decision must be made in each case regarding whether the best strategy is to use thick disguise; to ask the patient's consent; to limit the clinical illustration to process data without biographical details; to ask another colleague to serve as author; or to use composites" [4].

Oh, and—do remember the sleep test!

References

[1] Kantrowitz JL. Writing about patients, I: ways of protecting confidentiality and analysts' conflicts over choice of method. *J Am Psychoanal Assoc.* 2004;52:69-99. (Note: Kantrowitz has a series of articles and a new book on this subject.)
[2] Levine SB, Stagno SJ. The ethical dilemma of right to privacy versus pedagogical freedom. *J Psychother Pract Res.* 2001;10:193-201.
[3] Simon RI. *Concise Guide to Psychiatry and Law for Clinicians.* 2nd ed. Washington, DC: American Psychiatric Publishing; 1998:58.
[4] Gabbard GO: Disguise or consent: problems and recommendations concerning the publication and presentation of clinical material. International Journal of
[5] Psychoanalysis 2000;81:1071-1086.
[6] Gabbard GO, Williams P. Preserving confidentiality in the writing of case reports. *Int J Psychoanal.* 2001;82:1067-1068.

Acknowledgment

A slightly modified version of this piece appeared in the December 1, 2007, issue of *Psychiatric Times.* Thanks to Glen Gabbard MD for references to his work.

HOW AMERICAN PSYCHIATRY CAN SAVE ITSELF

Part I The Nature of the Beast

Charles Dickens might well say of American psychiatry, "These are the best of times and the worst of times." Certainly, our profession can point to some important accomplishments. In the past thirty years, the burgeoning fields of neuropsychiatry and behavioral neurology have begun to bridge the Cartesian rift between mind and body. Using new types of brain imaging, neuroscientists can now peer into the molecular and chemical mechanisms that underlie such basic human emotions as anger and grief. Devastating illnesses, such as schizophrenia and bipolar disorder, are slowly disclosing the subtle ways in which they affect the brain's structure and function [1]. And, in the past three decades, psychiatry has made notable progress in developing effective forms of both psychotherapy and "somatic" treatment. For example, the 1980s and 90s saw the growing use of cognitive-behavioral therapies for anxiety and depression; as well as the development of clozapine, arguably the most effective medication for schizophrenia. Technical refinements in the use of electroconvulsive therapy (ECT) have led to reduced cognitive side effects, while maintaining efficacy in the treatment of severe depression [2]. And we are increasingly making use of newer technologies and techniques, such as transcranial magnetic stimulation and ketamine infusion, for the treatment of depressive and other disorders.

And yet, this rather glossy synopsis omits many reasons why psychiatry as a profession finds itself in deep trouble. (Googling the phrase, "psychiatry is in trouble" brings up over 2100 hits). A spate of recent books by psychiatrists and other mental health professionals offers a range of "diagnoses" for psychiatry's present malaise: e.g., claims that psychiatry lacks a unified model of so-called "mental illness" (a term that is itself a sign of philosophical confusion in the field); that psychiatry has no "objective" criteria or biological markers for any of its principal diagnoses; that psychiatry has "medicalized" perfectly normal human reactions to stress and loss; and finally, that psychiatry has botched its system of diagnosis and classification—witness the recent debacle over the nature and development of the DSM-5.

Perhaps most damning is the charge that psychiatry has abandoned its most fundamental and sacred obligation: *to see the suffering patient as a whole person*, and not merely as a cerebral container in which a bunch of chemicals are sloshing around—a kind of neurochemical soup requiring an adjustment of ingredients. (Etymologically, our term, "patient" is related to the Latin *pati*, "to suffer.") Recently, several high-profile articles claiming that psychotherapy has nearly vanished from psychiatric practice [3] seem to have convinced the public that psychiatry's demise is all but certain—and all too often, this conviction is voiced in the spirit of, "Good-bye and good riddance!"

Each of these critiques contains at least a grain of truth—and some contain a few drams. Yet, in my view, each of these claims regarding what is wrong with psychiatry either oversimplifies the problem, or ignores more fundamental issues. In Part 1 of this essay, I consider each critique in some detail. In Part 2, I address what I believe are more central problems for American psychiatry, and some ways of redressing them.

- First: it is true that psychiatry lacks a unified model of so-called "mental illness." For critics such as psychiatrists Niall McLaren [4] and Dusan Kecmanovic [5], this "conceptual cacophony" is a serious, even a fatal, flaw. To be sure, any modern textbook of psychiatry is likely to explain conditions such as schizophrenia or major depressive disorder by invoking biological, psychological, social, and even spiritual factors, with greater weight usually given to the biological realm, for the most serious disorders. Yet there is nothing inherently "unscientific" in such pluralistic models; on the contrary, the testing and verification of these potentially complementary causal hypotheses is very much within the purview of the scientific method. Furthermore, many of the most important advances in the history of psychiatric treatment have occurred in the absence of any single, unifying "model" of mental illness—for example, the discovery that lithium is effective in stabilizing the mood swings of bipolar disorder, or the development of cognitive-behavioral therapy (CBT) for mood disorders. (The "fathers" of CBT—psychiatrist Aaron Beck and psychologist Albert Ellis—had to push back hard against the prevailing psychoanalytic model of mental illness.)
- The claim that modern-day psychiatry lacks "objective" criteria or biological markers for any of its principal diagnoses is only partly correct. Much depends on what we understand by the term "objective".* Scientists steeped in the philosophical tradition known as *logical positivism* insist that "objective" data are those obtained by direct observation and measurement—for example, by viewing bacteria under a microscope. But this model is hard to apply to many medical specialties, and the positivist notion of "objectivity" has been largely discredited or undermined by many modern-day philosophers of science. The neurologist who takes a careful history of the patient's head pain and makes a diagnosis of "migraine headache" sees nothing at all under a microscope: the relevant "data" consist almost entirely of the patient's narrative, in the presence of a normal neurological examination. This is entirely commensurate with the psychiatrist's method of arriving at a diagnosis, after a careful history and mental status exam and appropriate methods of ruling out medical or neurological disease that explains the patient's symptoms. In so far as their observations are systematic and replicable by other qualified practitioners, both the neurologist and the psychiatrist are carrying out "objective" investigations. Furthermore, there are no "lab tests" or imaging studies that allow the neurologist to "confirm" a diagnosis of migraine: like epilepsy and many chronic pain syndromes, the diagnosis is clinically based. Finally, while it is true that no psychiatric disorder has an office-ready, biological marker or "blood test" associated with it, it is incorrect to conclude that no progress has been made in this regard. Several biological markers of psychiatric illness have been repeatedly supported by careful studies over several decades; for example, abnormal smooth pursuit eye movements in schizophrenia [6], and derangements of hypothalamic-pituitary-adrenal function in certain types of severe ("melancholic") major depression [7]. Unfortunately, for a variety of practical and theoretical reasons, these tests have not found a useful place in everyday psychiatric practice. (Alas, even many psychiatrists are unaware of these biological findings, and spend inordinate time apologizing for psychiatry's supposed ignorance of biological mechanisms in the diseases we treat.)

- One of the most widely-bruited claims in recent years is that psychiatry has "medicalized" or "pathologized" various types of "normal" human behavior. This claim is sometimes voiced most forcefully by psychiatrists themselves, as several widely-publicized critiques by Dr. Allen Frances make clear [8]. (Dr. Frances, of course, was Chair of the task force that developed the DSM-IV.) The "medicalizing" claim has been made in relation to a variety of psychiatric conditions, including attention deficit/hyperactivity disorder (ADHD); incipient psychotic states, and major depression. For example, in their book, *The Loss of Sadness*, professors Jerome Wakefield and Allan Horwitz argued that recent "decontextualized" DSM criteria for major depression have created a false epidemic of depression in this country. (In fact, several epidemiological studies in the U.S. and Canada have shown that the incidence of major depression has remained largely the same over the past 50 years, when the same basic criteria are carefully applied [9].)

The problem with the notion that psychiatry is "medicalizing" normality is that it rests on certain assumptions about terms "disease", "disorder" and "normality"; for example, that there are relatively clear demarcations or veridical tests that define these terms. Seen from this perspective, any attempt at broadening the criteria for a particular disorder runs the risk of creating "false positives" or even "false epidemics." Yet in truth, terms such as "disease," "illness," "dysfunction," and "disorder" have been in flux throughout the history of clinical medicine. The philosopher Ludwig Wittgenstein cautioned us against so-called "essential definitions"—those specifying the necessary and sufficient conditions that define a term—and argued that words derive their meaning from the diverse ways in which they are used [10]. Thus, the term "disease" will acquire a variety of legitimate meanings, depending on whether the word is used by an epidemiologist, a psychiatrist, or your next-door neighbor.

Furthermore, since there are no universally agreed biological criteria for psychiatric disorders, the notion of a "false positive" becomes extremely difficult to explain, in a psychiatric context. Indeed, the term "false positive" was appropriated from fields such as microbiology, where, for example, we can point to the organism *treponema pallidum* as the causal agent of syphilis. It's easy to define a "false positive" in such cases—no bug, no disease. It becomes much harder when dealing with the diagnosis of, say, major depression. Much depends on what degree of suffering and incapacity we wish to impute to the realm of the "normal"—and this is only in part a matter of "objective" science. It is, in greater measure, an *existential decision*, involving very general ideas about health, disease, and how we choose to define what the ancient Stoics called "the flourishing life."

- On the claim that the APA has badly mishandled the entire DSM-5 process, much has been written, sometimes based on quite valid concerns. Dr. Allen Frances and others have complained, for example, that the DSM-5 work groups have reified new, untested diagnoses; that most members of the work groups lack "real world" clinical experience and have been isolated from much-needed input from everyday clinicians; and that lower thresholds for several diagnoses will lead to excessive prescription of psychotropics. (Dr. Frances has also called for an independent scientific review of the entire DSM-5 project [11], and on that issue, we were in agreement.)

But while each of these criticisms of DSM-5 is worthy of debate, they all miss the central problems with the most recent DSMs, which run much deeper than Dr. Frances's concerns. Fundamentally, the entire DSM approach to understanding and classifying psychiatric illness—while useful for researchers—is routinely ignored by many work-a-day clinicians, who use the DSM codes principally to satisfy insurers and third-party payers. As Dr. James Phillips advised psychiatrists, "Give up your expectations that the [DSM] should tell you what is essential in your assessment and treatment of your patient. Think of it rather as a crude guideline that, we hope, will land you in the right diagnostic ballpark—and not much more" [12].

To be sure, the DSM criteria sets help researchers by creating what is termed "good inter-rater reliability"; i.e., the specific categorical diagnoses can be readily agreed upon by multiple researchers. The DSMs have also helped establish "thresholds" of pathology (e.g., by stipulating interference with social or vocational function). There is also a great deal of valuable textual commentary and information in the new DSM-5, pertaining to demographics, course of illness, associated features, etc. But, in my experience, most clinicians have neither the time nor the inclination to follow the stringent inclusion and exclusion rules stipulated in the DSMs—nor do many clinicians believe that these criteria sets tell us much about the nature and "deep structure" of the patient's problem. In this sense, the "person" has been lost, amidst our diagnostic classifications, as Dr. Phillips has put it [12].

Indeed, even with DSM-5's many refinements, the overall schema presents the psychiatrist with a fundamental dilemma: by lacking either a sound biological basis, or a rich description of the patient's subjectivity, the DSM world-view leaves clinicians in a kind of diagnostic no-man's-land. On the one hand, without validated biomarkers for the major disorders, the DSM diagnoses remain only loosely moored to modern biological science (a complaint voiced by Dr. Thomas Insel, of the NIMH). On the other hand, the DSM-5 does not provide the deep understanding of the patient's "inner world" that existential, psychodynamic, and phenomenological approaches foster. The solution to this dilemma will not come easily, but I will try to sketch some radical ways in which our diagnostic system may need to change.

Part II: What Must Be Done?

So far, I have discussed problems with American psychiatry that, in my view, are largely peripheral to the central concerns of the average clinician—as well as to the average person who suffers from a serious psychiatric illness. In particular, the "loss of faith" in psychiatry that many in the general public evince stems from another set of concerns, both more pressing and more pragmatic than the academic debates swirling around the DSM-5.

I very much doubt that many Americans lose sleep over whether or not psychiatry has a "unified model" of so-called mental illness; nor do I believe that the public's animus toward psychiatry [13] stems primarily from concerns over the DSM-5's development or content (though harsh, well-publicized critiques of the DSM process have certainly not enhanced our profession's stature).

I believe the American public's jaundiced perceptions of psychiatry stem from the confluence of five main factors; specifically, (1) psychiatry's inability, thus far, to develop robustly effective, well-tolerated treatments for several major disorders, such as schizophrenia, autism, and most of the severe personality disorders (despite our having moderately effective treatments for bipolar disorder, major depressive disorder, panic disorder, and several other conditions); (2) psychiatry's inappropriately close ties with the pharmaceutical industry in recent decades; (3) the decline, over the past decade, in the use of psychotherapy among U.S. psychiatrists [14]; and the attendant public perception (even if unwarranted) that psychiatrists "no longer listen" to their patients; (4) a lack of understanding, among the general public, of the *benefits* of psychiatric treatments, and not simply the risks; for example, the erroneous belief that psychiatric medications are highly "addictive" or merely "cosmetic" in their effect [15]; (5) vituperative attacks on psychiatry by critics both within and outside the profession, often exacerbated by internet-based anti-psychiatry groups and lurid depictions of psychiatry in the media [13,15].

So, what *is* required to regain the confidence of the general public? On a concrete level, psychiatry needs to advance goals and initiatives that address each of the factors noted; for example, by (1) lobbying for more robust and better-funded research to develop more effective and better-tolerated treatments; (2) restraining the influence of pharmaceutical companies upon psychiatric education and practice, while seeking a healthier and more transparent relationship with such companies; (3) ensuring that comprehensive psychotherapy training is a central part of every psychiatric residency program; (4) bolstering "outreach" and public education efforts [13] as well as improving communication with non-psychiatric physicians; and (5) rebutting unwarranted attacks on psychiatry, while remaining receptive to constructive criticism from within and outside the profession [16].

And what about the DSM system? In retrospect, I believe that an objective, independent review of the DSM-5 process and its proposed changes would have been in the profession's best interest, and might have marginally enhanced the public's confidence in psychiatry. In my view, the National Science Foundation would have been best equipped to provide such a review. Perhaps, as the DSM-5 is updated electronically (DSM-5.1, 5.2, etc.), such an external review could be undertaken. However, I believe more radical changes are needed. In my view, the DSM framework is simply not serving everyday clinicians very well. As Aaron Mishara MD and Michael Schwartz MD recently observed, "...DSM-III's logical empiricist agenda inserted a wedge between clinician and clinical researcher which still has not been appropriately addressed" [17].

I appreciate the perils of re-thinking of a diagnostic system that has been in place, with many variations, for over thirty years. And, I realize that the likelihood of such fundamental change is low. Nevertheless, I believe that a very different kind of diagnostic model is needed. In brief, I am proposing the following:

1) Changing the name of our classification scheme. One possibility might be the *Manual of Neurobehavioral Disease*, or MND. This name helps eliminate the confusing Cartesian split implied in the present "mental disorders" designation—a problem explicitly acknowledged in the introduction to the original (1994) DSM-IV. The MND title would also allow for the (continued) inclusion of conditions such as Alzheimer's, Huntington's and Parkinson's Disease, which markedly alter behavior, cognition, and mood. I realize that many psychodynamically-oriented clinicians will not like the term "neurobehavioral," and I acknowledge that no single label adequately addresses the nature and complexity of the conditions psychiatrists treat.

(In lieu of the MND, I could also live with, simply, "Manual of Psychiatric Disease.")

2) Emphasizing the crucial importance of suffering *and* incapacity as hallmarks of disease (etymologically, *dis-ease*), and omitting from the MND any condition that lacks these features. This is a departure from the DSM's "either/or" criteria, which require "clinically significant distress *or* impairment." I believe the resultant categories of psychiatric disease would number far fewer than in the current classification—not in itself a virtue (see number 6), but probably a welcome change for those who believe psychiatry has invaded the territory of "normality" with its expanding nosology. (In fact, however, the DSM-5 does *not* increase the total number of disorders, beyond those in DSM-IV). My proposal doesn't mean that non-disease conditions or situations should not be within the purview of psychiatric care; for example, there is no reason a psychiatrist shouldn't help a family struggling with the death of a parent, or the break-up of a marriage--though neither situation constitutes "disease." Many of the DSM-5's "V" codes, such as Uncomplicated Bereavement, would still be well within the scope of clinical practice, but not within the category of *disease.*

3) Separating *clinical descriptions* of disease ("prototypes") from *research-oriented criteria,* while also ensuring that the two levels of descriptions are compatible. The prototypical descriptions would be aimed at giving the clinician a rich, holistic, phenomenological understanding of a disease—emphasizing the "inner world" of the patient—rather than a "one from column A, one from column B" list of criteria. The research-oriented "DSM type" criteria could appear as an appendix to the main MND text. This "two-tiered" system of diagnosis has its roots in the writings of Hughlings Jackson, and the clinical/research separation I advocate was also recently suggested by Prof. Joel Paris [18]. (The ICD classification of mental disorders also uses a modified prototype approach.)

4) Regarding psychiatric classification not as an end in itself, but as a *means* toward the effective relief of certain kinds of human suffering and incapacity. Thus, rather than viewing diagnostic categories as reified "objects"—like rocks or trees—they would be understood *instrumentally*; i.e., as *tools* in the service of medical-ethical goals. As Dr. Joseph Pierre has observed, "…clinicians do not in general fret over what does or does not constitute a disease…If, for example, a patient's arm is broken in a car accident, a doctor doesn't lose sleep pondering whether this represents 'broken bone disorder' or simply an expected response to an environmental stressor—the bone is set and the arm is casted… mental disorder or not, clinicians working in 'mental health' see it as their calling to try to improve the lives of whomever walks through their office door seeking help" [19]. Precisely!

5) Regarding biological data as *supporting*, but not *defining*, disease categories. In so far as "biomarkers" and biological data are found to correlate with specific disease categories, this information should become part of the supporting text of the MND. (DSM-5 does this to a limited extent already). But psychiatric diagnosis would remain essentially "clinical" (from Gk. *klinikos* "of the [sick]bed), much like diagnosis in many neurological and pain-related conditions.

6) Applying the principle of parsimony, usually expressed in terms of Occam's Razor; i.e., "entities should not be multiplied beyond what is necessary." This does not mean

deliberately reducing *or* increasing the number of diagnostic categories; but rather, retaining only those categories which are absolutely necessary, and which entail substantial suffering and incapacity. Thus, some conditions that involve merely "disapproved of" behaviors, without substantial suffering or functional impairment, would no longer count as instantiations of disease.

Reclaiming the High Ground

On an even more fundamental level, I believe psychiatrists must reclaim and reinvent our role as holistic healers—doctors who are as comfortable with motives as with molecules, and as willing to employ poetry as prescribe pills [20]. When guided by sound empirical evidence, this is not promiscuous eclecticism; but rather, what I have termed, "polythetic pluralism." I favor an expansion of the psychiatry residency to five years, so that residents may receive enhanced training in psychotherapy and the humanities; e.g., literature, comparative religion, and philosophy [21]. The added year could also be used to provide greater integration of psychiatric and neurobehavioral training. To be sure: this expansion would pose additional financial challenges and require greater sacrifice on the part of trainees; but I believe it would strengthen the foundations of psychiatric practice and enhance our stature as a medical specialty. (Ideally, I would also favor a concomitant reduction in medical school training from four to three years, with substantial streamlining and condensation of the pre-clinical curriculum—but I recognize some serious drawbacks to this proposal).

Finally, and most important, psychiatry must maintain a single-minded focus on our primary ethical and clinical mission: not the development of elegant conceptual models or ideal diagnostic criteria, but the relief of our patients' profound suffering and incapacity [22].

Note

*James Knoll IV, MD, has pointed out to me (personal communication, January 2, 2012) that several judicial decisions reflect the misleading view that psychiatry is "totally subjective." For example, Dr. Knoll notes that in Sheehan v. Metropolitan Life Ins. Co. 368 F.Supp.2d 228 (2005), which involved the recovery unpaid disability benefits, a high federal district court held: *"Unlike cardiologists or orthopedists, who can formulate medical opinions based upon objective findings derived from objective clinical tests, the psychiatrist typically treats his patient's subjective symptoms."*

Acknowledgments

I would like to thank Joseph Pierre MD and James Knoll IV, MD, for their helpful comments on this essay. A slightly modified version of parts 1 and 2 of this piece appeared in the February 8 and March 1, 20120, issues of *Psychiatric Times*, respectively.

References

[1] Arnsten AF. Ameliorating prefrontal cortical dysfunction in mental illness: inhibition of phosphotidyl inositol-protein kinase C signaling. *Psychopharmacology (Berl).* 2009;202(1-3):445-455.

[2] Kellner CH, Knapp R, Husain MM, et al. Bifrontal, bitemporal and right unilateral electrode placement in ECT: randomised trial. *Br J Psychiatry.* 2010;196:226-234.

[3] Harris G. Talk doesn't pay so psychiatry turns instead to drug therapy. *The New York Times.* 2011 March 5.

[4] McLaren N. Interactive dualism as a partial solution to the mind-brain problem for psychiatry. *Med Hypotheses.* 2006;66:1165-1173.

[5] Kecmanovic D. Conceptual discord in psychiatry: origin, implications and failed attempts to resolve it. *Psychiatr Danub.* 2011;23(3):210-22.

[6] Levy DL, Sereno AB, Gooding DC et al. Eye tracking dysfunction in schizophrenia: characterization and pathophysiology. *Curr Top Behav Neurosci.* 2010;4:311-347.

[7] Fink M, Taylor MA. Resurrecting melancholia. *Acta Psychiatr Scand Suppl.* 2007;433:14-20.

[8] Frances A. Good grief. *The New York Times.* 2010 August 14. Available from: http://www.nytimes.com/2010/08/15/opinion/15frances.html. Accessed March 1, 2014.

[9] Eaton WW, Kalaydjian A, Scharfstein DO, et al. Prevalence and incidence of depressive disorder: the Baltimore ECA follow-up, 1981-2004. Acta Psychiatr Scand. 2007;116(3):182-188.

[10] Wittgenstein L. The Blue and Brown Books: Preliminary Studies for the Philosophical Investigations. New York: Harper and Row; 1958.

[11] Frances A. DSM-5 will not be credible without an independent scientific review. Psychiatr Times. 2011 November 2. Available from: http://www.psychiatrictimes.com/dsm-5-0/dsm-5-will-not-be-credible-without-independent-scientific-review. Accessed March 1, 2014.

[12] Phillips J. The missing person in the DSM. *Psychiatr Times.* 2010 December 21. Available from: http://www.psychiatrictimes.com/dsm-5-0/missing-person-dsm. Accessed March 1, 2014.

[13] Friedman RA. The role of psychiatrists who write for popular media: experts, commentators, or educators? *Am J Psychiatry.* 2009;166:757-759.

[14] Mojtabai R, Olfson M. National trends in psychotherapy by office-based psychiatrists. *Arch Gen Psychiatry.* 2008;65:962-970.

[15] Sartorius N, Gaebel W, Cleveland HR, et al. WPA guidance on how to combat stigmatization of psychiatry and psychiatrists. *World Psychiatry.* 2010; 9:131-144.

[16] Pies R, Thommi S, Ghaemi SN. Getting it from both sides: foundational and anti-foundational critiques of psychiatry. *Association for the Advancement of Philosophy and Psychiatry (AAPP) Bulletin,* vol. 18, No. 2, 2011. Accessed at: http://alien.dowling.edu/~cperring/aapp/BulletinVol18No2.pdf

[17] Mishara A, Schwartz MA. Who's on first? Mental disorders by any other name? *Association for the Advancement of Philosophy and Psychiatry (AAPP) Bulletin* 2010;17:60-63. Available from: alien.dowling.edu/~cperring/aapp/bulletin_v_17_2/37.doc. Accessed March 9, 2014.

[18] Paris J. Commentary in : The Six Most Essential Questions In Psychiatric Diagnosis: A Pluralogue. Part 3. In: Phillips J, Frances A, editors. *Philosophy, Ethics, and Humanities in Medicine (PEHM)* 2012; 7: 9. Available from: http://www.ncbi.nlm.nih.gov/pmc/articles/PMC3403926/

[19] Pierre J. Commentary in The Six Most Essential Questions In Psychiatric Diagnosis: A Pluralogue. Part 1. In: Phillips J, Frances A, editors. *Philosophy, Ethics, and Humanities in Medicine (PEHM)*, 2012; **7**:3 Available from: http://www.peh-med.com/content/7/1/3

[20] Pies R. Reclaiming our role as healers: a response to Prof. Kecmanovic. *Psychiatr Danub*. 2011;23:229-231.

[21] Pies R, Geppert CM. Psychiatry encompasses much more than clinical neuroscience. *Acad Med*. 2009;84:1322.

[22] Knoll JL IV. Psychiatry: awaken and return to the path. *Psychiatr Times*. 2011 March 21. Available from: www.psychiatrictimes.com/display/article/10168/1826785. Accessed March 1, 2014.

Chapter 5

PSYCHIATRY AND HUMANE VALUES

PSYCHIATRISTS, PHYSICIANS, AND THE PRESCRIPTIVE BOND

Sir Launcelot smiled and said, hard it is to take out of the flesh what is bred in the bone.— Heywood Dialogue of Proverbs ii. viii. K2 (1546)

Almost the first memory I have of a physician is our family doctor at my bedside, leaning over to press his warm fingers against my neck and beneath my jaw. I'm five, maybe six years old. I have a fever and a sore throat, and Dr. Gerace is carefully palpating my cervical and submandibular lymph nodes. In my family, Dr. Gerace's opinion carried a lot of weight. It was the 1950s, and my mother did not quite trust those new-fangled antibiotics. She usually tried to haggle with the doctor over the dose—"Can't the boy take just half that much?"—but even my mother would ultimately bow to Dr. Gerace's considered opinion. Doctors counted for a lot in our family. I knew that if I wanted to stay up late to watch a television show, I first had to persuade my mother that it was a show "about a doctor." Growing up with two MDs in the family—my Uncle Morris, the ENT specialist, and Uncle Elmer, the surgeon—I could say that I was "scripted" to become a doctor. But I never felt pushed to enter the profession. Doctoring always felt like something, well—bred in the bone.

Twenty years later, I'm a medical intern, bounding down the corridor at Upstate Medical Center, trying to keep up with my two testosterone-crazed medical residents, Frank and Dave. When "Code Red! Code Red!" sounded over the income—an indication that somebody, somewhere, had just keeled over—Frank and Dave always raced to be the first ones on the scene: the ones who would "run the code." For Frank and Dave, a myocardial infarction was an invitation to adventure, mastery, and derring-do. Sure, they wanted to save the patient, and often did. But you also knew that these two young doctors were testing themselves against some unseen God of Chaos. They were hard to work with, and nearly impossible to please— but if you were the one keeling over with an MI, you wanted Frank and Dave running your code.

Three decades later, I am in the harvest years of my trade and calling. And I find my profession, psychiatry, riven by competing ideologies, rival theories, and divided loyalties. Yes, we have many critics outside the profession. But it sometimes feels that the real threat to psychiatry—and much of the rancor directed at it--comes from within our own ranks. Our internecine squabbles often bring to mind Yeats's line from "The Second Coming : *"The best lack all conviction, while the worst/ Are full of passionate intensity."* How can we hold out hope for psychiatry, when it is regularly disparaged by some who continue to call themselves psychiatrists?

To be clear: psychiatry has many sincere and well-intentioned critics whose voices need to be heard, and whose criticism is often justified. It is true, for example, that some psychiatrists have become too enamored of the so-called biomedical model and the ubiquitous "pills for ills" that often promise more than they deliver. Some of us—ignoring our better angels—have allowed market forces to pull us far from our heritage of listening, understanding, and healing. At the same time—somewhat paradoxically—some psychiatrists have lost touch with their medical roots and allowed their skills as physicians to deteriorate. We sometimes hear the charge—false, to be sure—hat "psychiatrists never do physical exams." Unfortunately, many within the profession have played into the hands of these critics. I suspect that the number of psychiatrists who routinely check the patient's blood pressure and pulse, or do a circumscribed neurological exam when the patient complains of "muscle twitches," is much smaller than it should be. In many respects, we have actually widened the rift anthropologist Tanya Luhrmann described in her book, *Of Two Minds: The Growing Disorder in American Psychiatry*" [1]. There, Lurhmann described two competing models of psychiatric illness and treatment: roughly, the *biomedical* and the *psychodynamic*. Luhrmann does not take sides—but she correctly observes that

> "These two ideals embody different moral sensibilities, different fundamental commitments, different bottom lines... The differences become part of the way the young psychiatrist imagines himself with patients, the way he comes to empathize with patients, and, ultimately, the way he comes to regard his **patients as moral beings**" [1 p. 158].

In my view, the gap between these two models and cultures has widened into a chasm—hastened, perhaps, by the economic stresses and professional competition faced by psychiatrists, in the decade since Lurhmann's book appeared. How can we bridge this formidable divide? Some see the solution in a kind of "doubling down" strategy: one that urges psychiatrists to become even more focused on neurobiology, neural circuits, and neurotransmitters, leaving "talk therapy" to the psychologists and social workers. Others have gone to the opposite extreme: belittling the real strides we have made in understanding the biology of mental illness; denouncing medication as nothing more than "covering up symptoms"; and even suggesting that psychiatry should no longer be a specialty within general medicine.

Indeed, *t*he recent controversy over "prescribing privileges" for psychologists has revealed to me an even more fundamental dichotomy than the one Luhrmann describes. Having exchanged ideas with psychiatrists both for, and against, so-called prescribing privileges for psychologists, I have reluctantly concluded that psychiatrists (with many exceptions, of course) fall into two main camps, divided by radically different self-identities. There are those who see themselves as *psychiatrists first, and physicians second*—if, indeed, they view themselves as physicians at all. Then there are those who see themselves as *physicians first, and psychiatrists second*—I sit squarely in this camp. Some in the first camp have spoken quite candidly of their basic discomfort, going back many years, with their identity as physicians—discomfort experienced almost from the day they were told to put on that heavily symbol-laden "white coat." I respect colleagues who feel this way, and I have no reason to believe that they are not fine, decent, and effective clinicians. But I am also saddened by them, as I see them tugging our profession as far from our core values as those who think only in terms of neurotransmitters and brain circuitry.

There is nothing more emblematic of the split within psychiatry than the debate over that deceptively simple piece of paper, the prescription. To some psychiatrists, uncomfortable with assuming the historical role of the physician, the prescription has come to symbolize the worst elements of psychiatry: "pushing pills;" selling out to "Big Pharma"; and—worst of all—refusing to deal with the complexities of the patient's inner life. Of course, no group is homogeneous, and it is a mistake to assume that all psychiatrists in this camp think alike. Some, for example, will acknowledge the need for medication in certain "extreme" cases, such as florid psychosis or severe bipolar disorder. Most will acknowledge that, on occasion, medication can be helpful in the short run, even if it merely "covers over the problems of living" the patient must ultimately confront. Even so, one finds among these psychiatrists a kind of patronizing tolerance of pharmacotherapy—as if it were some slovenly, ne'er-do-well in-law, sacked out uninvited on the living room couch.

Of course, there is more than a grain of truth in their complaints. Unfortunately, many prescriptions for psychotropics are written in haste—often after the infamous "15-minute med check—and without any real understanding of the patient's inner life or psychopathology. But this is only one side of that piece of paper—the flip side proves to have moral, symbolic and psychological meanings usually ignored by critics.

Those who see the prescription as merely an exercise in biological psychiatry do not understand the complexity and strength of what I call the prescriptive bond. To understand this bond, we first need to acknowledge the multi-layered meanings and symbolism patients attach to psychotropic medications themselves. In a seminal article, Metzl and Riba observe that

> "...Symbolically speaking, medications convey a host of connotative implications that are difficult to recognize, let alone to quantify. These range from preconceived beliefs about drugs that patients carry with them into the examination room, to unspoken messages of nurturance at play when doctors prescribe (or choose not to prescribe) psychotropic medications... *understanding the symbolic functions of the medications is as important as knowing their elimination half-lives or suggested dosing regimens*" (italics added) [2].

For some patients, being handed a prescription may convey, on an unconscious level, the therapist's role as "nurturing figure"; whereas for others, that same prescription may represent the overbearing authority of the punitive parent. Patients may also have idiosyncratic associations with specific drugs. I recall treating a profoundly psychotic patient who would take only one antipsychotic—the brand name of thiothixene, *Navane*. This drug was no more effective than other antipsychotics he had taken, but in his psychotically-concrete thinking, "Navane" had been symbolically fused with an over-the-counter, bromide-based, sedative he had taken in the 1940s, called *"Miles' Nervine."* Nervine was nurturance for him—and thus, he would consent to Navane.

In addition to the symbolism and meanings of psychotropic medications, there is also the meaning of that piece of paper itself. The prescription embodies more than a drug name and dosage. It is something that bears the physician's name and signature. It is, in a sense, a tiny part of the physician that the patient takes home—in short, a kind of *transitional object*, with all the powers and valences associated with these objects. Following Donald Winnicott and other object relations theorists, Metzl and Riba describe transitional objects as "...imbued with meaning because they symbolize a transition from dependency to autonomy" [2].

And, of course, there are counter-transference implications to the prescription: for some psychiatrists, writing a prescription may reflect unconscious anxiety about the patient's prognosis, or doubts regarding the psychiatrist's grasp of the case. For others, the prescription may represent the physician's hope for the patient's recovery. As Metzl and Riba observe, "...the act of prescription involves a merging of the expectations of the patient and of the doctor and thus shapes the clinical dialogue of both parties" [2].

There is also an important *ethical dimension* to placing one's signature on that little piece of paper. I may not see Hippocrates looking over my shoulder when I sign that prescription, but I am keenly aware of a host of physician forebears, scrutinizing my decision. In my mind's eye, there is Dr. Gerace, his fingers still warm on my neck; and there is Uncle Morris and Uncle Elmer, asking, "*Are you sure about that? Have you double-checked the dose? Will that medicine do more good than harm?*" The perverse notion—once voiced by a well known psychologist, but echoed recently by some psychiatrists—that "prescribing is no big deal" reflects profound ignorance not only of psychopharmacology, but also of the *moral dimensions* of the prescribing act. When I put my signature on that piece of paper, I am putting my name and that of my family behind an unspoken oath. That oath is a critical part of the prescriptive bond. That oath implicitly says to the patient,

> "*I accept medical responsibility for your life and health. I affirm that I understand not only the nature of the medication I am giving you, but also the medication's interaction with your medical and psychiatric diagnoses; other medications you are taking; and your body's physiology. I affirm that I know both the benefits and risks of this medication, which, in good faith, I have discussed with you. I also affirm that I know how to manage these risks safely; and that, to the best of my knowledge, these risks are outweighed by this medication's benefits. I accept that you have placed your faith in me, and placed your life in my hands. I am honored by your trust, and, in turn, I trust you to take this medication responsibly.*"

Any clinician who cannot inwardly utter this oath, with confidence and conviction, has no business picking up a prescription pad—whatever the clinician's profession.

Biology versus psychology; brain vs. mind; pills versus skills; molecules versus motives—I say, enough of this Manichean mind-set, and enough balkanizing of human personhood! Somehow, we need to bridge these widely separated islands of oversimplification. Perhaps such a bridge will follow the contours of psychiatrist-philosopher Karl Jaspers' approach, which Nassir Ghaemi, MD, has called, "biological existentialism" [3]. For Jaspers, there was no contradiction between explaining the patient's problem at the level of neurobiology; and also *understanding* it at the level of existential meanings. As Ghaemi observes of Jaspers, "...His approach to spiritual and existential notions...built on, rather than negated, an appreciation for science" [3].

These days, such integration is a daunting task for psychiatrists, who are hard-pressed to find even a half-hour to see patients—much less to achieve what the poet John Keats called "negative capability": in essence, the ability to entertain two seemingly contradictory or competing concepts at once.

So here I stand, alongside Dr. Gerace; my physician uncles; and my crazed residents, Frank and Dave. Whatever and wherever I may be twenty years from now, I know I will always remain a physician. And for all the uncertainties in American psychiatry, I am certain of one thing: if psychiatry is to survive as a profession, we need to become physicians of the body who are also willing to plumb the depths of the soul.

Acknowledgment

Thanks to Glen Gabbard, MD, for his helpful comments on this paper, and for his seminal work toward a pluralistic model of psychiatric illness and treatment. A slightly modified version of this piece appeared in the April 16, 2012, issue of Psychiatric Times.

References

[1] Luhrmann T. Of Two Minds: An Anthroplogist Looks at American Psychiatry. New York: Vintage; 2001.
[2] Metzl JM, Riba M. Understanding the symbolic value of medications: a brief review. Primary Psychiatry. 2003;10:45-48.
[3] Ghaemi SN. On the nature of mental disease: the psychiatric humanism of Karl Jaspers. Existenz. 2008;3:1-9.

For Further Reading

Gabbard G, Bartlett A. Selective serotonin reuptake inhibitors in the context of an ongoing analysis. *Psychoanalytic Inquiry.* 2000;18:673-701.

~~~~~~~~~~~~~~~~~~~~

HEALTH CARE IS A HUMAN RIGHTS ISSUE

Some see health care as a political or economic issue. They are correct, of course, on one level. But I believe that health care is fundamentally a *moral* issue; indeed, a matter of basic human rights. I do not believe that a nation as rich as ours (albeit with most wealth concentrated among the upper income levels) can shirk its moral responsibilities in the matter of providing basic health care for all its citizens. This doesn't mean that everybody who wants a face-lift should get one on the taxpayer's dime: I am talking about providing all citizens with the most basic health care, required to sustain life and limb. And, yes: I believe this is a right that any citizen may claim, particularly in a country purporting to be "civilized."

I am hardly alone in this view, nor is my position new. In 1948, the General Assembly of the United Nations adopted The Universal Declaration of Human Rights, article 25 of which states:

> "Everyone has the right to a standard of living adequate for the health and well-being of himself and of his family, including food, clothing, housing and medical care and necessary social services, and the right to security in the event of unemployment, sickness, disability, widowhood, old age or other lack of livelihood in circumstances beyond his control."

I don't pretend to be an expert on health care economics, and I am aware of significant logistical problems in some countries that provide health care to all their citizens; e.g., very long waiting lists for elective procedures. I am not advocating the infamous "government takeover" of health care that has been so much a part of recent political diatribes from some quarters. Rather, I favor a *single-payer national health insurance system*. One ambitious proposal describes this as

> "...a system in which a single public or quasi-public agency organizes health financing, but delivery of care remains largely private. Under a single-payer system, all Americans would be covered for all medically necessary services, including: doctor, hospital, preventive, long-term care, mental health, reproductive health care, dental, vision, prescription drug and medical supply costs. Patients would [retain] free choice of doctor and hospital, and doctors would [retain] autonomy over patient care." [from website of Physicians for a National Health Program, http://www.pnhp.org/facts].

I would urge all psychiatrists to read over the FAQ section of this website. The PNHP site also notes the following:

> "A number of studies (notably a General Accounting Office report in 1991 and a Congressional Budget Office report in 1993) show that there is more than enough money in our health care system to serve everyone if it were spent wisely. Administrative costs are at 31% of U.S. health spending, far higher than in other countries' systems. These inflated costs are due to our failure to have a publicly financed, universal health care system. We spend about twice as much per person as Canada or most European nations, and still deny health care to many in need. A national health program could save enough on administration to assure access to care for all Americans, without rationing."

On the specific issue of mental health care, we have a long way to go as a nation. For example, many patients with depression—particularly some minority groups—are not being provided adequate care. Contrary to the much-ballyhooed claim that "depression is over-treated" in this country, a recent study [1] suggests that many Americans with clinical depression are not getting *any kind of care at all*. As the lead author, Hector Gonzalez MD, put it in an interview with the Wall Street Journal, "Few Americans with depression actually get any kind of care, and even fewer get care consistent with the [best practice] standards of care" [2]. Gonzalez et al. found, in particular, that Mexican American and African American individuals meeting 12-month major depression criteria "...consistently and significantly had lower odds for any depression therapy and guideline-concordant therapies" [1].

In this country, according to a 2002 study by the Institute of Medicine, 18,000 Americans die every year because they don't have health insurance [3]. Almost certainly, some of these individuals die by their own hand, owing to untreated major depression. This is simply unconscionable, particularly in the nation with the highest GDP in the world. Recent changes in health care coverage—i.e., through the Affordable Care Act—will improve things for millions of Americans [4], but much more must be done. A publicly financed, universal health care system, while not without its own costs and problems, is worth trying—and is surely preferable to our current health care debacle. It is also the right thing to do.

Acknowledgment

A slightly modified version of this piece appeared in the November 15, 2010, issue of Psychiatric Times.

References

[1] González HM, Vega WA, Williams DR, et al. Depression care in the United States: too little for too few. *Arch Gen Psychiatry*. 2010;67:37-46.

[2] Wang SS. Studies: Mental ills are often overtreated, undertreated. *Wall Street Journal*. 2010 January 5. Available from: http://online.wsj.com/article/SB10001424052 748703580904574638750777038042.html. Accessed March 1, 2014.

[3] Institute of Medicine. Care Without Coverage: Too Little, Too Late [online]. Available from: http://www.iom.edu/Reports/2002/Care-Without-Coverage-Too-Little-Too-Late.aspx. Accessed February 25, 2014.

[4] The Affordable Care Act. Available from: http://www.healthcare.gov/law/introduction /index.html. Accessed March 1, 2014.

~~~~~~~~~~~~~~~~~~~~~

TWO ROOMS A PHYSICIAN SHOULD NEVER ENTER

Keep far away from a bad neighbor.—Talmud (Pirke Avot 1:7)

Medicine has not yet solved the problem of how to balance the particular good of the identified patient against the general good of the unidentified masses. We lose our practical ethical guideline when we try to serve such greater good.—Alan Stone, MD [1]

There are two rooms a physician should never enter, or even go near: the executioner's chamber and the interrogator's cell. I'm speaking figuratively, but I have very concrete circumstances in mind. Indeed, in recent years, psychiatrists have been drawn into controversies related to both these "rooms"—one involving the physician's role in capital punishment cases; the other, in cases related to the interrogation of suspected terrorists.

Capital Punishment

The issue of capital punishment is emotionally charged and legally complicated. I recognize that there are well-meaning individuals who sincerely believe that capital punishment is justified under certain circumstances. I happen to oppose the "death penalty" on ethical grounds; for example, I am unwilling to risk killing a potentially innocent person, when permanent incarceration of the "death-row" inmate would provide adequate protection to society. But such personal views are beside the point. The American Medical Association has clearly ruled that a physician's involvement in an execution is not ethically permissible. The AMA states that,

> "A physician, as a member of a profession dedicated to preserving life when there is hope of doing so, should not be a participant in a legally authorized execution. Physician participation in execution is defined generally as actions which would fall into one or more of the following categories: (1) an action which would directly cause the death of the condemned; (2) an action which would assist, supervise, or contribute to the ability of another individual to directly cause the death of the condemned; (3) an action which could automatically cause an execution to be carried out on a condemned prisoner" [2].

And yet, in a letter to the New York Times (December 21, 2009), two psychiatrists argue that the AMA has not gone far enough. Abraham L. Halpern, MD, is Professor Emeritus of Psychiatry at New York Medical College and former President of the American Academy of Psychiatry & The Law. His son, John H. Halpern MD, is Assistant Professor of Psychiatry at Harvard Medical School. They write that

> "If doctors and nurses did not participate in the death penalty, there would be practically no executions at all. Unfortunately, this can't happen because it is virtually impossible to discipline health professionals who are involved directly in the execution or in the training of technicians to do the killing...The American Medical Association's Council on Ethical and Judicial Affairs [CEJA]...refuses to remove the ambiguities in its ruling that prohibits physician participation in executions" [3].

I contacted Dr. John Halpern and asked him what "ambiguities" he and his father had in mind. He called my attention, first, to a statement in the CEJA's Opinion 2.06 that reads, "When a condemned prisoner has been declared incompetent to be executed, physicians should not treat the prisoner for the purpose of restoring competence unless a commutation order is issued before treatment begins" [3; Paragraph 5 Section 2.06].

But Dr. Halpern then pointed out a problem with the CEJA's ruling. In the same paragraph, the ruling states that,

> "No physician should be compelled to participate in the process of establishing a prisoner's competence or be involved with treatment of an incompetent, condemned prisoner if such activity is contrary to the physician's beliefs. Under those circumstances, physicians should be permitted to *transfer care of the prisoner to another physician*" (italics added) [3].

Both Dr. John Halpern and Dr. Abraham Halpern believe that this "transfer" option opens the door to unethical behavior. Their interpretation is that the CEJA "... is approving the involvement of 'another physician,' thereby sanctioning physician participation" in the overall process of capital punishment. Thus far, their attempts to elicit clarification from the CEJA have not met with success.

Not all experts are convinced that "...if doctors and nurses did not participate in the death penalty, there would be practically no executions at all..." After all, the state could probably find, or train, non-physician "executionists" to take over any matters now in the purview of physicians. (My colleague Alan Stone, MD, a scholar in this area, believes that medical technician phlebotomists are already involved in executions [personal communication, January 5, 2010]). But predictions aside, I agree that Halpern and Halpern have identified a genuine "ambiguity" in the AMA's ethical code.

The AMA spoke more clearly in their amicus curiae brief, filed in a capital punishment case before the Supreme Court of North Carolina. The AMA's brief noted that,

> "Physicians are fundamentally healers, not instruments of death... when they mix those roles, the perception of the profession changes and patient trust erodes. And when that trust erodes, the physicians' ability to care for the patient is diminished. Physician participation in executions, even if legally sanctioned, interferes with the ability to care for patients in wholly different settings" [4].

I would venture even further than this. In my view, psychiatrists would be well advised by their professional organizations to refrain from offering any opinions on a prisoner's "competence to be executed," *even though such opinions may be sought and sanctioned by the legal system*. I believe our role in capital cases should be limited solely to clinical diagnosis and treatment; that is, *to the identification and mitigation of suffering and incapacity*. In this role, we are within proper ethical bounds when providing the legal system with our *diagnostic assessment* and *treatment recommendations*, so long as our doing so is (a) intended to reduce the suffering and incapacity of the prisoner-patient; and (b) not used by the legal system to further the goal of executing the prisoner. If the latter condition requires a commutation order, so be it.

But wait—isn't there an argument to be made for psychiatric involvement in "competence to be executed" determinations, if—at least potentially—lives can be saved? Suppose, for example, that a psychiatrist in the prison system sincerely believes, on the basis of a professional evaluation, that the condemned individual would *not* meet legal criteria for "competence to be executed"? (Although the precise definition of "competence to be executed" is still in flux, a recent U.S. Supreme Court decision (*Panetti v Quarterman*, 127 SCt 2842 [2007]) emphasized that the condemned prisoner must evince a "rational understanding" of both the nature of the punishment and the reasons why it is being applied; see Applebaum [5]). Would it not be legally and morally incumbent on that psychiatrist to express that judgment—thus preserving the prisoner's life, or at least delaying an execution?

Under our current legal system, I think the answer is yes. After all, as my colleague Dr. Alan Stone rightly points out, medical ethics "...is a mix of deontology and consequentialism" (personal communication, December 24, 2009). That is, medical ethics invokes both "duty-based" (cf. *deon*, Gk. "duty") and "consequence-based" judgments. Dr. Stone argues specifically that "...once declared incompetent, prisoners are rarely executed" (personal communication, December 24, 2009). Thus, given the aforementioned scenario, a consequentialist view of medical ethics might urge psychiatric involvement in the "competence to be executed" process on humanitarian grounds—but this is not to endorse the existing *policy* of psychiatric involvement in such determinations. On the contrary, I believe it is bad medical ethics and bad public policy to drag psychiatrists into *any* aspect of the capital punishment process in the first place. In the long run, prohibiting such involvement on the part of physicians will nullify the consequentialist argument. (And let's bear in mind that, in principle, one psychiatrist's determination of incompetence could be overturned in a few days by another psychiatrist, or psychiatric "expert panel.")

Yet another argument asserts that psychiatric involvement in "competence to be executed" determinations is fundamentally no different than our offering an opinion on, say, whether a patient is competent to refuse medical treatment, such as antipsychotic medication. Indeed, to invoke linguist Noam Chomsky's terminology, the "superficial structures" of the phrases, "competence to refuse medication" and "competence to be executed" are quite similar. But, from a moral and existential standpoint, these two determinations have radically different "deep structures."

This may be revealed by trying to re-formulate the two phrases as, "competence to make medication decisions" and "competence to make execution decisions." When psychiatrists engage in determinations of whether a patient understands the risks and benefits of taking an antipsychotic agent, they are indeed assessing the patient's *ability to make informed medication decisions*. But when we participate in "competence to be executed" determinations, we most certainly are *not* assessing the prisoner's ability to make informed execution decisions! Rather, we are assessing—solely at the behest of the potential executioner—*whether the prisoner is cognizant of the impending execution and why society has justified it.*

As my colleague James Knoll points out (personal communication, January 4, 2010), the "…ability to understand the relevant legal constructs" is one legitimate sense of the term "competence"—which is fundamentally a *legal*, not a psychiatric, term of art. But this is not at all the sense embodied in competency determinations *pertaining to medical treatment.* Judged by the usual operational definition of "competence"—namely, "the mental capacity to make a decision *in accordance with the patient's goals, concerns, and values*" (italics added) [6]—the phrase, "competence to be executed" is a linguistic somersault of Orwellian perversity.

The reason for this is not hard to discern. The determination of *competence to refuse treatment* has, as its underlying ethical basis, the safeguarding of the patient's autonomy and the potential for restoring the patient's psychic and bodily integrity. In contrast, the determination of *competence to be executed* is indifferent or antithetical to the prisoner's autonomy, and has the potential for literally *annihilating* the prisoner's psychic and bodily integrity. The deep structures of these two kinds of "competency" determinations could hardly be more different. To put it in more concrete terms: if a patient is not competent to make antipsychotic medication decisions, a "substituted judgment" is rendered by the court, aimed at determining what the patient would desire if he or she *were* competent. But if a patient is deemed not competent to be executed, nobody renders a substituted judgment as to what the patient would wish ("Let's see…would Joe want to be executed or not?") if he were competent!

Yes—we must acknowledge that these are extremely complex issues, and that humane and reasonable individuals will differ in their conclusions [7]. Nobody should luxuriate in a sense of self-righteous certitude on these matters. But my personal take as a bioethicist remains simply this: the executioner's room is a "bad neighborhood" for physicians, and we should keep far away from it!

At first glance, the *interrogation* of prisoners—such as those held at Guantanamo Bay—may seem to be in a different moral category than the execution of prisoners. After all, such interrogation, in cases involving national security, may be aimed at preventing injury or death on a massive scale—as has been argued in the now-famous (or infamous) "ticking bomb" scenario. And yet, the ethical rationale for avoiding any involvement in interrogations is essentially the same as that prohibiting the physician's involvement in executions: physicians are fundamentally *healers*, not support staff for military or civilian interrogators. Nonetheless, as Prof. John Thomas describes in Psychiatric Times [8], both psychologists and (initially) physicians have been involved to varying degrees in the interrogation of suspected terrorists. (The physicians, evidently, were not considered cooperative enough, and were dropped from the "team" after 2004, as Prof. Thomas describes).

Let me be clear: I mean no disrespect to military or civilian authorities charged with investigating crime or suspected acts of terror. Indeed, preventing mass casualties—as might well occur with an act of terror—is clearly an ethically defensible goal. The use of non-coercive interrogation techniques, *consistent with the Geneva conventions*, represents a vital tool in law enforcement's armamentarium. However, *the lawful goals of police, professional interrogators and military personnel are not necessarily commensurate with the ethical responsibilities of the physician*. Indeed, in my view, our moral imperatives require that physicians stay "far away" from the neighborhood of the interrogator. This means that no psychiatrist should cooperate in any *non-medical* matter, with respect to any kind of military or police interrogation—coercive, non-coercive, or otherwise. Aside from providing general, scientific information to appropriate authorities, regarding specific psychiatric disorders; or undertaking the diagnosis and treatment of a detainee's psychiatric symptoms in order to relieve suffering and incapacity, *psychiatrists should have nothing to do with either military or civilian interrogations.* As the American Psychiatric Association states in their May, 2006, position statement,

> "Psychiatrists providing medical care to individual detainees owe their primary obligation to the well-being of their patients, including advocating for their patients, and should not participate or assist in any way, whether directly or indirectly, overtly or covertly, in the interrogation of their patients on behalf of military or civilian agencies or law enforcement authorities" [9].

Moreover, as Halpern et al. argue:

> "...not only forensic psychiatrists, but all psychiatrists, must remain constantly alert to the danger of being drawn into unethical conduct in the service of an elusive and not infrequently unjust "justice." It has long been recognized that in countries where misuse of psychiatry has been, and in some countries still is, rampant, such as the former Soviet Union, China, Romania, South Africa and others, psychiatrists justified their unethical conduct on the grounds that they were furthering the interests of their countries' justice" [10].

Physicians are healers. Psychiatric physicians are ethically bound to ensure the well being of their patients. We need to keep far away from neighborhoods in which we are urged to violate or compromise that obligation.

Acknowledgments

I wish to thank James Knoll, MD, Alan Stone, MD, Eugene Kaplan, MD, Howard Zonana, MD, John Halpern, MD, and Abraham Halpern, MD, for their comments, criticisms, and suggestions. However, unless otherwise noted, the author alone is responsible for the views expressed in this editorial. A slightly modified version of this piece appeared in the January 26, 2010, issue of *Psychiatric Times*.

References

[1] Stone AA. The ethical boundaries of forensic psychiatry: a view from the ivory tower. *J Am Acad Psychiatry Law*. 2008;36:136-172. Available from: http://www.jaapl.org/cgi/content/full/36/2/167. Accessed March 1, 2014. (Originally published *Bull Am Acad Psychiatry Law*. 1984;12:209-219.)

[2] American Medical Association Council on Ethical and Judicial Affairs. Opinion 2.06—Capital punishment. Available from: http://www.ama-assn.org/ama/pub/physician-resources. Accessed February 26, 2014.

[3] Halpern AL, Halpern J. [Letter to the Editor]. *The New York Times*. 2009 December 20. Available from: http://www.nytimes.com/2009/12/21/opinion/l21death.html. Accessed February 26, 2014.

[4] Amicus Curiae Brief of American Medical Association. *North Carolina Department of Correction v North Carolina Medical Board*. 2 June 2008. Supreme Court of North Carolina. [online]. Available from: http://www.ama-assn.org/ama1/pub/upload/mm/395/nc_captialpunishment.pdf. Accessed February 26, 2014.

[5] Appelbaum PS. Death row delusions: when is a prisoner competent to be executed? *Psychiatr Serv*. 2007;58:1258-1260.

[6] Simon RI, Shuman DW. *Clinical Manual of Psychiatry and Law*. Washington DC: American Psychiatric Press; 2007: 64.

[7] Zonana HV. Competency to be executed and forced medication: *Singleton v. Norris*. *J Am Acad Psychiatry Law*. 2003;31:372-376.

[8] Thomas J. Mental health professionals in the "enhanced" interrogation room. *Psychiatr Times*. 2009 October 28. Available from: http://www.psychiatrictimes.com/display/article/10168/1481838. Accessed March 1, 2014.

[9] American Psychiatric Association. Position paper on psychiatric participation in interrogation of detainees. 2006 May. Available from: http://www.psychiatry. Accessed March 1, 2014.

[10] Halpern AL, Halpern JH, Doherty SB. "Enhanced" interrogation of detainees: do psychologists and psychiatrists participate? *Philosophy, Ethics, and Humanities in Medicine*. 2008;3:21. Available from: http://www.peh-med.com/content/3/1/21#B2. Accessed March 1, 2014.

WHY PSYCHIATRISTS MUST CONFRONT GUN-RELATED VIOLENCE

During my recent stay in Scotland, I had a most peculiar experience while walking through the streets of Edinburgh, Glasgow, and Stirling, late at night: *I felt safe*. This is a sensation I almost never have while walking at night in American cities of comparable size. As my wife and I learned during our stay there, Scotland has a violent and bloody history, going back many centuries. And, to be sure, modern-day Scots—a remarkably friendly and civil people—must deal with crime, drugs, and violence, just as Americans do. But they do not worry much about gun-related violence. According to the London-based Gun Control Network, there were a grand total of *four* gun-related homicides in Scotland, between 2009 and 2011 [1]. That's right: *four*. Leaving aside per capita comparisons for the moment, keep in mind that there were over 20,000 gun homicides in the U.S. during the period of 2009-2010 alone [2].

And lest you suppose that the Scots are stabbing or bludgeoning each other in droves—i.e., committing thousands of *non-gun*-related homicides—Scotland's average total homicide rate between 2006 and 2008 was less than half the average for the U.S. homicide rate during this same period [3, 4].

I don't want to draw any sweeping conclusions from this one comparison—I simply want to introduce an international perspective to the issue of firearms regulation. I also want to argue that this contentious issue is of urgent relevance to psychiatry, as several articles in *Psychiatric Times* have demonstrated [5-7].

Why should psychiatrists care about firearms regulation? The reason that might first come to mind—the putative role of "mental illness" in several recent mass shootings—is actually the least important. Aurora, Colorado-type mass shootings—horrific though they are—actually amount to a minuscule percentage of gun-related deaths in the U.S. There are more compelling reasons why psychiatrists should be involved in the gun control debate.

First, psychiatrists are experts in assessing risk factors for suicide, and gun possession is a major risk factor for completed suicide. In fact, *the majority of gun-related deaths in the U.S. are suicides,* and the U.S. has a *firearm-related* suicide rate almost six times higher than comparison countries [8]. One study of handgun possession in California found that, in the first week after the purchase of a handgun, the rate of firearms suicide among purchasers is about 57 times as high as the adjusted rate in the general population [9].

Similarly, a recent review concluded that

> "There are at least a dozen U.S. case–control studies in the peer-reviewed literature, all of which have found that a gun in the home is associated with an increased risk of suicide. The increase in risk is large, typically 2 to 10 times that in homes without guns, depending on the sample population" [10].

Second, psychiatrists are frequently called upon to assess "dangerousness" to others. Such requests may originate in emergency settings; on inpatient units, or in the context of a forensic evaluation. While persons with psychiatric illness comprise only a small fraction of those involved in gun violence, gun possession per se is an important factor in any determination of dangerousness to others—particularly in this country. Compared with other high-income countries, firearm homicide rates in the U.S. are nearly 20 times higher; and in the population aged 15 to 24, firearm homicide rates are almost 43 times higher here than in other high-income countries [8].

These extraordinary rates of gun-related killing cannot be written off as artifacts of faulty study methods or misinterpretation of the data. For example, the claim that other high-income countries have higher *overall* homicide rates than the U.S., owing to *non-gun-related* homicides (via stabbings, blunt objects, etc.) is not borne out by the best available data. Thus, Table 4 shows overall intentional homicide rates and intentional gun-related homicide rates in the U.S. and 3 other high-income countries for 2009 [4]. (The United Nations Office on Drugs and Crime defines "intentional homicide" as "...*unlawful* death purposely inflicted on a person by another person.") It also shows percentage of homicides due to firearms:

Table 4. Homicides per 100,000 by Country

	U.S.	France [*2007]	Canada	Australia
Overall intentional homicide rate per 100,000	5.0	1.1	1.8	1.2
Intentional gun homicide rate per 100,000	3.3	0.1	0.5	0.1
Percent of homicides due to firearms	66.9%	9.6%	32%	11.5%

Source: UNODC (United Nations Office on Drugs and Crime) [4]

Simply stated, the extraordinarily high rate of intentional homicides in the U.S. compared with these other countries is driven by the high percentage of homicides *due to guns*. The weapon of choice makes a huge difference in *lethality*.

Gun Violence in the U.S.

What about the relationship of gun ownership, firearms laws, and violent crime in the U.S.? Of course, proving *causal* connections (vs. mere associations) between gun regulations and violent crime rates is exceedingly difficult, given the multitude of confounding variables. Yet one myth that continues to be proffered by those who oppose any and all regulation of firearms is that gun ownership decreases crime rates and "keeps people safe." In truth, there is little credible evidence to support these claims, and considerable evidence against them. Thus, a recent review in the *New England Journal of Medicine* concluded that

> "Americans have purchased millions of guns, predominantly handguns, believing that having a gun at home makes them safer. In fact, handgun purchasers substantially increase their risk of a violent death. This increase begins the moment the gun is acquired—suicide is the leading cause of death among handgun owners in the first year after purchase—and lasts for years....Gun ownership and gun violence [rates] rise and fall together...[Moreover] permissive policies regarding carrying guns have not reduced crime rates, and permissive states generally have higher rates of gun-related deaths than others do (see map)" [11].

These conclusions are consistent with a study from the Violence Policy Center (VPC), based on 2008 data from the Centers for Disease Control and Prevention. The VPC study found that

> "States with higher gun ownership rates and weak gun laws have the highest rates of gun death... The analysis reveals that the five states with the highest per capita gun death rates were Alaska, Mississippi, Louisiana, Alabama, and Wyoming. Each of these states had a per capita gun death rate far exceeding the national per capita gun death rate of 10.38 per 100,000 for 2008. Each state has lax gun laws and higher gun ownership rates. By contrast, states with strong gun laws and low rates of gun ownership had far lower rates of firearm-related death" [12].

Voices opposed to firearms regulation often point to John R. Lott's book, *More Guns, Less Crime: Understanding Crime and Gun Control Laws* (3rd ed., 2010). This work purports to show an inverse relationship between gun ownership and violent crime; e.g., it claims that states allowing citizens to carry concealed weapons ("right to carry") show decreased rates of violent crime. Lott's claims and methods, however, have been vigorously challenged—if not discredited—by many scholars. A recent (2009) comprehensive review by Yale Law school professors Ian Ayres and John J. Donohue III found that "right to carry" (RTC) laws were clearly associated with an *increase in aggravated assaults*; and possibly with *higher rates of murder and robbery*, although the latter findings were not statistically significant [13]. Again: association does not prove causality, but these findings lend no support to the claim that right-to-carry laws reduce violent crime.

Of course, laws have other purposes, beyond the expectation that they will actually reduce or prevent a specific injurious or antisocial act. Laws also represent society's moral values, and our intention to set limits on certain types of behavior. Laws may also reflect society's wish to reduce the likelihood of certain types of injurious behavior, even while realizing that this wish may not be fulfilled. There are, of course, always people with evil intentions who will ignore the law--but that is no reason to omit or expunge the law. Research might show, for example, that laws against private citizens possessing bazookas or shoulder-fired missiles do not, by themselves, prevent certain people from illegally obtaining and firing these weapons. Nevertheless, in my view, there is strong ethical justification for keeping such laws on the books, as a matter of sound public policy. Similarly, even if we could not demonstrate that laws banning production and private ownership of rapid-fire, semi-automatic weapons actually reduced mass shootings, a civilized society would still have sound ethical reasons for retaining these laws. That is, these laws legitimately reflect society's value judgment that no good will come from the possession of such destructive lethal weapons by private citizens—and that much harm may ensue. But, as it turns out, there *is* credible (though not conclusive) evidence that *nationally-promulgated laws*—not state-by-state regulations—may reduce the incidence of mass shootings. Thus, as my colleague, forensic psychiatrist Dr. James Knoll has observed,

> "Countries with less stringent gun control laws have been observed to have a higher risk of mass murder than countries with stricter laws. One Australian observational study compared mass murders before and after 1996, the year of a widely publicized mass murder in Tasmania. Australia quickly enacted gun law reforms that included removing semiautomatic, pump-action shotguns and rifles from civilian possession. In the 18 years

before the gun laws, the Australian authors reported 13 mass shootings. In the 10.5 years after the gun law reforms, there were none" [14].

Indeed, the authors of the Australian study concluded that "Removing large numbers of rapid-firing firearms from civilians may be an effective way of reducing mass shootings, firearm homicides and firearm suicides." Furthermore, contrary to a popular notion that says, "If you remove dangerous firearms, people will just find other ways of killing themselves or others"—the so-called "substitution" hypothesis—these authors found "...*no evidence of substitution effect for suicides or homicides*" [15].

It is crucial to note that the Australian firearms regulations were *nationally* applied and enforced. *A piecemeal approach to firearms regulation that affects only some cities or states cannot reasonably be expected to produce a robust effect on gun-homicides or mass shootings*. For example, the recent spike in gun homicides in Chicago, IL—which mandates strict regulation of firearms—emphatically does *not* prove that nationally-enforced firearms regulations are bound to fail. Chicago's tough firearms statutes are seriously undermined by guns brought in from suburban areas; guns from neighboring states with less stringent regulations; and by "...a well-funded gun lobby and an underfunded federal enforcement effort" [16] that impedes crackdowns on Cook County gun dealers who sell to "straw buyers"—people without criminal records who buy guns for felons.

Finally, there is another reason psychiatrists are well-equipped to address the issue of gun control: we are experts in recognizing irrational fears. Many people in this country are, quite understandably, very concerned about their safety. But the notion that even reasonable regulation of firearms and ammunition represents the first step in "disarming" the populace is an unwarranted fear, based on flawed historical analogies [7]. We can agree, as a society, that an individual "right to bear arms" should be respected, under recent U.S. Supreme Court interpretations of the second amendment. Yet we may still insist that stockpiling semi-automatic weapons against a hypothetical totalitarian state is no answer to the here-and-now reality of the carnage on our streets. Placing sensible restrictions on firearms—such as eliminating production and sale of semi-automatic weapons—has been advocated by groups as politically diverse as the American Psychiatric Association and the International Association of Chiefs of Police [17]. Contrary to some fear-mongering, eliminating production and sales of semi-automatic weapons does *not* mean that currently owned weapons would be "confiscated." (Voluntary "buy-back" programs to remove semi-automatic weapons from the street is an option worth considering, though the effectiveness of these programs has been questioned) [18].

Psychiatrists, like all physicians, have an ethical duty to protect the health and safety of the general public. We simply cannot claim to do so, if we oppose reasonable limits on firearms and ammunition in this country. Guns, by and large, do not keep people safe. And if we, as a people, foolishly sacrifice genuine security for a false sense of freedom, we shall find ourselves in a nation neither secure nor free.

Acknowledgments

I wish to thank James L. Knoll IV, MD; Garen J. Wintemute, MD, MPH; and David Hemenway, PhD, for their helpful comments on this essay; however, the positions advocated here reflect my own views. A slightly modified version of this piece appeared in the October 26, 2010, issue of *Psychiatric Times*.

References

[1] Gun Control Network. Firearms offenses: Scotland [online]. Available from: http://www.gun-control-network.org/GF04.htm. Accessed March 9, 2014.

[2] United Nations Office on Drugs and Crime. Homicides by firearms. Available from: http://www.unodc.org/documents/data-and-analysis/statistics. Accessed March 9, 2014.

[3] Statistical Bulletin Crime and Justice Series: Homicide in Scotland, 2009-10 http://www.scotland.gov.uk/Publications/2010/12/10110553/3

[4] United Nations Office on Drugs and Crime. UNODC homicide statistics. Available from: http://www.unodc.org/documents/data-and-analysis/statistics/Homicide/Globa_study_on_homicide_2011_web.pdf. Accessed April 3, 2014.

[5] Robertson R. POINT: The Case for Gun Control. *Psychiatr Times*. 2012 October 5. Available from: http://www.psychiatrictimes.com/display/article/10168/2106376. Accessed March 9, 2014.

[6] Frances A. Mass murders, madness, and gun control. *Psychiatr Times*. 2012 July 30. Available from: http://www.psychiatrictimes.com/blog/frances/content/article /10168/2093233. Accessed March 9, 2014.

[7] Horwitz J. COUNTERPOINT: Gun Control and the Second Amendment. *Psychiatr Times*. 2012 October 5. Available from: http://www.psychiatrictimes.com/display-old/article/10168/2106371. Accessed March 9, 2014.

[8] Richardson EG, Hemenway D. Homicide, suicide, and unintentional firearm fatality: comparing the United States with other high-income countries, 2003. *J Trauma*. 2011;70:238-243.

[9] Wintemute GJ, Parham CA, Beaumont JJ, et al. Mortality among recent purchasers of handguns. *N Engl J Med*. 1999;341:1583-1589.

[10] Miller M, Hemenway D. Guns and suicide in the United States. *N Engl J Med*. 2008;359:989-991.

[11] Wintemute GJ. Guns, fear, the Constitution, and the public's health. *N Engl J Med*. 2008; 358:1421-1424.

[12] Violence Policy Center. States with higher gun ownership and weak gun laws lead nation in gun death [online]. 2011 October 24. Available from: http://www.vpc.org /press/1110gundeath.htm. Accessed March 9, 2014.

[13] Ayres I, Donohue JJ. More guns, less crime fails again: the latest evidence from1977 – 2006. *Econ Journal Watch*. 2009;6:218-238. Available from: http://works.bepress.com /cgi/viewcontent.cgi?article=1065&context=john_donohue. Accessed March 9, 2014.

[14] Knoll JL. The "pseudocommando" mass murderer: Part II, The language of revenge. *J Am Acad Psychiatry Law*. 2010;38:263-272. Availble from: http://www.jaapl.org /content/38/2/263.full.pdf. Accessed March 1, 2014.

[15] Chapman S, Alpers P, Agho K, et al. Australia's 1996 gun law reforms: faster falls in firearm deaths, firearm suicides, and a decade without mass shootings. *Injury Prev*. 2006;12:365-372.

[16] Main F. Chicago gangs don't have to go far to buy guns. *Chicago Sun-Times*. 2012 August 26. 2012. Available from: http://www.suntimes.com/news/crime/14715658-418/chicago-gangs-dont-have-to-go-far-to-buy-guns.html. Accessed March 9, 2014.

[17] International Association of Chiefs of Police. Violent Crime in America: Recommendations of the IACP Summit on Violent Crime. Available from: https://www.ncjrs.gov/App/Publications/abstract.aspx?ID

[18] Irons ME. Success of gun buyback programs is debated. *The Boston Globe*. 2014 February 13.

For further reading

Miller M, Azrael D, Barber C. Suicide mortality in the United States: the importance of attending to method in understanding population-level disparities in the burden of suicide. *Annual Review of Public Health*. 2012;33:393-408.

Harvard Injury Control Research Center [online]. Available from: https://www.hsph.harvard.edu/research/hicrc/index.html. Accessed March 9, 2014. (An extremely useful source of reliable data on gun-related violence.)

~~~~~~~~~~~~~~~~~~~~

THE EIGHT-FOLD PATH OF INTERNET ETHICS: A PRIMER FOR HEALTH CARE PROFESSIONALS

Anyone who has written blogs or published articles on line knows that the Internet is the new "Wild West," so far as etiquette is concerned. As a physician who has blogged on several different websites, or responded to postings by other health care professionals, I have been astounded by the level of bile and vitriol that infects so many communications among "colleagues." Worse still, many websites aimed at health care professionals permit anonymous postings—a sure-fire invitation to the "flaming" e-mail, in which someone purporting to be a physician or other professional berates a colleague in terms that would embarrass the proverbial fishmonger's wife (my apologies in advance to fishmongers and their spouses).

As Neil Swidey recently wrote in the *Boston Globe*,

> "Anonymous commentary is a push and pull between privacy and trust... Online postings can sway political opinion and heavily influence whether products or businesses thrive or fail. They can make or break reputations and livelihoods. On one side, anonymous comments give users the freedom to be completely candid in a public forum. On the other, that freedom can be abused and manipulated to spread lies or mask hidden agendas" [1].

Recently, there has been a movement toward restricting or prohibiting anonymous (or pseudonymous) postings on the internet—and not only on professional websites. For example, mass media papers like the *Washington Post* are said to be re-assessing their own posting rules [1]. There has also been a good deal of discussion in legal circles regarding the "unmasking" of anonymous bloggers who clearly defame another individual. Thus, according to Joel Reidenberg, founder of the Center on Law and Information Policy at Fordham Law School, the judicial trend has been to "…permit unmasking of anonymous bloggers when there is a strong showing that the statement is defamatory and that the victim would be likely to prevail in a defamation lawsuit" [2].

To be sure: there are extremely rare instances in which an anonymous posting may be justifiable; for example, when someone exposing a genuine social evil or criminal act risks retaliation, revenge, or even death, by providing his or her real name. But in my view, it is not enough that an anonymous health care professional wishes to avoid "embarrassment", or finds it "inconvenient" to provide his or her name. I find it especially deplorable—and cowardly-- when one physician hides behind the safety of a pseudonym while attacking a *named* colleague. Yet this goes on all the time, on numerous "medical" websites.

That said, my aim in this piece is not to engage in still more adversarial exchanges. Rather, I'd like to suggest some ethical guidelines for health care professionals (or anyone else) who post blogs and comments on line. In addition to urging my colleagues to provide their full name and degree (MD, PhD, etc.) in all online communications, I would also encourage them to build their critiques on a foundation of collegiality, respect and fairness. In my view, this is not a matter of "Emily Post" etiquette, but of ethical and professional responsibility. And so—with apologies to the "Noble Eightfold Path" of Siddhartha Gautama [3]—here are my eight principles of ethical online conduct:

1) When criticizing a colleague, try to begin your critique with something appreciative and positive—or at least neutral—such as, "Dr. X. raises some very timely and important questions in his/her thoughtful essay."
2) Try not to write anything about your colleague that you would not feel justified in saying to his or her face, at a professional conference (and bear in mind, that's where the two of you may meet next!).
3) Never—ever—dash off an e-mail or blog comment in a fit of anger; rather, write a draft version "off line"; reflect upon it; revise if necessary (it usually is); and send only after a suitable "cooling down" period. (Yes, this degree of restraint is hard—and I have violated this rule once or twice, myself—only to regret it later).
4) Always consider having a colleague read over any critique that leaves you feeling uneasy or slightly "guilty," regarding statements about another person. (And keep in mind: there are still laws against libel.)
5) Always phrase your criticism in terms of *ideas* or *behaviors*, not your opponent's *character* or *mentality*; e.g., say, "The notion that we should use that approach is misguided, in my opinion," not "Dr. X is totally out of his mind!"
6) Try to include some points of agreement with your opponent, if you can legitimately find any (and look hard for them!).
7) Hard as it may be, try to attribute a benign intention or motivation to your opponent; e.g., "Dr. X clearly intends to protect the welfare of the general public; however, in my view, her approach may lead to serious problems." ("In my view" is a good mantra to recite.)

8) Always try to summarize your opponent's view in a fair and convincing manner, while allowing for the possibility that you have misunderstood his position. (In the Talmud, the School of Hillel garnered more approval than did its opponents, the School of Shammai, because in writing their opinions, the Hillelites typically began by accurately stating the Shammaites' point of view.)

As one commentator has observed, in discussing the Buddha's concept of "right speech": "The importance of speech in the context of Buddhist ethics is obvious: words can break or save lives, make enemies or friends, start war or create peace" [3]. Surely, those of us whose livelihood and calling depend on the power of words must take this counsel to heart.

A slightly modified version of this piece appeared in the January 5, 2011, issue of Psychiatric Times.

References

[1] Swidey N. Inside the mind of the anonymous online poster. *The Boston Globe*. 2010 June 20. Available from: http://www.boston.com/bostonglobe/magazine/articles/2010/06/20/inside_the_mind_of_the_anonymous_online_poster. Accessed March 9, 2014.

[2] Karni A. End of Internet anonymity. Fordham University School of Law. Available from: http://law.fordham.edu/faculty/18870.htm. Accessed March 9, 2014.

[3] The Noble Eightfold Path. Available from: http://www.beyondthenet.net/dhamma/nobleEight.htm

~~~~~~~~~~~~~~~~~~~~

PSYCHIATRY AND THE HEART OF DARKNESS

...wrongs darker than death or night...—Percy Bysshe Shelley, *Prometheus Unbound*

The press reported it in various ways—either as a "brutal gang rape" or, more forensically, as a "2 1/2-hour assault" on the Richmond High School campus. Any way you look at it, the horrendous attack on a 15-year-old girl raises troubling questions for theologians, criminologists and, of course, psychiatrists. How do we understand an act as brutal as rape? What factors and forces in the rapist's development can possibly account for such behavior? And how on earth do we explain the apparent indifference of the large crowd that watched the attack in Richmond, Calif, and allegedly did nothing to stop it—or even, to report it?

In a thoughtful analysis on CNN, Stephanie Chen provides a range of "expert opinions" on this last question. Essentially, the various hypotheses asserted that:

- Bystanders in large groups are unlikely to take appropriate action in such cases, because they assume that others have already done so or because "doing nothing becomes the norm" (the so-called bystander effect).

- Witnesses who might have phoned 911 may have feared retaliation from the perpetrators.
- Bystanders do not feel a "bond" with the victim, and may actually identify with the perpetrator, who is perceived as "more important" than the victim.

The CNN report speculated at length on the so-called Genovese syndrome, named for the woman stabbed to death in Queens, NY, in 1964—supposedly after 38 witnesses to the attack did nothing to help her. The facts, however, are almost certainly otherwise, as an article in the *American Psychologist* argues. Indeed, the authors concluded that "there is no evidence for the presence of 38 witnesses, or that witnesses observed the murder, or that witnesses remained inactive."

Even in the case of the Richmond High rape, it now appears that at least one person—Margarita Vargas—*did* notify the police [1]. However, as ABC News reported it, Vargas was not a witness to the rape. Rather, "...the 18-year-old mother and former Richmond High School student was at home watching a movie when her brother-in-law came home and said he had seen a girl getting raped." It is remarkable that this man seems to have brought the news to Vargas with the same sense of urgency as someone who had just witnessed a fender-bender. Reportedly, he was "scared"—so perhaps we ought to allow for some degree of shock, and perhaps fear of retaliation.

Nevertheless, media reports on the Richmond High rape have largely ignored the moral implications of the bystanders' failure to aid the rape victim. Thus, the forensic experts, quoted in the CNN piece, took a predictably "objective" point of view. None ventured the opinion that the crowd at Richmond High School failed to help because many human beings often act in a selfish, callous, and cowardly manner.

Nobody put forth the view of rabbinical Judaism that we are all born with two primal inclinations, constantly at war with one another. The "good inclination" (*yetzer hatov*) is usually considered a kind of later "add-on" to the more powerful "evil inclination" (*yetzer hara*), which often gains the upper hand. The *yetzer hara* seems to have been alive and well at Richmond High—and nobody there lifted a finger to stop it. Rabbi Bruce Kadden, however, points out that the *yetzer hara* is not some "devil" external to our own selves, rather it is very much a part of us, and we have a responsibility to tame, control and modulate this inclination [2].

The problem of human evil, however defined, has arisen in a number of recent events that have been subject to lengthy psychological analyses; e.g., the mass shooting at Fort Hood and the attack on a 15-year-old boy, who was set on fire by 5 other teenagers [3]. Yet many psychiatrists, it seems to me, have been reluctant to venture into the obscure headwaters of evil—the territory explored so vividly in Josef Conrad's 1902 novella, *The Heart of Darkness*. Many in our profession have taken the "scientific" view that matters of good and evil are best left to theologians and clergy, and that clinicians should limit themselves to analyzing and correcting the developmental, biological, and psychological precursors of so-called antisocial behavior.

That's all very sensible, of course—but also a dodge, in my view. It's true that, as mental health professionals, we may rightly insist on examining any behavior, however heinous, in terms of its psychopathological roots. And in so doing, we may invoke any number of biological, social, and psychological "explanations." Yet psychiatrists and other mental health professionals cannot avoid moral issues, or moral narratives, when considering violent antisocial acts. After all, the constructs of good and evil are very real, and matter very deeply, to most of our patients. Should they not also matter to us?

Indeed, a woman who presents in therapy with a rape-related traumatic syndrome may be said to *embody the problem of human evil:* even her physiological responses to trauma-related stimuli have been altered by her experience. But more than that, the patient (male or female) who has suffered a brutal assault may need to explore the moral dimensions of the act and its consequences: "How could another human being do such a horrible thing? And—why me, Doctor? Was I being punished by God? Am I somehow responsible for what happened? What should I do with all the hatred and rage I feel toward this monster? Is it right that I want him to suffer as much as I have—and even have thoughts of killing him? Does this make *me* evil, too, Doctor?"

These understandable moral questions do not arise for all victims of trauma; but when they do, psychiatrists must be prepared to engage the patient in a serious "I-Thou" dialogue, to use Martin Buber's term. Similarly, philosopher and ethicist Margaret U. Walker has written of the need for "moral repair" after an act of wrongdoing. As therapists, we help effect such repair by establishing trust—the first step in mending the torn fabric of the traumatized patient's moral universe. But to gain the patient's trust, we must be ready to talk frankly and comfortably about good and evil. This doesn't mean proselytizing the patient. But it often means engaging in a moral dialogue with the patient, and confronting the enormity of acts such as those that occurred at Richmond High.

Acknowledgment

A slightly modified version of this piece appeared in the November 30, 2009, issue of *Psychiatric Times*.

References

[1] Ishimaru H. Richmond rape: good Samaritan speaks [online]. ABC7 News. 2009 November 4. Available from: http://abclocal.go.com/kgo/story?section=news/local/east_bay&id=7101419. Accessed March 9, 2014.
[2] Kadden B. The Vocabulary of Jewish Life: Yetzer Tov and Yetzer Ra. Sermon, July 16, 2010. Available at:
[3] http://www.templebethel18.org/images/stories/The_Vocabulary_of_Jewish_Life_-_Yetzer_Tov_and_Yetzer_Ra.pdf
[4] Associated Press. Mom of teen set on fire describes "nightmare" [online]. NBC News. 2009 October 15. Available from: http://www.msnbc.msn.com/id/33325007. Accessed March 9, 2014.

THE MADNESS OF A STRANGER—IN OUR HOUSE

Be not forgetful to entertain strangers: for thereby some have entertained angels unawares. —Hebrews 13:2

The knock on the door came just after 1 in the morning, as my wife and I were getting ready for bed. In the small, Central New York town where we spend summers, "ordinary" people do not knock at that hour, save for the rare tourist with a broken down car and a dead cell phone. Shuffling barefoot into our kitchen, I approached the front door with trepidation and asked, "Who is it?" A young woman's panicky voice, muffled through the glass, replied, "I'm looking for my brother's house! Do you know where he lives?" I pulled back the curtain with the door still locked, and saw a sweaty, disheveled figure, standing next to what looked like a child's scooter. The young woman was stuffed into a short skirt, 2 sizes too small for her zaftig physique. "My car broke down!" she said, her eyes dark with tear-smudged mascara, "I had to ride here on my scooter! Please, can I use your phone?"

I realize now that the bizarre scene at that hour should have prompted more caution on my part. Wisdom would have dictated keeping a safe distance from this late-night intruder. But my gut told me that here was a young woman in distress; and my religious beliefs—whispering from somewhere deep in my subconscious—must also have been working within me. After all, doesn't the Bible tell us that Abraham and Sarah welcomed three strangers into their tent, bringing them food and kindness? (*Genesis* 18) For all Abraham knew, the strangers were thieves or murderers!

In the Jewish faith, hospitality toward strangers is a *mitzvah*—a commandment. On the other hand, my 30 years of psychiatric training should have had a stronger voice in the matter. Individuals with psychiatric illnesses are not, for the most part, given to violence. In fact, they are more often the target of violent attacks—especially persons with serious mental illness who are also homeless. Yet untreated psychosis, especially when accompanied by substance abuse, is associated with an increased risk of violence. No doubt, I should have been more wary of someone who had just ridden a child's scooter to my house, at 1 in the morning.

Sighing deeply, I said, "Okay, you can use my phone." I opened the door and let the young woman into my house.

At first, things went reasonably well. She gave me a number to call—apparently, her brother's—but there was no answer. The young woman was sweating profusely and became increasingly more agitated. I thought I smelled alcohol on her breath, but her state of mind suggested a more complex set of problems. "I was just in the hospital," she blurted, "and my heart stopped! They had to revive me twice. I'm bleeding internally! I have ovarian cysts. I know I'm supposed to take my medication but I don't like the side effects—and besides, I like my natural highs! Can I have some water or some juice? My blood sugar is low . . ." And on and on her narrative went, in what emergency department physicians and psychiatrists usually describe as "talking ragtime." If you are not actually in a florid manic state, it's almost impossible to mimic the "flight of ideas" that this phase of bipolar disorder provokes—a kind of staccato, *rat-a-tat-tat* of loosely connected thoughts, often delivered in a loud, insistent manner. Okay, I thought, I have just let a floridly manic patient into my house. How foolish was that? My wife—a retired psychiatric social worker—had wisely scurried upstairs, to the relative safety of our bedroom.

Over the course of the next 20 minutes or so, I did my best to calm down our young visitor, but there really is no calming down a manic patient, short of medication and a quiet, dimly lit room. And yet, something curious happened to me as I listened to this distressed young woman regale me, at breakneck speed, with her tales of woe: I began to feel less fearful. And I began to see that beneath the sweating, speeding, mascara-smeared mess of her acute illness, a decent human being longed for a more stable life. I offered her a glass of fruit juice, and she gratefully drank it.

Her name was Kara. She lived in the poorer section of town, and—at age 18—had already been in and out of psychiatric hospitals for several years. She knew she needed help, but she never stayed on her medications: "Too many side effects!" But the side effect of her going off medication was the ruination of her life, and the enmity of others. Kara had been in trouble with the local police, who saw her as a troublemaker and a menace—which was not entirely inaccurate.

I later learned that, the same night as her visitation, Kara had gone to the firehouse and claimed that someone had placed a bomb in her grandmother's house. This led to an expensive wild goose chase by our town's tiny police force and volunteer firemen, diverting them from a major brushfire. I suspect Kara had not acted maliciously, and that the false report was the product of her delusions. Still, her actions did not endear her to the local authorities. To make matters worse, she was known to run around with kids who had "been into bath salts," the latest supercharged hallucinatory mix, out on the streets. It later occurred to me that Kara's manic symptoms and behavior might have been due, in part, to this nasty chemical brew.

"It sounds to me like you could use some medical help, Kara," I said at last. "I'm going to call 911." She did not protest. In fact, she said, "Yeah, I could use a doctor." Within a few minutes, two police officers and a fireman showed up at our door, followed shortly by an ambulance. The fireman argued a bit with the police, urging the young policewoman in charge to "have that girl arrested!" I felt obligated to interject something vaguely professional, and said, "Officer, this young woman really needs medical attention, not jail." The officer agreed. Within a few minutes, Kara walked peacefully out of our house and was taken to a nearby hospital for evaluation.

Kara's intrusion into my home life left me reflecting on how so many individuals with serious psychiatric disorders are ill-served in this country. Many lack health care insurance. Many patients with so-called "dual diagnoses" (major psychiatric illness plus substance abuse) lack access to comprehensive care. The very small minority of patients who represent a danger to themselves or others, but who refuse treatment, often have few alternatives to involuntary hospitalization—only a few states have so-called "outpatient commitment" laws, which can lead to successful (albeit involuntary) treatment. Finally, given the broad, unmonitored discretion of police officers in such cases, Kara might well have wound up in jail—a problem that requires our urgent attention.

I don't believe I'll allow any more late night visitors into our home. But I am not quite prepared to say that letting Kara in was entirely a mistake. Oh, yes—about those three visitors Abraham and Sarah entertained: one biblical interpretation suggests that they were heavenly messengers. And sometimes, even when the messenger is decidedly of this earth, the message she brings us is still worth heeding.

Acknowledgments

My thanks to James L. Knoll, IV, MD, for his helpful comments on this piece. A slightly modified version of this piece appeared in the July 18, 2012, issue of *Psychiatric Times*.

Author Contact Information

Dr. Ronald William Pies, MD
Professor of Psychiatry
Lecture on Bioethics & Humanities
SUNY Upstate Medical University
Syracuse, NY
Tel: 781-862-8124
ronpies@massmed.org

INDEX

#

20th century, 58

A

Abraham, 98, 132, 170, 174, 185, 186
abstraction, 41
abuse, 35, 37, 131, 133, 136, 137, 141
access, 39, 145, 168, 186
actuality, 1, 8
acute schizophrenia, 2
acute stress, 87
AD, 27
adaptation, 87, 106, 107, 112
adaptations, 104, 117
ADHD, 73, 78, 99, 155
adjustment, 89, 153
adolescents, 109, 136
adulthood, 34
advertisements, 32, 36
advocacy, 3, 39
affective disorder, 119
Afghanistan, 133
age, ix, x, 41, 55, 85, 114, 133, 150, 186
agencies, 173
aggression, 51
aging process, 107
AIDS, ix, 7
Alaska, 177
allergist(s), 25
allergy, 25
amenorrhea, 100
American Psychiatric Association, ix, 60, 61, 73, 83, 91, 173, 174, 178
amine(s), 33, 34, 35, 36, 115
amygdala, 63
anatomy, 24, 101, 118, 122

anemia, 70
anger, 55, 80, 81, 100, 153, 181
angina, 16
angiogram, 28
angiography, 30
anorexia, 21, 97, 98
anorexia nervosa, 21
anthropologists, 17
anthropology, 17, 19, 29
antidepressant(s), 20, 24, 34, 35, 36, 37, 41, 93, 94, 95, 108, 112, 114, 116, 119, 129, 136, 136, 137
antidepressant medication, 129
antigen, 30
Antipsychiatry, 135
antipsychotic, 12, 52, 53, 65, 93, 94, 99, 136, 137, 165, 172
antipsychotic drugs, 137
antisocial acts, 100, 184
antisocial behavior, 183
antithesis, 41
anxiety, 33, 55, 59, 63, 64, 74, 85, 87, 88, 101, 112, 137, 153, 166
anxiety disorder, 55, 88
APA, 31, 85, 135, 155
apathy, 125, 126
appetite, 103, 113, 124, 126
Aristotle, 115
assault, 46, 47, 50, 100, 182, 184
assessment, ix, 16, 18, 19, 24, 26, 38, 40, 42, 43, 90, 119, 121, 136, 142, 156, 171
assessment tools, 90
assets, 44
atoms, 8, 50
atrophy, 13, 136
attitudes, 99
atzvut, 125, 127
authorities, 108, 142, 145, 173
authority, 17, 112, 141, 165
autism, x, 6, 157

autobiographical memory, 112
autonomy, 47, 49, 80, 147, 166, 168, 172
avoidance, 41, 51
awareness, 100, 107, 126

B

bacteria, 154
bacterium, 69
bad behavior, 8, 44, 94
baggage, 38
ban, 84
bank fraud, 86
base, 15, 70, 136
BD, 112
Beck Depression Inventory, 90, 120
behavioral disorders, 97
behaviors, 8, 15, 20, 21, 23, 51, 70, 100, 141, 143, 159, 181
Belarus, 125
beneficial effect, 13, 35
benefits, 25, 93, 98, 103, 104, 105, 107, 108, 157, 159, 166, 172
benign, 96, 101, 114, 136, 181
Bereavement, v, 75, 103, 111, 118, 119, 122, 123, 128, 129, 130, 158
bias, 98, 99, 100, 101, 102, 110, 137, 140, 141, 142, 143, 144
Bible, 73, 127, 185
Big Bang, 60
Bigotry, 71, 98
bile, 126, 180
biochemistry, 81
biological markers, 153, 154
biological psychiatry, 29, 38, 165
biomarkers, 2, 21, 24, 25, 58, 68, 70, 81, 96, 121, 156, 158
Biomarkers, 57
biopsy, 96
Biopsychosocial, 32, 62
bipolar disorder, x, 28, 31, 35, 36, 37, 55, 56, 57, 61, 71, 74, 76, 82, 88, 120, 122, 137, 138, 147, 153, 154, 157, 165, 185
blame, 33, 82, 124
bleeding, 185
blogger, 78, 82
blogs, xii, 32, 36, 84, 135, 138, 139, 180, 181
blood, 16, 25, 40, 46, 57, 71, 92, 134, 154, 164, 185
blood pressure, 40, 46, 57, 71, 134, 164
body weight, 92
bonding, 110
bonds, 46
bone(s), 104, 125, 158, 163

bounds, 171
brain, ix, x, 7, 8, 9, 10, 11, 15, 22, 27, 31, 32, 33, 34, 35, 36, 42, 45, 46, 47, 48, 49, 50, 51, 53, 59, 63, 67, 104, 108, 111, 134, 153, 160, 165, 166
brain abnormalities, x
brain chemistry, 33, 34
brain tumor, 10, 15, 23
breathing, 15
Buddhism, vii
burn, 15, 142
businesses, 180
buyers, 178
bystander effect, 182

C

calcium, 24
calculus, 112
cancer, 7, 13, 58, 96, 104, 113, 116
candidates, 99
capital punishment, 169, 170, 171, 172
cardiovascular disease, 92, 104
caregivers, 138
caricature, xi
caricatures, 31
Carnap, 17
case study, 151
cash, 46, 64, 71, 104
catatonia, 23
catatonic, 21, 23
category a, 56
causality, 33, 45, 50, 51, 91, 118, 177
causation, 35, 45, 63
central nervous system (CNS), 13, 15, 133
central obesity, 100
cerebrospinal fluid, 47
challenges, 79, 81, 104, 132, 159
character traits, 7, 12
chemical(s), vii, xi, 30, 31, 32, 33, 34, 35, 36, 153, 186
Chicago, 5, 11, 12, 16, 73, 84, 92, 102, 104, 178, 180
childhood, 31, 35, 37
children, 6, 55, 136
China, 173
chronic fatigue, 2, 26
chronic fatigue syndrome, 2, 26
citizens, 167, 177
City(ies), 137, 175, 178
civil law, 45
civil liberties, 4
Civil War, 97
clarity, 104

classification, 1, 13, 24, 26, 27, 37, 67, 68, 71, 93, 97, 153, 157, 158
clinical application, 43
clinical assessment, 21, 85, 121
clinical depression, 64, 75, 110, 125, 168
clinical diagnosis, 23, 26, 29, 60, 171
clinical holistic medicine, 61
clinical judgment, 18, 129
clinical problems, 72
clinical syndrome, 72
clinical trials, 147
clothing, 168
clozapine, 136, 153
clusters, 98
CNN, 182, 183
cocaine, 90, 133, 136
coercion, 52, 84
cognition, 9, 10, 11, 72, 157
cognitive abilities, 3
cognitive capacity, 136
cognitive deficit(s), 104
cognitive flexibility, 108
cognitive function, 21, 107, 108
cognitive process, 107
cognitive psychology, 31
cognitive skills, 108
cognitive therapists, 31
cognitive-behavioral therapy, 12, 109, 154
collateral, 135
collateral damage, 135
commodity, 98
common sense, 76, 85, 114
common symptoms, 58
communication, 35, 126, 130, 148, 157, 171
community(ies), 30, 53, 83, 99, 114, 116, 143
community service, 53
comorbidity, 70
compassion, 100, 138
compatibility, 46
competence, 141, 170, 171, 172
competing interests, 141
competition, 164
complement, xi, 117
complex partial seizure, 80, 133
complexity, 39, 41, 43, 67, 75, 157, 165
compliance, 53
complications, 152
composites, 152
computer, 41, 51
computing, 115
conception, 33, 58, 127
conceptual model, 159
Concise, 152

concordance, 36, 57, 71, 84
concrete thinking, 165
condensation, 159
conduct disorder, 99
conduction, 21
conference, 181
confidentiality, 149, 151, 152
confinement, 3
conflict(s), vii, 37, 42, 59, 72, 86, 131, 132, 139, 140, 141, 142, 143, 144, 145, 146, 147, 152
conflict of interest, 140, 141, 142, 143, 144, 145, 146, 147
confounding variables, 176
Congressional Budget Office, 168
consciousness, 64
consensus, 86
consent, 136, 147, 148, 149, 150, 151, 152, 165
consequentialism, 171
constipation, 41
constituents, 104
Constitution, 179
construct validity, 60
construction, 18, 29, 68
consumers, 76, 139
context, xi, 7, 15, 37, 77, 83, 85, 86, 87, 88, 89, 90, 91, 92, 99, 113, 114, 116, 117, 128, 129, 149, 155, 167, 175, 179, 182
contextualists, 89
contingency, 10
contradiction, 71, 109, 166
controlled studies, 13, 47, 117
controversial, x, 5, 22, 40, 45, 55, 76, 97, 108
controversies, xii, 26, 28, 63, 101, 114, 132, 133, 169
convention, 3
convergence, 2, 140
conviction, 153, 164, 166
cooling, 181
cooperation, 112
coronary arteries, 3
coronary artery disease, 3, 14, 106
correlation, 57, 71, 91
cortex, 106
cortisol, 68, 88
cosmetic, 136, 157
cost, 104
counsel, 117, 139, 182
counseling, 33, 94, 121
covering, 128, 164
CPT, 81
criminal justice system, 53, 99
criticism, 39, 137, 157, 164, 181
CT, 68, 81
CT scan, 68, 81

cues, 110
cultural imperialism, 97
cultural influence, 97
culture, 97
cure(s), 7, 16
curriculum, 159
cycling, 36

D

danger, 60, 173, 186
dangerousness, 81, 175
David Hume, 44
death penalty, 170, 171
death rate, 177
deaths, 175, 176, 179
decay, 125
defamation, 181
defects, x
deficiencies, 39
deficiency, 70
deficit, 155
delirium, 21, 135
delusion(s), 2, 50, 64, 86, 174, 186
delusions of grandeur, 64
dementia, 21, 136
democracy, 134
demonstrations, 28
deontology, 171
depressive symptoms, 87, 89, 107, 112, 113, 114, 115, 117, 121, 128, 129
depth, viii, 49, 65, 74, 75, 80, 120
despair, ix, 123, 129
detachment, 130
detainees, 173, 174
detectable, 142
determinism, 44, 45, 46, 48, 49, 50, 51
deterrence, 53
developmental process, 72
deviation, 10, 22
diabetes, 92, 93, 94, 95, 104
Diagnosis, v, 3, 14, 43, 56, 58, 61, 67, 72, 79, 118, 127, 133, 161
Diagnostic and Statistical Manual of Mental Disorders, 61, 73, 83, 92
diagnostic criteria, 38, 39, 56, 93, 94, 96, 98, 102, 116, 129, 159
dichotomy, 164
diet, 117
differential diagnosis, 59, 90
dignity, 82
direct observation, 17, 154
disability, 43, 52, 72, 89, 94, 105, 108, 159, 168

disclosure, 142, 145, 147
discomfort, 2, 15, 164
discrimination, 82, 83
disease(s), x, 1, 2, 6, 8, 9, 10, 13, 14, 15, 20, 21, 23, 24, 26, 38, 56, 58, 68, 69, 70, 71, 76, 97, 98, 99, 101, 133, 154, 157, 177
dislocation, 68
disorderness, 79, 85, 86, 89, 90
distortions, 70, 109, 115
distress, 49, 72, 78, 89, 93, 95, 158, 185
dizziness, 85, 87
doctors, 32, 33, 34, 78, 93, 105, 135, 138, 159, 163, 165, 168, 170, 171
dopamine, 34, 136
dorsolateral prefrontal cortex, 108
dosage, 165
dosing, 165
draft, xii, 23, 42, 83, 99, 121, 181
drug abuse, 135
drug action, 36
drug therapy, 160
drugging, 135
drugs, 20, 24, 26, 36, 92, 135, 136, 137, 143, 144, 145, 165, 175
DSM, v, 37, 38, 39, 40, 56, 57, 64, 67, 71, 74, 75, 76, 77, 79, 85, 87, 89, 97, 99, 102, 114, 116, 117, 120, 155, 156, 157, 158
DSM-5, ix, x, xii, 25, 26, 27, 28, 29, 38, 54, 55, 56, 57, 60, 62, 63, 67, 71, 72, 73, 74, 75, 76, 77, 79, 80, 83, 85, 86, 87, 88, 90, 91, 92, 93, 94, 95, 100, 116, 119, 123, 124, 127, 128, 129, 130, 132, 133, 134, 153, 155, 156, 157, 158, 160
DSM-IV-TR, 4, 60
dualism, 7, 160
due process, 81, 136
Dunbar, 101, 102
dysphoria, 36
dysplasia, 26
dystonia, 2

E

economic evaluation, 147
economics, 168
editors, 4, 12, 14, 43, 44, 79, 102, 112, 118, 143, 146, 161
education, 39, 93, 139, 157
educators, 160
egoism, vii
EKG, 16
electron, 96
e-mail, 180, 181
emergency, 16, 136, 175, 185

emotion, 17, 36, 51, 62, 72, 81, 87, 112
emotion regulation, 72
emotional responses, 120
empathy, 64, 104
Empathy, 117
empirical methods, 81
empirical studies, 93
employment, 39, 99
encouragement, xii
endangered, 87
endocrine, 15
endocrinologist, 42
endophenotypes, 2, 61
enemies, 182
energy, 111, 126, 149
enforcement, 178
Engel, 39, 41, 43, 137
engineering, 25, 93
environment, 31, 35, 37, 38, 58, 91, 105
environmental stress, 158
Epictetus, 49, 54, 85
epidemic, 36, 113, 116, 117, 155
epidemiologic, 116
epidemiologic studies, 116
epilepsy, 23, 24, 26, 57, 82, 154
episteme, 2, 3
epistemology, 28
equilibrium, 64
Erklären, 59
ethical issues, 132
ethics, xi, 48, 171, 182
ethnicity, 97, 101, 150
etiology, 2, 9, 34, 70
etiquette, 180, 181
Europe, 125
evidence, 10, 13, 14, 15, 25, 28, 29, 31, 35, 36, 39, 41, 42, 47, 49, 52, 53, 56, 57, 68, 70, 77, 81, 87, 91, 93, 97, 106, 107, 108, 109, 110, 111, 114, 118, 136, 159, 176, 177, 178, 179, 183
evil, 46, 49, 138, 177, 181, 183, 184
evolution, x, 69, 71, 87
Evolutionary, 106
exclusion, x, 60, 74, 79, 91, 93, 113, 118, 119, 124, 127, 128, 130, 133, 156
execution, 170, 171, 172, 173
executive function, 108
exercise, 3, 28, 140, 165
expertise, 133
exposure, 116
eye movement, 2, 21, 154

F

fabrication, 141
facial expression, 29, 110, 112
facial pain, 2, 23
fairness, 103, 181
faith, 5, 77, 103, 156, 166, 185
false positive, 76, 77, 85, 87, 90, 91, 92, 93, 116, 155
family environment, 35
family history, 29, 41, 56, 129
family members, 33, 151
family physician, 44, 58
family system, 134
fasting, 92
fatalism, 45
FDA, 94
fear(s), ix, x, 33, 35, 47, 49, 80, 87, 88, 135, 178, 179, 183
feelings, ix, 21, 45, 53, 63, 73, 100, 109, 121, 124, 125, 126, 128, 150
fever, x, 163
fiber(s), 69, 89
fibromyalgia, 26, 27
field theory, 38
financial, 140, 141, 142, 143, 144, 145, 146, 147, 159
financial resources, 146
financial support, 144
firearms, 175, 176, 177, 178, 179
fixation, 78
flaws, 29, 132
flexibility, 21, 23
flight, 87, 88, 185
fluid, 75
fMRI, 36
food, 25, 27, 168, 185
force, 16, 25, 27, 28, 53, 81, 84, 155, 186
formation, 14, 81
formula, 19
Fort Hood, 183
Foucault, 2, 3, 5, 17
foundations, 50, 71, 159
France, 79, 176
fraud, 16, 32, 36, 84
free choice, 168
free will, 44, 45, 46, 47, 48
freedom, 44, 45, 46, 47, 48, 49, 50, 52, 53, 152, 178, 180
freedom of will, 46
Freud, 148
friendship, 138
frontal lobe, 108
funding, 61, 145

fuzziness, 57, 95, 96

G

GABA, 34
Gabbard, xi, xii, 39, 43, 132, 139, 152, 167
gangs, 180
GDP, 168
General Accounting Office, 168
general adaptation syndrome, 87, 88
genes, 35
genetic defect, 95
genetic factors, 34
genetics, 35
genocide, 53
Genovese, 183
Germany, 115, 116
Ghaemi, xi, xii, 1, 4, 5, 17, 19, 24, 28, 29, 30, 31, 32, 39, 42, 43, 44, 50, 54, 57, 60, 61, 62, 65, 71, 72, 73, 75, 94, 95, 112, 118, 122, 132, 136, 137, 147, 160, 166, 167
gifted, vii
glucose, 92, 106, 112, 136
glucose tolerance, 92
glutamate, 34
gnosis, 80, 133
God, vii, 96, 104, 163, 184
google, 106
goose, 186
Grief, v, 91, 103, 111, 119, 121, 122, 124, 127, 130
growth, 27, 35, 82, 107
Guantanamo, 173
guardian, 30, 84
guessing, 113
guidance, 160
guidelines, 99, 101, 128, 142, 181
guilt, 63, 105, 126
guilt feelings, 63
guilty, 33, 52, 109, 131, 181
gun control, 175, 177, 178, 179

H

hair, 62, 69, 75
hallucinations, 3, 15, 16, 47, 51, 57, 59, 64, 65, 70, 71, 80
happiness, 105, 130
hate crime, 99
hatred, 98, 99, 100, 132, 137, 138, 139, 184
haze, 31
headache, 8, 16, 23, 26, 27
healing, 37, 40, 41, 42, 164

health, viii, 3, 15, 16, 19, 22, 24, 27, 42, 43, 54, 78, 81, 93, 98, 104, 115, 121, 125, 129, 133, 138, 139, 140, 143, 146, 155, 166, 167, 168, 170, 174, 178, 179, 180, 181, 183, 186
health care, viii, 81, 129, 138, 140, 146, 167, 168, 180, 181, 186
health care professionals, 81, 138, 180, 181
health care system, 129, 168, 169
health insurance, 168
health risks, 93, 104
heart attack, 117
heart disease, 104
height, 61
helplessness, 105
hemodialysis, 13
hemoglobin, 105
heroin, 136
high school, 6, 98
histology, 2
history, x, 2, 6, 21, 23, 32, 57, 61, 63, 68, 78, 85, 97, 100, 101, 114, 115, 125, 129, 135, 147, 148, 149, 154, 155, 175
HM, 14, 169
hobby, 46
homes, 35, 175
homicide, 51, 52, 53, 54, 175, 176, 179
homicide rates, 175, 176
Hong Kong, 97
hopelessness, 125, 126, 129
hormone, 42
horses, 81
Horwitz, 72, 86, 91, 113, 114, 115, 116, 117, 118, 155, 179
hospitality, 185
hospitalization, 53, 120, 186
host, 165, 166
hostility, 101
House, xi, 131, 184
housing, 39, 134, 168
human, 6, 18, 29, 40, 41, 42, 47, 51, 60, 62, 63, 68, 69, 74, 76, 77, 78, 81, 87, 90, 98, 99, 104, 105, 120, 129, 131, 153, 155, 158, 166, 167, 183, 184, 186
human behavior, 155
human brain, 51
human condition, 42
human experience, 40, 76
human perception, 18
human psychology, 62
human reactions, 153
human right(s), 167
human sciences, 81
human subjects, 47

Index

humanism, viii, 72, 73, 122, 167
humanistic perspective, xi, 132
Hume, 44, 45
husband, 6
hybrid, 59, 62
hydrogen, 8
hyperactivity, 155
hypertension, 100
hypothesis, 33, 34, 35, 36, 45, 55, 56, 81, 98, 103, 104, 108, 178
hypothesis test, 108
hypothetico-deductive, 55
hypothyroidism, 41, 147

I

ice pack(s), 8
ID, 147, 180
ideal(s), 6, 74, 76, 149, 159, 164
identical twins, 35
identification, 26, 38, 55, 80, 101, 150, 171
identity, vii, 12, 82, 142, 147, 148, 149, 150, 151, 152, 164
ideology, 42
idiopathic, 23
idiosyncratic, 165
Illness, xii, 4, 5, 10, 11, 12, 16, 65, 72, 97, 98, 127
illusions, 24
image(s), 30, 62, 107, 126, 184
imagery, 13
imagination, vii
Imbalance, xi, 30, 32, 36
imbalances, 36
impaired immune function, 115
impairments, 9, 108
imperialism, 76, 77
impulses, 51, 62, 121, 124
impulsivity, 90
incarceration, 170
incidence, 116, 118, 155, 160, 177
income, 143, 163, 167, 175, 176, 179
incompatibility, 42
independence, 101
individuals, xii, 5, 8, 25, 34, 44, 45, 51, 64, 73, 78, 99, 100, 101, 104, 108, 110, 112, 114, 125, 131, 132, 138, 168, 169, 172, 186
induction, x, 18, 29
industry, x, 137, 143, 145, 146, 147, 157
infancy, 54
infection, 58
inflammatory responses, 121
informed consent, 4, 136, 148, 149, 150, 151
ingredients, 153

inheritance, 70
inhibition, 108, 110, 160
injections, 47
injury, 9, 52, 89, 173
inner world, 23, 39, 42, 64, 65, 90, 121, 156, 158
inositol, 160
insane, 2, 3
insanity, 3, 52
insomnia, 113, 124, 128
insulin, x
integration, 159, 166
integrity, 172
intelligence, 62
intentionality, 50
interference, 115, 156
internalizing, 82
internet, viii, ix, 45, 53, 69, 73, 135, 157, 180
internist(s), 78, 96, 133
interpersonal skills, 108, 110
interrogation(s), 169, 173, 174
intervention, 26, 94, 107, 129, 135
intoxication, 90, 133
intracranial pressure, 134
iron, 70
irritability, 61
islands, 166
issues, 5, 11, 17, 20, 44, 62, 64, 67, 74, 78, 79, 83, 84, 91, 113, 134, 139, 146, 153, 159, 172, 183

J

Jaspers, 40, 42, 43, 44, 50, 54, 59, 63, 71, 73, 74, 166, 167
Jews, 98
joints, 57, 74, 80, 96, 129
justification, 177

K

Kendler, 4, 5, 86, 87, 91, 114, 118
kidnapping, 50
kill, 100, 147
Kontos, 38, 39, 41, 42, 43

L

labeling, 87, 94
laboratory studies, 15, 42, 43
laboratory tests, 25, 81, 99, 134
later life, 35
law enforcement, 173
laws, 45, 47, 176, 177, 179, 181, 186

lead, 15, 25, 31, 33, 34, 35, 69, 92, 93, 94, 98, 111, 112, 119, 125, 126, 140, 155, 168, 179, 181, 186
learning, 35, 95, 104
legend, 30, 31, 32, 36
legs, 68
Lehrer, 103, 106
leisure, 39
lens, 37, 68
leprosy, ix
lesions, 1, 9, 15, 68
lethargy, 41
life course, 75
lifetime, vii, 107
light, 2, 3, 5, 15, 57, 82, 95, 96, 119, 127, 143
limbic system, 63
linguistics, 29
lithium, 36, 136, 147, 154
liver, 18
lobbying, 157
local authorities, 186
locus, 101
Louisiana, 177
love, 98, 129, 138
Luhrmann, x, 40, 43, 132, 164, 167
lupus, 133
lymph, 163
lymph node, 163

M

magnetic resonance, 12
magnetic resonance imaging, 12
major depression, vii, x, 16, 26, 28, 37, 41, 64, 73, 74, 85, 92, 103, 104, 105, 107, 108, 109, 110, 111, 112, 114, 117, 118, 120, 121, 122, 123, 124, 125, 127, 128, 129, 130, 154, 155, 168
Major depression, 118
major depressive disorder, x, 35, 41, 56, 57, 76, 77, 93, 94, 95, 103, 106, 107, 112, 116, 120, 121, 124, 128, 130, 154, 157
majority, 34, 78, 101, 107, 175
malaise, 153
malaria, 105
malignancy, 89
man, 39, 41, 43, 44, 47, 74, 85, 104, 156, 181, 183
management, 3, 25, 121
mania, 33, 90, 133
manic, 21, 35, 55, 133, 185, 186
manic episode, 21, 35, 133
manic symptoms, 186
manipulation, 93
manslaughter, 52
Marfan syndrome, 147

marketing, 34
marriage, 158
mass, 173, 175, 177, 178, 179, 181, 183
mass media, 181
materialism, 12
matter, 6, 8, 13, 35, 44, 45, 52, 56, 57, 67, 68, 78, 96, 105, 108, 116, 135, 151, 152, 155, 167, 173, 177, 181, 184, 185
MB, 16, 92, 118, 122
measurement, 154
media, 73, 157, 160, 183
median, 114, 145
medical care, 42, 95, 168, 173
medical history, 15, 38, 115
medical science, 41, 42, 59, 60
Medicalization, 76
medication, xi, 31, 33, 40, 52, 53, 65, 76, 77, 86, 93, 94, 99, 133, 135, 136, 153, 164, 165, 166, 172, 174, 185, 186
medicine, vii, 2, 3, 4, 7, 13, 16, 18, 20, 21, 23, 26, 27, 37, 39, 41, 55, 56, 57, 59, 61, 67, 70, 77, 81, 85, 89, 96, 100, 115, 129, 155, 164, 166
melancholia, 71, 127, 160
melancholy, 125, 126
membership, 41
memory, 7, 15, 21, 65, 70, 163
memory loss, 70
mental capacity, 172
mental disorder, xi, 3, 30, 32, 61, 67, 68, 69, 72, 73, 84, 88, 91, 99, 113, 115, 118, 157, 158
mental health, ix, 3, 14, 27, 53, 93, 97, 99, 101, 103, 104, 112, 125, 128, 133, 134, 143, 153, 158, 168, 183
mental health professionals, 97, 99, 125, 133, 153, 183
mental illness, viii, ix, x, xi, 3, 5, 6, 7, 8, 9, 10, 11, 12, 15, 16, 20, 31, 32, 36, 44, 67, 69, 73, 79, 83, 84, 92, 97, 98, 99, 102, 112, 138, 153, 154, 156, 160, 164, 175, 185
mental life, 120
mental processes, 29, 108
mental state, 52, 63
mentor, vii
Mercury, 54, 56
merirut, 125, 127
mesothelioma, 116
messages, 165
messengers, 186
meta-analysis, 12, 136, 137
metabolism, 34, 106, 112
metaphor, 2, 5, 6, 7, 8, 10, 11, 61, 68, 74
methodology, 28, 29, 56, 81
microscope, 58, 68, 69, 154

migraine headache, 8, 15, 22, 23, 26, 82, 154
military, 173
mind-body, 7, 12
miniature, 6
minority groups, 99, 168
misconceptions, 91
mission, ix, 159
misunderstanding, 20, 33, 43
misuse, 93, 173
models, x, 24, 38, 40, 41, 43, 74, 84, 136, 137, 154, 164
modifications, 54
mold, vii
molecular biology, 17, 71
molecules, xi, 31, 42, 59, 132, 159, 166
mood disorder, x, 32, 33, 34, 37, 72, 103, 106, 107, 112, 118, 122, 128, 154
mood states, 33, 90
mood swings, 33, 35, 154
moral imperative, 173
morbidity, 93, 109
morphology, 18, 98
mortality, 93, 180
motivation, 99, 142, 181
MRI, 16
multiple sclerosis, 57
murder, 138, 177, 183
music, 124
mutual respect, 138
myocardial infarction, 117, 163
myocardial ischemia, 88

N

narratives, 2, 32, 59, 63, 131, 135, 183
National Public Radio, 128, 130
National Research Council, 106
national security, 173
natural science, 40, 42, 43, 59
natural sciences, 43
Naturalism, 48, 49, 51, 54
nausea, 15, 23, 87
negative emotions, 149
neglect, 31, 78
nerve, 21, 62, 63, 136
nerve growth factor, 63, 136
nervousness, 79
neural network(s), xi
neurobiology, 114, 164, 166
neurogenesis, 137
neuroimaging, 23
neuroleptics, 136
neurological disease, 154

neurologist, 15, 22, 23, 26, 154
neuronal circuits, 51
neurons, 136
Neuropathology, 12, 13, 14
neuropsychiatry, 59, 153
neuroscience, 31, 35, 38, 66, 161
neurosyphilis, 134
neurotransmitters, x, 29, 164, 165
neurotrophic factors, 137
neutral, 114, 116, 181
New England, 20, 176
norepinephrine, 33, 34
normal children, 55
Normality, 77, 88
nurses, 126, 134, 170, 171
nursing, 38, 42
nursing care, 38
nurturance, 165

O

obedience, 23
obesity, 56, 61
objectivity, 3, 14, 15, 16, 18, 19, 24, 29, 43, 140, 141, 154
obsessive-compulsive disorder, 57, 101
obstacles, 126
occipital lobe, 62
offenders, 54
officials, 135
olanzapine, 136
old age, 107, 168
oppression, 2, 81
opt out, 152
optic chiasm, 62
optic nerve, 62
optimism, x, xi, 83, 126
organ, 168
organism, 15, 58, 87, 155
outpatient(s), 101, 104, 186
outreach, 157
ovarian cysts, 185
overlap, 57, 71, 87
oversight, 151
ownership, 176, 177, 179
ox, 6
oxygen, 8

P

pain, 8, 15, 16, 20, 57, 67, 83, 87, 89, 90, 95, 96, 123, 129, 154, 158

paints, xi, 47
pallor, 21
palpitations, 85
Panic, 85, 86, 88, 91
panic attack, 59, 85, 86, 87, 88, 89
panic disorder, 57, 74, 86, 88, 91, 135, 157
panic symptoms, 88, 101
paralysis, 68
paranoia, 98
paranoid schizophrenia, 51, 99, 134
parenting, 35
parents, x, 99
paresthesias, 15, 87
participants, 109, 142
pasture, 81
pathogenesis, 22
pathologist, 5, 13, 68, 69, 71, 84
pathology, 4, 9, 11, 13, 14, 22, 23, 26, 28, 45, 58, 68, 86, 88, 89, 90, 96, 101, 156
pathophysiological, 2, 9, 13, 26, 59
pathophysiology, 1, 2, 9, 25, 26, 27, 34, 70, 71, 72, 82, 95, 101, 116, 127, 160
pathways, 51
patient care, 39, 168
Paxil, 34
PBPI, 75, 119, 120, 121, 123
peace, 182
peer review, 142
permission, 48, 70, 139, 147, 148, 149, 151, 152
permit, 111, 120, 129, 180, 181
perpetrators, 183
personal autonomy, 136
personal communication, 7, 8, 23, 42, 50, 52, 60, 78, 80, 88, 115, 116, 117, 139, 143, 148, 149, 151, 159, 171, 172
personal history, 63
personal relations, 141
personal relationship, 141
personal responsibility, 45
personal views, 170
personality, x, 29, 31, 36, 50, 51, 76, 102, 134, 157
personality disorder, 76, 157
personality traits, 134
personhood, 51, 166
PET, 29
PET scan, 29
pharmaceutical, x, 30, 34, 131, 137, 143, 144, 145, 146, 157
pharmacology, 31
pharmacotherapy, x, 40, 59, 93, 108, 165
phencyclidine, 133
phenomenology, 23, 43, 54, 63, 64, 66, 68, 70, 71, 72, 75, 96, 118, 119, 120, 122, 123

phenotype, 31
pheochromocytoma, 59, 87
Philadelphia, 14
photophobia, 23
physical chemistry, 17, 25
physical features, 150
physical health, 3, 103
physical laws, 47, 51
physical sciences, 81
physicians, 2, 7, 15, 16, 22, 28, 32, 34, 38, 39, 42, 57, 58, 60, 74, 76, 78, 90, 91, 93, 94, 95, 96, 99, 100, 115, 116, 117, 129, 131, 133, 134, 136, 138, 145, 146, 151, 157, 164, 167, 170, 171, 172, 173, 178, 185
physics, 29, 47, 81
physiology, 9, 34, 68, 88, 166
placebo, 94, 144
plaque, 3
plasticity, 36
Plato, 74, 80, 96
Platonic, 58, 74, 75, 96
plausibility, 21
pleasure, 105
pluralism, x, 29, 37, 38, 40, 41, 44, 54, 60, 159
poetry, 17, 31, 82, 159
polarity, 18
police, 173, 183, 186
policy, 142, 147, 171
politics, 133
Polythetic, x, 37, 40, 41
population, 104, 133, 175, 176, 180
portraits, 125
positive mood, 112
positivism, vii, 1, 4, 17, 22, 28, 29, 30, 54, 58, 68, 81, 154
positivist, 2, 3, 17, 21, 58, 154
postmodernism, 2, 135
post-traumatic stress disorder, 89, 97, 98
postural hypotension, 134
potential benefits, 94
poverty, 114
pragmatism, 29
praxis, 3, 86
precancer, 26
predators, 100
prefrontal cortex, 108
prejudice, ix, xii, 82, 99, 138
prescription, 33, 92, 93, 119, 155, 165, 166, 168
president, ix, 17, 170
prestige, 54
prevention, 112
principles, 136, 181
prisoners, 171, 173

private ownership, 177
probability, 96, 140, 141
problem-solving, 35, 38, 103, 104, 105, 107, 108, 109, 112
problem-solving skills, 103, 104, 105, 109
professionals, 134, 138, 170, 174, 180, 183
profit, 138
prognosis, 58, 101, 166
project, 54, 155
proposition, 9, 10, 77, 95
prostate cancer, 28
prostate specific antigen, 28
protection, 142, 149, 170
protein kinase C, 160
prototype(s), 74, 75, 76, 80, 120, 122, 158
Prozac, 34
PST, 108
psychiatric diagnosis, 1, 3, 4, 13, 16, 20, 22, 30, 37, 39, 41, 42, 44, 54, 55, 58, 73, 74, 75, 76, 77, 79, 80, 82, 83, 95, 99, 116, 130, 158
psychiatric disorders, x, 5, 13, 20, 45, 47, 49, 51, 53, 56, 59, 67, 71, 96, 101, 133, 155, 173, 186
psychiatric hospitals, 186
psychiatric illness, vii, 4, 9, 20, 21, 32, 33, 34, 35, 38, 65, 138, 154, 156, 164, 167, 175, 185, 186
psychiatric patients, 82
psychiatrist, ix, xi, 15, 17, 18, 22, 30, 39, 42, 50, 52, 59, 63, 64, 74, 82, 86, 100, 101, 111, 133, 139, 143, 148, 150, 154, 155, 156, 158, 159, 164, 166, 171, 172, 173, 177
psychodynamic perspective, 80
psychologist, 71, 73, 131, 133, 134, 154, 166
psychology, 35, 39, 67, 74, 80, 81, 132, 166
psychopathology, 29, 38, 43, 44, 51, 54, 62, 74, 86, 87, 88, 91, 101, 133, 165
psychopharmacology, 166
psychosis, 33, 52, 80, 94, 95, 101, 126, 135, 165, 185
psychosocial interventions, 37
psychosocial stress, 89
psychotherapy, x, xi, xiii, 7, 31, 40, 41, 51, 59, 72, 84, 86, 99, 101, 118, 122, 129, 132, 136, 137, 153, 157, 159, 160
psychotropic medications, 135, 136, 137, 165
PTSD, 88, 97
public awareness, 116
public education, x, 157
public health, 93, 94, 145
public opinion, 10
public policy, 53, 93, 171, 177
public safety, 53
publishing, 148
punishment, 49, 54, 170, 171, 174

Q

quality of life, 42
quantum mechanics, 45
questioning, vii
questionnaire, 90, 92, 123

R

race, 100, 101
racial minorities, 137
racism, ix, 99, 101
radio, 135
rape, 182, 183, 184
rating scale, 53, 54, 120
rationality, 50
RE, 73
reactions, ix, 33, 35, 103, 114
reactivity, 126
reading, xii, 5, 23, 62, 95, 96, 110, 119, 124, 149, 151, 180
realism, 46, 72, 118, 122
reality, 1, 3, 7, 9, 10, 14, 64, 67, 99, 101, 105, 178
reasoning, 15, 52, 53, 89, 140
recall, 21, 105, 114, 129, 165
reception, 63
receptors, 36, 136
recognition, 46, 60, 70, 97, 99
recommendations, 152, 171
recovery, 82, 83, 84, 111, 149, 159, 166
recurrence, 114
reductionism, 39, 43
reflexes, 21
reform(s), 4, 138, 177, 179
regulations, 176, 177, 178
rehabilitation, 46, 51, 53
rejection, 59
relatives, 58, 61
relevance, 175
reliability, 14, 24, 30, 38, 40, 56, 74, 93, 96, 156
relief, x, 15, 105, 158, 159
religion, 100, 159
religious beliefs, 185
religious traditions, vii
remorse, 63
repair, 184
reporters, 6
repression, 3
requirements, 22, 150
researchers, 16, 33, 74, 75, 88, 142, 146, 156
resentment, 81
resilience, 105

resistance, 137
resources, 51, 174
respiratory rate, 87
response, 16, 26, 53, 56, 57, 62, 70, 71, 87, 88, 93, 100, 101, 110, 111, 113, 114, 115, 116, 120, 126, 128, 158, 161
Responsibility, 52
restitution, 53
restoration, 53
restrictions, 121, 178
retaliation, 181, 183
retardation, 21, 113, 120, 121, 126
retribution, 53, 54
rewards, 52
rhetoric, ix, 10, 131, 132, 137
rights, 151
risk(s), 10, 35, 41, 52, 92, 93, 94, 95, 106, 114, 120, 128, 139, 155, 170, 157, 166, 172, 175, 176, 177, 181, 185
risk factors, 114, 175
risperidone, 136
Romania, 173
roots, 111, 158, 164, 183
rules, 6, 17, 43, 74, 128, 156, 181
Rumination, 107, 109, 110, 112

S

sadness, 64, 72, 78, 86, 91, 113, 114, 115, 117, 118, 123, 126, 128, 129, 155
safety, 9, 138, 178, 181, 185
salts, 186
sanctions, 52, 53
Sartorius, 118, 139, 160
schema, 44, 71, 80, 101, 115, 156
schizophrenia, x, 1, 2, 3, 5, 6, 8, 9, 11, 12, 13, 14, 16, 21, 23, 31, 35, 40, 45, 47, 53, 54, 56, 57, 60, 61, 64, 66, 71, 74, 82, 84, 94, 101, 133, 134, 137, 153, 154, 157, 160
Schizophrenia, 9, 12, 13, 43, 64, 65, 102
Schlick, 17, 44, 45
scholarship, vii
school, 22, 58, 92, 159, 177
science, vii, x, 2, 13, 17, 18, 19, 25, 26, 28, 29, 30, 40, 42, 43, 45, 48, 49, 50, 54, 55, 56, 57, 58, 59, 60, 61, 63, 65, 67, 68, 81, 82, 83, 84, 93, 94, 137, 146, 147, 154, 155, 156, 166
Science, x, xii, 4, 17, 19, 28, 29, 30, 32, 36, 37, 43, 54, 55, 56, 62, 65, 72, 81, 85, 118, 122, 157
scientific method, 18, 28, 56, 60, 154
scientific observation, 56
scientific understanding, x, 49
scientific validity, 55

scientism, 59, 62, 81
scope, 9, 39, 45, 158
security, 168, 178
sedative, 165
Seddon, 50, 52, 54
seizure, 23
self-control, 47
self-esteem, 63, 82, 125
self-improvement, 126
self-interest, 142
self-promotion, ix
semantics, 135
sensation(s), 88, 109, 175
senses, vii, 8, 129
sensitivity, 15, 59, 76, 93, 96, 116
serotonin, 33, 34, 136, 167
serum, 68, 88
services, 143, 168
sexual activity, 21, 110
sexual behavior, 70
shape, 56, 80, 97
shock, x, 97, 183
shock therapy, x
showing, 52, 54, 67, 93, 94, 108, 114, 120, 128, 181
shyness, 41, 76
sickle cell, 105
side effects, 40, 52, 135, 136, 153, 185, 186
signs, 20, 21, 22, 23, 37, 56, 58, 70, 89, 90, 95, 99, 100, 135
Singapore, 91
skills training, 94
skin, 57, 71
slavery, 132
smoking, 117
social benefits, 39
social context, 99
social control, 3
social dilemma, viii
social norms, 10
social organization, 2
social problems, 107, 110
social sciences, 59
social services, 168
social skills, 110
social support, 134
social workers, ix, 133, 134, 164
society, vii, ix, 3, 22, 26, 42, 52, 68, 70, 72, 170, 172, 177, 178
Socrates, vii
solar system, 6
solution, 26, 58, 156, 160, 164
somatization, 92
South Africa, 173

Soviet Union, 173
specialists, 23, 25, 69, 99, 103, 134
species, vii, 77, 78, 90, 104
speculation, 13, 23
speech, 3, 5, 6, 10, 14, 21, 22, 29, 85, 182
spending, 168
sputum, 58
SS, 36, 169
stability, 71
standard of living, 168
statistics, 147, 179
statutes, 178
stenosis, 28
stereotypes, 44
sterile, 132
stigma, xii, 83, 84, 105
stimulation, 153
stock, 142
stockpiling, 178
Stoics, 49, 51, 52, 155
stomach, 78, 137
stress, xiii, 76, 88, 91, 117, 153
stress response, 88
stressful events, 119
stressful life events, 118
stressors, 115, 119, 134
structural changes, 129
structure, 23, 29, 60, 63, 64, 65, 80, 120, 143, 153, 156
stupor, 21
style, 46, 51
subgroups, 101
subjective experience, 95, 120
subjectivity, 3, 18, 40, 42, 71, 96, 156
subpoena, 150
substance abuse, 150, 185, 186
substance use, 21
substitution, 178
substitution effect, 178
substrate, 31
Suffering, 77, 90
suicide, 21, 104, 105, 107, 114, 118, 120, 121, 128, 130, 175, 176, 179, 180
suicide attempts, 21, 121
suicide rate, 107, 128, 175
Sun, 56, 180
supervisor(s), 37, 38, 134, 143, 144
support staff, 173
Supreme Court, 171, 174, 178
survival, 105
survivors, 37
Sweden, 116
swelling, 20, 21, 22

symbolism, 165
sympathy, 41, 44, 58, 131, 137
symptoms, 20, 23, 27, 37, 56, 58, 70, 75, 78, 85, 88, 89, 90, 92, 95, 97, 99, 100, 101, 109, 113, 114, 120, 124, 129, 136, 154, 159, 164, 173
synaptic plasticity, xi
syndrome, 26, 67, 70, 71, 72, 73, 88, 91, 95, 100, 101, 102, 112, 183, 184
synthesis, 125
syphilis, 116, 155
Szasz, 1, 2, 3, 4, 5, 10, 11, 12, 13, 16, 72, 73, 84, 92, 102

T

tachycardia, 87, 88
takeover, 168
talk therapy, 33, 36, 164
Talmud, 14, 105, 131, 169, 182
tardive dyskinesia, 136
target, 1, 20, 28, 185
taxon, 87
taxonomy, 5
taxons, 87
teachers, xii, 132
technician, 171
techniques, 13, 51, 81, 153, 173
technology(ies), 10, 30, 153
temporal lobe, 13, 59, 133, 134
tension, 59, 63, 142
tenure, xii
territory, 76, 158, 183
terrorism, 53
terrorists, 89, 169, 173
testing, 9, 10, 14, 15, 18, 29, 30, 58, 59, 61, 81, 85, 101, 154, 163
testosterone, 163
textbook(s), 11,13, 58, 154
thalamus, 62
therapeutic practice, 139
therapist, 149, 165
therapy, xi, 35, 64, 94, 108, 112, 147, 149, 153, 168, 184
thoughts, 43, 45, 100, 109, 121, 123, 124, 125, 126, 184, 185
threats, 80, 132
thyroid, 41, 134
time periods, 118
tincture, 113
tonic, 23
top-down, 35, 36
torsion, 2
toxic effect, 138

toxicity, 133
trade, 37, 163
traditions, 4
trainees, 159
training, 93, 103, 133, 134, 157, 159, 170, 185
traits, 100, 104
trajectory, 129
transference, 150, 166
transformation, xi
transmission, 101
trauma, 35, 87, 89, 90, 101, 184
treatment, x, xi, 2, 3, 4, 7, 15, 16, 26, 27, 31, 36, 37, 38, 39, 41, 42, 44, 53, 56, 57, 58, 59, 62, 70, 71, 77, 80, 84, 86, 89, 90, 92, 93, 94, 95, 99, 101, 106, 108, 111, 114, 115, 116, 117, 119, 121, 128, 129, 130, 135, 136, 147, 148, 149, 150, 151, 153, 154, 156, 164, 167, 170, 171, 172, 173, 186
tremor, 57, 71
trial, 160
TSH, 41
tuberculosis, 7
tumor, 58, 59, 133, 134
twins, 35, 36
type 2 diabetes, 92
typhoid, 58
typhoid fever, 58

U

underwriting, 144, 145
uniform, 26, 101
United Kingdom (UK), 11, 13, 145
United Nations, 167, 176, 179
United States, 69, 169, 179, 180
Universal Declaration of Human Rights, 167
universe, 18, 45, 49, 60, 184
unmasking, 181
urban, 30, 32
urine, 23, 58
urologist, 96

V

validation, 37, 56
Validity, 43, 56, 62
Values, v, 3, 67, 163
vapor, 14
variables, 121
variations, 31, 157
varieties, 140
vertebrae, 68
Vice President, xii
victims, 184

Vietnam, 97
Viking, 48
violence, viii, 52, 175, 176, 180, 185
violent crime, 99, 176, 177
vision, 168
voicing, 77
VPC, 177
vulnerability, 110

W

Wakefield, 72, 86, 87, 91, 92, 113, 114, 115, 116, 117, 118, 123, 155
walking, 68, 92, 98, 175
war, 81, 182, 183
warts, 74
Washington, xiii, 61, 73, 83, 99, 102, 106, 135, 152, 174, 181
water, 8, 185
weakness, 22, 100
wealth, 114, 167
weapons, 177, 178
web, 179
websites, 132, 137, 180, 181
weeping, 126
weight gain, 41, 136
weight loss, 21, 120, 128
welfare, 141, 144, 181
well-being, 16, 19, 24, 43, 95, 98, 142, 168, 173
wellness, 7
white matter, 57, 61
William James, 46, 64, 71, 104
windows, 62, 90
withdrawal, 126
witnesses, 23, 51, 52, 183
Wittgenstein, 2, 5, 6, 11, 17, 19, 40, 50, 54, 57, 61, 68, 73, 75, 76, 89, 92, 95, 96, 100, 102, 135, 137, 155, 160
World Health Organization, 90, 97
worldview, 1
worry, 85, 175
wrongdoing, 143, 146, 184

Y

yield, 55, 58, 70, 109

Z

Zisook, xii, 64, 65, 79, 83, 91, 107, 111, 114, 116, 117, 118, 119, 121, 122, 123, 127, 130
Zoloft, 34